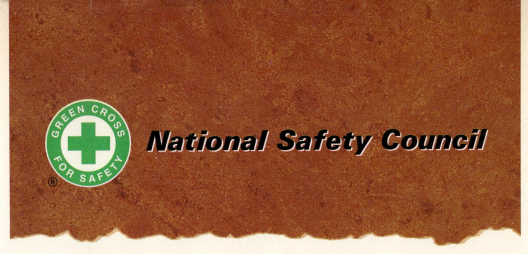

National Safety Council

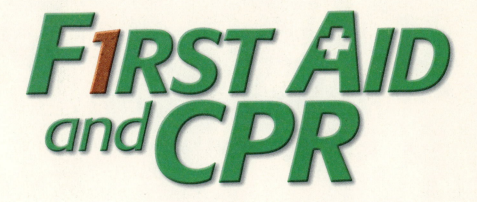

F1RST AID and CPR

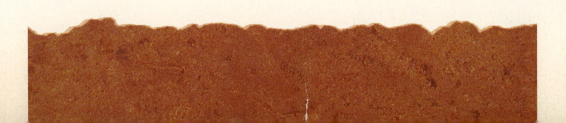

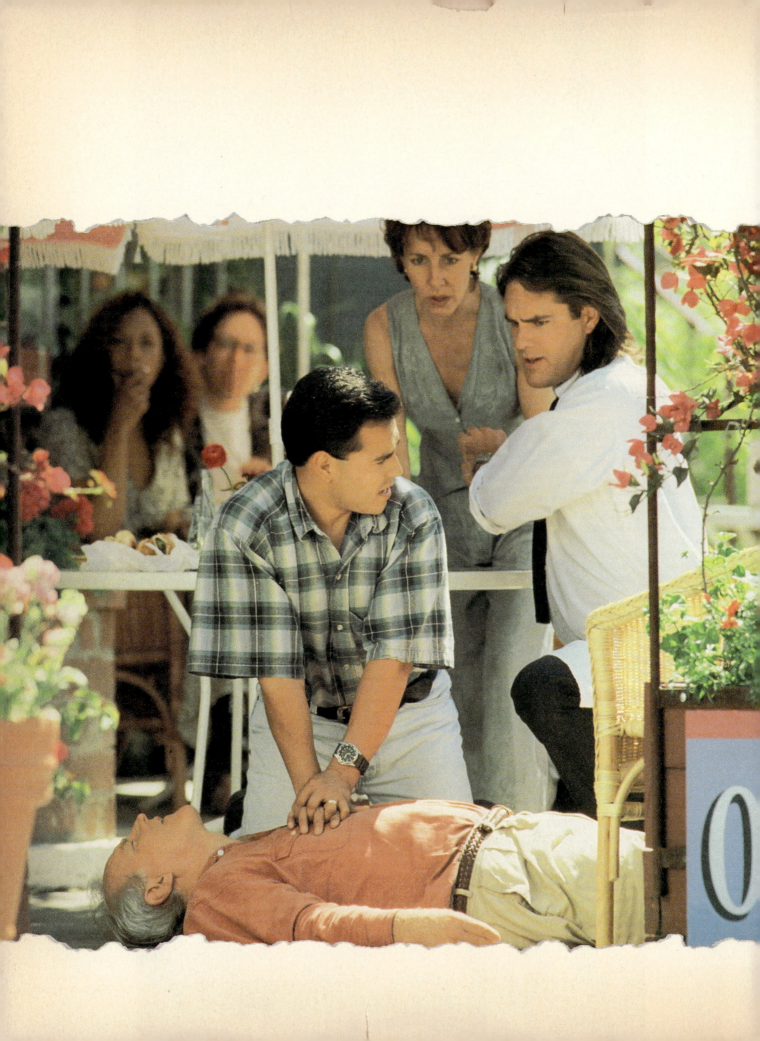

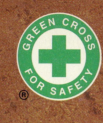

National Safety Council

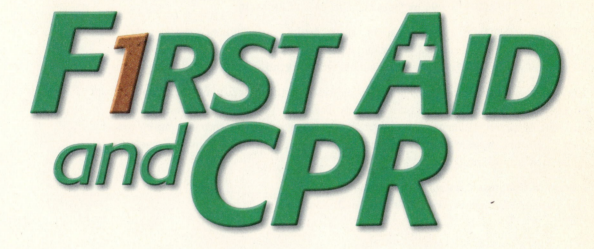

FIRST AID and CPR

THIRD EDITION

Jones and Bartlett Publishers
Sudbury, Massachusetts

Boston   London   Singapore

Editorial, Sales, and Customer Service Offices

Jones and Bartlett Publishers
40 Tall Pine Drive, Sudbury, MA 01776
508·443·5000, 1·800·832·0034
Internet: http://www.jbpub.com/nsc/, email: nsc@jbpub.com

Jones and Bartlett Publishers International
Barb House, Barb Mews
London W6 7PA, UK

The first aid and CPR procedures in this book are based on the most current recommendations of responsible medical sources. The National Safety Council and the publisher, however, make no guarantee as to, and assume no responsibility for the correctness, sufficiency or completeness of such information or recommendations. Other or additional safety measures may be required under particular circumstances.

Library of Congress Cataloging-in-Publication Data
First Aid and CPR: advanced / National Safety Council. — 3rd ed.
      p.   cm.
    Includes index.
    ISBN 0-7637-0183-1
      1. First aid in illness and injury.   2. CPR (First aid)
   I. National Safety Council.
   RC86.7.F5592   1996
   616.02'52 — dc20   96-21029
                             CIP

Chief Executive Officer: Clayton E. Jones
Chief Operating Officer: Donald W. Jones, Jr.
Executive Vice President and Editor-in-Chief: Tom Walker
Vice President, Production and Manufacturing: Paula Carroll
Vice President, Sales and Marketing: Rob McCarry
Emergency Care Editor: Tracy Murphy
Technical Consultant: Alton L. Thygerson
Production Administrator: Anne S. Noonan
Manufacturing Manager: Dana L. Cerrito
Text Design: Martucci Studio, Inc.
Editorial Production Service: Books By Design, Inc.
Illustrations: Rolin Graphics
Principal Photographer: Richard Nye
Photo Research: Tanya Barrett, Anne S. Noonan
Typesetting & Pre-press: Pre-Press Company, Inc.
Cover Design: Marshall Henrichs
Cover Photographs: ©Bruce Ayres, Tony Stone; ©Bob Daemmrich, Stock Boston;
                   Steve Ferry, P&F Communications
Printing and Binding: Metropole Litho, Inc.
Cover Printing: John P. Pow Company

Additional illustration and photo credits appear on page 467, which constitutes a continuation of the copyright page.

Printed in Canada
00 99 98 97 96   10 9 8 7 6 5 4 3 2 1

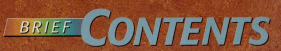
BRIEF CONTENTS

CONTENTS

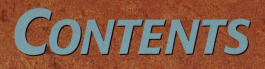

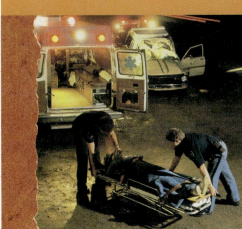

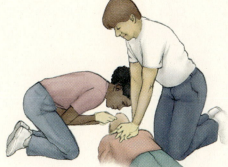

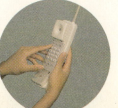

CONTENTS

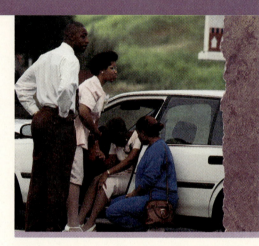

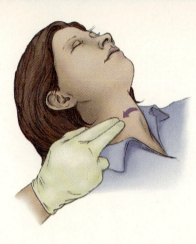

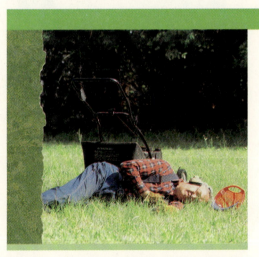

0–4 minutes: Brain damage unlikely if CPR started.

4–6 minutes: Brain damage possible.

6–10 minutes: Brain damage probable.

More than 10 minutes: Severe brain damage or brain death certain.

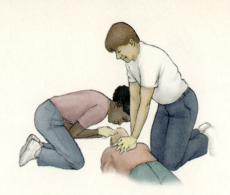

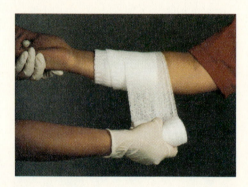

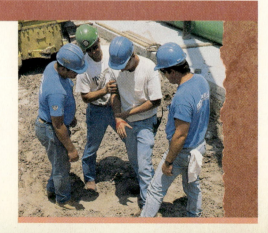

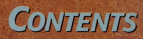

CONTENTS

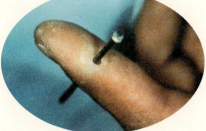

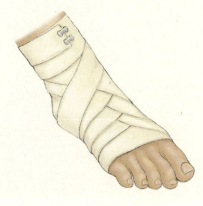

CONTENTS

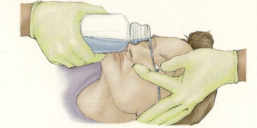

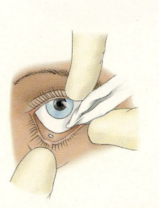

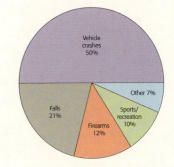

Chapter 12
Bone, Joint, and Muscle Injuries 220

Chapter 13
Extremity Injuries 228

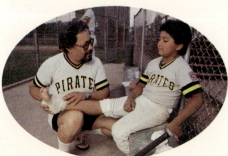

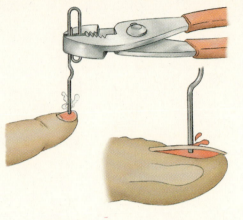

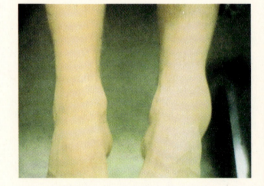

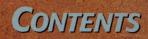

CONTENTS

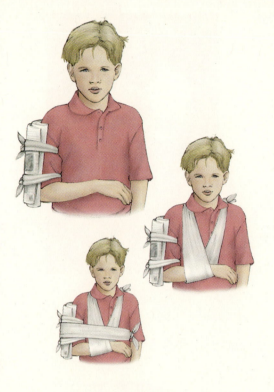

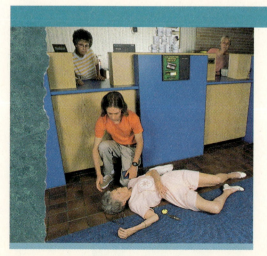

CONTENTS

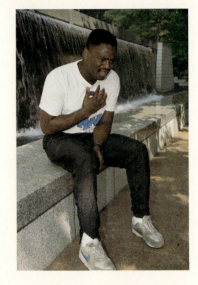

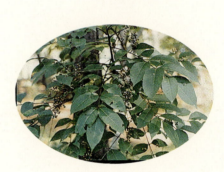

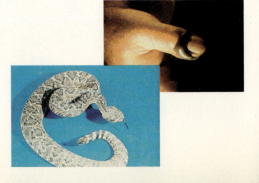

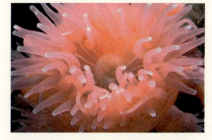

Areas infested with imported fire ants

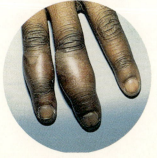

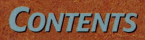

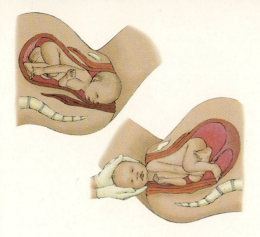

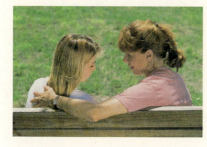

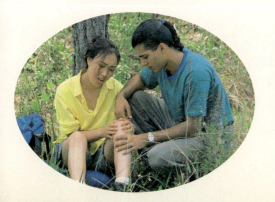

CONTENTS

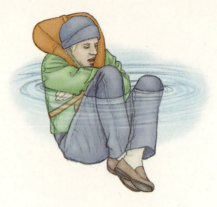

Chapter 23
Rescuing and Moving Victims   422

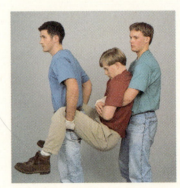

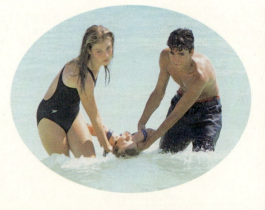

ABOUT THE NATIONAL SAFETY COUNCIL PROGRAM

Congratulations on selecting the National Safety Council's First Aid and CPR program! You join good company, as the National Safety Council has successfully trained over 2 million people worldwide in first aid and cardiopulmonary resuscitation (CPR). The National Safety Council's training network of nearly 10,000 instructors at over 2,500 sites worldwide has established the National Safety Council programs as the standard by which all others are judged.

In setting the standards, the National Safety Council has worked in close cooperation with hundreds of national and international organizations, thousands of corporations, thousands of leading educators, dozens of leading medical organizations, and hundreds of state and local governmental agencies. Their collective input has helped create programs that stand alone in quality. Consider just a few of the National Safety Council's current collaborations:

World's Leading Medical Organizations

The National Safety Council is currently working with both the American Academy of Orthopaedic Surgeons (AAOS) and the Wilderness Medical Society (WMS) to help bring innovative, new training programs to the marketplace. The National Safety Council and the AAOS are developing a new First Responder program and the National Safety Council and the WMS are developing the first-of-its-kind wilderness first aid program.

United States Government

The National Safety Council has developed an innovative computer-based training program for first aid that is currently being used to train United States Postal Service employees.

World's Leading Corporations

Thousands of corporations including Westinghouse, Disney, Exxon, General Motors, Pacific Bell, Ameritech, and U.S. West have selected many of the National Safety Council emergency care programs to train employees.

World's Leading Colleges and Universities

Hundreds of leading colleges and universities are working closely with the National Safety Council to fully develop and implement the Internet Initiative that will establish the National Safety Council as the leading on-line provider of emergency care programs.

Most importantly, in selecting the National Safety Council programs, you can feel confident that the programs are accepted and approved worldwide. You can rely on the National Safety Council. Founded in 1913, the National Safety Council is dedicated to protecting life, promoting health, and reducing accidental death. For more than 80 years, the National Safety Council has been the world's leading authority on safety/injury education.

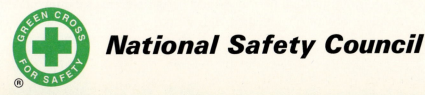

National Safety Council

ABOUT THE COURSE

Knowing what to do in an emergency situation is perhaps the most important skill anyone can learn. How many other courses teach you skills that could save a life? The National Safety Council's FIRST AID AND CPR course provides the most accurate, comprehensive, and up-to-date materials available. Instructors have access to a wide array of instructor supplements such as videos, slides, and CD-ROMs that have been carefully prepared to enhance your understanding of this important subject. Registered National Safety Council instructors can issue course completion cards for first aid and CPR.

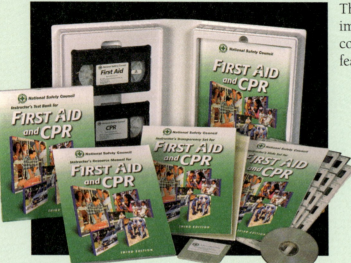

This textbook is perhaps the most important component of the course and includes the important features described below.

FIRST AID and CPR
Third Edition

When we published the first edition of *First Aid and CPR*, educators universally acclaimed the text as the finest book ever published in first aid. Over the past ten years, we have listened carefully to the users' feedback and we have been committed to improving the text. Now in its third edition, *First Aid and CPR* is even better!

The following enhancements have been made to the third edition:

Reorganization   A logical, student-oriented presentation of topics allows for increased proficiency and understanding of key skills and topics. For example, the bandaging chapter follows the wounds chapter and the splinting chapter follows the chapter on extremity injuries.

New Content   Responding to past users, we have added four new chapters on wilderness emergencies, the human body, bites and stings, and action at an emergency.

New Design   An outstanding new four-color design presents carefully planned pedagogy, and hundreds of new photographs, illustrations, charts, boxes, and flowcharts. Key elements of the design that will facilitate student learning and understanding of first aid and CPR include:

American Heart Association guidelines The latest guidelines for cardiopulmonary resuscitation and emergency cardiac care are presented in an easy-to-understand format.

Flowcharts Over 35 full-page flowcharts depict decision-making and appropriate first aid procedures.

SKILL SCAN: Bleeding Control

1. Direct pressure stops most bleeding. Wearing disposable gloves, place sterile gauze pad or clean cloth over wound. If bleeding does not stop in 10 minutes, press harder over a wider area.
2. A pressure bandage can free you to attend to other injuries or victims.
3. Do not remove a blood-soaked dressing. Add more on top.
4. If disposable gloves are not available, use another barrier or extra gauze pads or cloths.
5. If bleeding persists, use elevation to help reduce blood flow. Combine with direct pressure over the wound.
6. If bleeding still continues, apply pressure at a pressure point to slow blood flow. Locations are: (a) brachial or (b) femoral. Use with direct pressure over the wound.

Bleeding 113

SNAKEBITES

Ch 17 ▸ Bites and Stings

SKILL SCAN pages Over 20 skill scan pages present key first aid skills in a format that enhances student comprehension.

CAUTION: DO NOT
• try to warm the victim.
• give the victim anything to eat or drink. It could cause nausea and vomiting, which could result in aspiration. It could also cause complications if surgery is needed. Sucking on a clean cloth soaked in water will relieve a victim's dry mouth.

Highlighted *Do Not* procedures It is important to know what *not* to do as well as to know what to do.

STUDY QUESTIONS End-of-chapter self-tests and case studies help evaluate student mastery of the subject. Perforated pages allow students to hand in completed materials to the instructor.

STUDY QUESTIONS 18

Name _____ Course _____ Date _____

Activities

Activity 1
Mark each statement as true (T) or false (F).

T F 1. Shivering is a method the body uses to generate heat.
T F 2. You should massage frostbitten parts.
T F 3. Blisters may form as a result of frostbite.
T F 4. Smoking intensifies the harmful effects of cold.
T F 5. Frostbite is more severe if the injured area is thawed and then refrozen.
T F 6. In frostbite, the parts should be rewarmed rapidly, since rewarming reduces pain.
T F 7. Break the blisters that may develop in frostbite.
T F 8. Hypothermia can occur only in below-freezing temperatures.

Activity 2
Mark each action yes (Y) or no (N). Which of the following actions are proper first aid for frostbite?

___ 1. Rewarm a frostbitten part by exposing it to a fire or open flame.
___ 2. Rewarm a frostbitten part by using warm water (102°–105°F).
___ 3. Placing frostbitten hands in another person's armpits is as effective as using warm water.
___ 4. Rub the frostbitten part to restore circulation.
___ 5. Rub the frostbitten area with snow.
___ 6. A victim with frozen lower extremities should be carried, if possible, to the nearest medical facility.
___ 7. If a victim with a severely frostbitten foot cannot be carried to medical aid, keep the part frozen and assist him in walking.
___ 8. Break any blisters that have formed.

Activity 3
Check (✔) the appropriate action(s). Which of the following actions are proper first aid for hypothermia?

___ 1. Give hot coffee or hot chocolate to rewarm a victim.
___ 2. Treat the victim gently.
___ 3. Replace wet clothing with dry clothing.
___ 4. Get the victim out of the cold environment.

For mild hypothermia:

___ 5. Apply chemical heat pads to the head, neck, chest, and groin first.
___ 6. Place in a tub of hot water.
___ 7. Use your body heat against the victim's body while both of you are in a sleeping bag.

For profound hypothermia:

___ 8. Check the victim's breathing and pulse for at least 30 to 45 seconds.
___ 9. Quickly rewarm the victim even if you are near a medical facility.
___ 10. Arrange transportation to a medical facility.

Case Situations

Case 1
It is 5:30 P.M. on a Saturday in midwinter, and an 18-year-old female has been in the woods for most of the afternoon. She complains that her toes are numb. You find that they look grayish-blue and feel hard and frozen.

___ 1. This victim is most likely experiencing
a. deep frostbite (also called freezing)
b. frostnip
c. superficial frostbite
d. hypothermia

Study Questions **361**

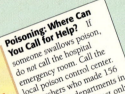

Poisoning: Where Can You Call for Help? If someone swallows poison, do *not* call the hospital emergency room. Call the local poison control center. Researchers who made 156 "test calls" to 52 hospital emergency departments in Illinois found that the advice given was correct only 64 percent of the time. Calls to the same emergency department on different days for the same problem did not consistently produce the same advice. In contrast, poison control centers gave correct advice in 17 out of 18 test calls (94 percent).

Source: H. N. Wigder et al., "Emergency Department Poison Advice Telephone Calls," *Annals of Emergency Medicine* 25:349 (March 1995).

FYI boxes These features present additional information that a student might like to know, including simplified medical journal articles for better understanding.

Hero CITATION

Roger Lindsay saved David Triplett from drowning, Isleta, New Mexico, May 7, 1990. Triplett, 37, attempted to swim across Sunrise Lake but began to struggle midway. He yelled for help. Fishing nearby from the bank, Lindsay, 30, was alerted to Triplett's plight. Although he had not swum for several years, following an accident which resulted in a leg being amputated below the knee, Lindsay, wearing a prosthesis, dived into the lake and swam about 150 feet to Triplett, who had by then submerged. Lindsay pulled Triplett to the surface of the water and began to swim back to the bank, towing him. He tired en route, his prosthetic leg pulling him down, and began to struggle. When he reached the bank, others pulled Triplett out of the water. He was revived and taken to the hospital for treatment.

Hero **CITATIONS** Real-life accounts about citizens saving lives are interspersed throughout the book.

FIRST AID TIPS

Insect in an Ear

Do not try to kill a lodged insect by poking something into the victim's ear. Insects are attracted to light, so it may be coaxed out with light. Outdoors, pull the ear lobe gently to straighten the canal and turn the ear toward the sun. Indoors, turn off all lights, then shine a flashlight into the ear while pulling gently on the ear lobe. This may induce the insect to crawl out toward the light.

If the light method fails, a little mineral oil may cause the insect to float out. Do not use this method if you are not *absolutely* sure that the foreign body in the ear is an insect. If the object is vegetable matter (e.g., a bean, popcorn), the object may swell and be difficult to remove. Do not use mineral oil if there is any sign of eardrum rupture.

Do not go into the ear canal to remove foreign objects.

• **FIRST AID TIPS** Tricks of the trade help the student become a more complete, well-rounded first aider.

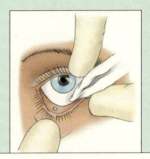

• **Outstanding illustrations** Accurately depicted graphics allow students to better understand proper procedures.

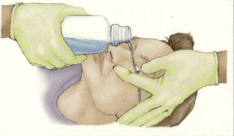

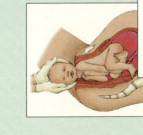

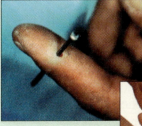

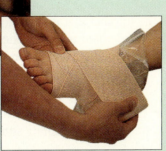

• **Injury photographs** Real injury photographs help prepare students to handle an actual real-life emergency.

We thank you for supporting the National Safety Council programs. For additional information on any aspect of this program, please contact Jones and Bartlett Publishers at **1-800-832-0034**, through e-mail at **nsc@jbpub.com** or via our homepage at **http://www.jbpub.com/nsc/**

TO THE INSTRUCTOR

The National Safety Council welcomes you to its family of instructors and congratulates you on selecting *First Aid and CPR,* Third Edition. You made the right choice! You join nearly 10,000 instructors who have already discovered the advantages of the National Safety Council. The National Safety Council firmly believes that the most important aspect of its program is the quality of instructors. The National Safety Council has designed an instructor-friendly program and invested heavily in state-of-the-art instructor resources. Key features of this exciting new program include:

Ease of Administration   Academic departments with registered First Aid and CPR instructors can internally administrate their own courses. Once approved as a National Safety Council Educational Training agency, your department will no longer be subject to the difficulties of an off-campus certifying organization.

Complete Academic Freedom   The National Safety Council's First Aid and CPR course is like other academic courses. Using the National Safety Council teaching materials, instructors determine the most appropriate course content, course length, and course structure best suited to their students.

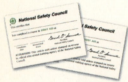

FREE National Safety Council Course Completion Cards   All students who successfully complete a course using *First Aid and CPR* receive FREE National Safety Council course completion cards for both first aid and CPR. The first aid cards are valid for three years and the CPR cards are valid for one or two years depending on your specific state requirements.

First Aid and CPR Internet Resources   The National Safety Council, in close association with leading colleges and universities, has developed an array of instructor resources designed to enhance and improve the course. These exciting resources, FREE to all adopters, include:

•**Online departmental approval** All departments seeking Educational Training Agency status can submit an electronic form to apply for departmental approval.

•**Online instructor credentialing** This new service allows instructors at educational institutions to qualify and maintain official instructor status. The credentialing process consists of basic questions that test an instructor on first aid procedures and teaching strategies. Instructors complete and submit an online exam via the Internet that is graded, and an e-mail response indicating the status of the approval is returned to the applicant. Instructors passing the minimum requirements receive accreditation and are sent an instructor card via surface mail. All instructors issuing National Safety Council course completion cards will be required to participate in this instructor credentialing process.

•**Instructor e-mail newsletter** Registered instructors receive a monthly, electronic instructor newsletter with the latest National Safety Council information, teaching strategies, and other first aid and CPR updates.

•**Instructor bulletin board** Instructors can post comments, ask questions and exchange ideas with other members of the National Safety Council community. You can access this service by visiting http://www.jbpub.com/nsc/ and choosing the bulletin board option.

•**Online electronic supplements** Electronic instructor supplements can be downloaded directly to your own personal computer.

All Internet resources can be accessed through the Jones and Bartlett Publishers homepage at http://www.jbpub.com/nsc/

The following FREE Instructor Supplements are provided to all qualified adopters:

Interactive First Aid: A Scenario Based Approach
This new CD-ROM covers all the key first aid topics and allows for classroom presentation and/or individual student usage through learning labs. This interactive CD-ROM includes full motion video, charts, boxes, illustrations, photographs, and key content from the text. The CD-ROM has been developed to challenge students' mastery of first aid through scenario-based learning. A student workbook is also available. ISBN 0-7637-0254-4

Instructor's Resource Manual
This new manual includes lesson plans, teaching strategies, proficiency tests, supplemental information, transparency masters, and answers to all study questions in the text. This manual helps you utilize all of the outstanding instructor resources. ISBN 0-7637-0200-8

First Aid Video (VHS, 55 minutes)
This new, full-feature video, designed in a topical format, corresponds with the material in the text. ISBN 0-7637-0196-3

CPR Video (VHS, 38 minutes)
This outstanding video applies to all CPR training and follows the latest American Heart Association standards as published in the JAMA supplement. An outstanding combination of dramatic, real-life emergencies with a proven lecture format make this video essential for all courses covering basic life support. ISBN 0-7637-0303-6

Instructor's Transparency Set
An all-new set of 40 full-color acetate transparencies depicting the most important boxes, charts, illustrations, and diagrams from the text. ISBN 0-7637-0298-6

Instructor's Slide Set
An all-new set of 80 35mm color slides depicting key first aid topics and actual injuries. The topical slides outline the most important information in the text while the injury slides prepare your students to handle real-life emergencies. ISBN 0-7637-0198-X

Instructor's Test Bank
An all-new, 1,500 test question manual that corresponds to the chapters in the text. ISBN 0-7637-0199-8

Instructor's Computerized Test Bank
A computerized version of the above test bank, available in both IBM and Macintosh formats. ISBN 0-7637-0201-3 IBM version ISBN 0-7637-0202-1 Macintosh version

Call 1-800-832-0034 for more information.

A PROGRAM FOR ALL YOUR NEEDS

Program	Description
First Aid and CPR, 3/E 0-7637-0183-1, 496 pp., Paper	The best-selling program on first aid and CPR is appropriate for all colleges, universities, and high schools. Includes the latest American Heart Association CPR guidelines as well as contributions and reviews from over 70 national organizations. The most definitive first aid textbook available.
First Aid 0-86720-755-8, 176 pp., Paper	This program is suited for courses in colleges, universities, and high schools where CPR is not covered. The student text includes the latest information and procedures on emergency care.
CPR, 2/E 0-7637-0213-7, 128 pp., Paper	A comprehensive program, based on the 1992 AHA CPR guidelines, suitable for all colleges, universities, and high schools. Including complete coverage of basic life support for adults, children, and infants as well as additional coverage of two-rescuer CPR and highlights of the OSHA bloodborne pathogens standards.
First Aid and CPR: **Infants and Children** 0-86720-211-0, 208 pp., Paper	A one-of-a-kind program developed for students and teachers in the childhood education field. Accidental injuries are the leading health problem in children, and this program helps prepare the participant for accidents involving children. This program is designed to meet all state, local, and federal requirements for first aid and CPR training of child care providers.
Infant and Child CPR 0-7637-0211-0, 64 pp., Paper	Based on the latest AHA guidelines. Suitable for child care providers in all settings.
Bloodborne Pathogens, 2/E 0-7637-0315-X, 88 pp., Paper	A comprehensive new training program to meet the needs of all students entering the health-related fields as well as those at risk of occupational exposure. Over 5 million workers in health care related fields are at risk of exposure to bloodborne pathogens, such as HIV and HBV. Includes a new chapter on airborne pathogens.
First Responder, 2/E 0-86720-541-5, 440 pp., Paper	A joint program developed by the National Safety Council and the American Academy of Orthopaedic Surgeons based on the 1995 DOT First Responder curriculum. This new edition provides the framework around which first responders can gain the knowledge, skills, and confidence needed to care for victims of sudden illnesses and accidents. Suitable for courses offered through training academies, colleges, and universities.
Oxygen Administration 0-86720-983-6, 35 pp., Paper	An essential element of emergency care consists of providing supplemental oxygen. This outstanding new program effectively outlines the importance and proper use of portable medical oxygen equipment.
National Pool and Waterpark **Lifeguard/CPR Training** 0-86720-848-1, 272 pp., Paper	A joint program of the National Safety Council, Ellis & Associates, and the National Recreation and Park Association for use in colleges, universities, and high schools. Guidelines developed by this program have revolutionized the aquatic safety industry.
Stress Management 0-86720-980-1, 72 pp., Paper	A state-of-the-art training program designed to provide the latest, most comprehensive approach to identifying and controlling stress. Ideal for classroom use by students in colleges, universities, and high schools.
Scuba Diving First Aid 0-86720-944-5, 54 pp., Paper	A new program, extensively reviewed by noted scuba diving physicians and diving medical technician trainers, ideal for teaching scuba diving first aid.
Primeros Auxilios y RCP 0-86720-847-3, 92 pp., Paper	A Spanish version of the best-selling **First Aid and CPR** program.
Good Samaritan: **Helping in an Emergency** 0-86720-544-X, 32 pp., Paper	A new program that provides the basics of emergency care to individuals not interested in a formal course. Covers recognizing an emergency, getting help, and practical information on how to handle dozens of common emergencies.

ACKNOWLEDGMENTS

We owe our deepest gratitude to the following members of the National Safety Council Educational Advisory Board. Their commitment and dedication to this program is surpassed only by their dedication and commitment to their students.

Sharon Adams
Spokane Community College

Frank Amato
Indian River Community College

Michael Ballard
Morehead State University

Carol Bond
Southern California Safety Training Center

Lori Carter
University of North Florida

Franklin Carver
Ohio University

Frank Chapman
University of North Carolina—Wilmington

Les Chatelain
University of Utah

Harvey Clearwater
University of Maryland, College Park

Vonnie Clovin
University of Kentucky

Kate Cunningham
Valencia State Community College

Caprice Dodson
Houston Community College

Greg Goebel
Southeast Community College

Robin Gurgainus
James Sprint Community College

John Healey
Lane Community College

Bert Hood
Arizona Chapter, National Safety Council

Kathy Hudson
Hudson County Public Schools

Dalia Jeziorski
Triton College

Tim Kayhill
Eastern Kentucky University

Jogoon Kim
Michigan State University

Marian King
North Atlanta High School

Laura Kitzmiller
Texas A&M

Frank Lagotic
Santa Fe Community College

Harold Leibowitz
Brooklyn College

Paula Linder
University of Maine, Orno

Brent Mangus
University of Nevada, Las Vegas

Dwaine J. Marten
University of Idaho

Debbie Moffett
Miami Dade Community College—Kendall Campus

Debra Murray
University of North Carolina, Chapel Hill

Jerry Nauman
Winona State University

Bruce Norris
West Chester University

Sharon Ogle
Brevard Community College

Glen Payton
Texas Christian University

Allan Peterson
Gordon College

Ron Pfeiffer
Boise State University

Joy Quanrud
National Safety Council

Scott Richter
University of Montana

D.J. Rowley
Utah Valley State College

Donna Siegfried
National Safety Council

Sherm Sowby
California State University, Fresno

David Spiro, EMT-P
Hartsdale, NY

Larry Starr
SOS Technologies

Jessie Stoner
Florida Community College at Jacksonville

Jeannie Stream
Danville Area Community College

Lance Tatum
Gordon College

Alton Thygerson
Brigham Young University

Maggie Tucker
University of Florida, Gainesville

Harry Tyson
Bowling Green University

Andrew Weinberg, MD
Harvard University

Deitra Wengert
Towson State University

C. Newton Wilkes
Northwestern State University

John Wingfield
Ball State University

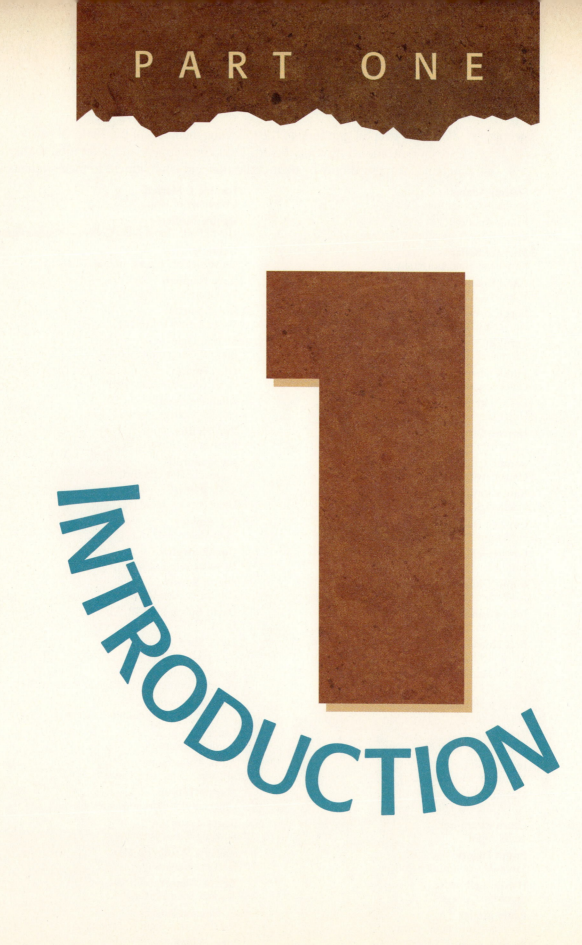

PART ONE

1

INTRODUCTION

CHAPTER 1
Background Information

CHAPTER 2
**Action at an
Emergency**

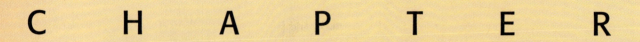

1

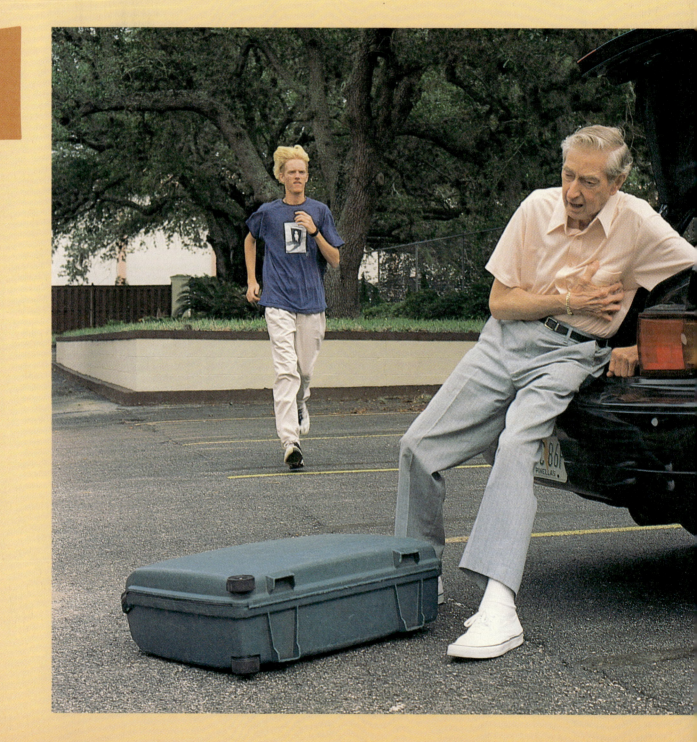

BACKGROUND INFORMATION

Need for First Aid Training

A large truck swings around a corner, crashes into an automobile, and pushes it over an embankment. Bystanders rush to the rescue. They remove the driver of the car, stop a passing car, lift him to his feet, and send him in a sitting position to a nearby hospital. Because of this unskilled and ignorant handling, the man's spinal cord was punctured by the sharp edge of a broken vertebrae so that he will remain paralyzed for the rest of his life—all of this might have been avoided by a knowledge of what to do in an emergency.

A backcountry hiker is bitten by a rattlesnake. Her frantic companion "cuts and sucks" the bitten area, not realizing that this is an obsolete and harmful procedure. A trained first aider would have known the proper procedures for taking care of the victim.

A swimmer is pulled unconscious from the water. No one helps because no one knows cardiopulmonary resuscitation (CPR). The emergency medical service (EMS) ambulance arrives too late to revive the swimmer. Giving CPR would have served as a holding action in preserving life for the few minutes needed for an ambulance to arrive.

Late at night, a man who had earlier smashed a fingernail in a car door can't stand the excruciating pain caused by the pressure of blood accumulating underneath the fingernail. He drives himself to the hospital emergency department where the blood clot is relieved. He later receives a bill for over $100. Knowing the proper first aid procedure, he could have relieved the pain sooner and saved money.

These cases clearly point out the need for first aid training. *It's better to know it and not need it than to need it and not know it.* Everyone should be able to perform first aid since most people will eventually find themselves in a situation requiring it, either for another person or for themselves.

A delay of as little as four minutes when a person's heart stops can mean death. Therefore, what a bystander does can mean the difference between life and death. However, most injuries do not require life-saving efforts. During their entire lifetime, most people will see only one or two situations involving life-threatening conditions. While saving lives is important, knowing what to do for less severe injuries demands greater attention and more first aid training.

Throughout the world, injuries are the leading cause of death during the first half of the human life span. Yearly, one in four people suffers a nonfatal injury serious enough to need medical attention or to restrict activity for at least a day. Few escape the tragedy of a fatal or permanently disabling injury to

> " *Whatever can go wrong, will.* "
>
> Murphy's Law

> " *Whatever can happen to one man can happen to every man.* "
>
> Lucius Annaeus Seneca (4 B.C.?–A.D. 65)

a relative or a friend. This does not include those requiring care for less severe injuries and sudden illness at home, work, or play. Tables 1-1, 1-2, and 1-3 describe just how often minor injuries happen in a single year.

Despite increased attention and progress in recent years, many people still lack an acceptable level of knowledge and proficiency in first aid. These skills are greatly needed.

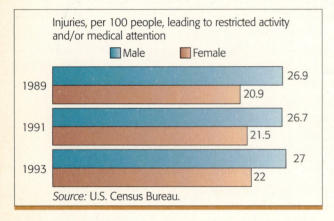

Injuries, per 100 people, leading to restricted activity and/or medical attention

	Male	Female
1989	26.9	20.9
1991	26.7	21.5
1993	27	22

Source: U.S. Census Bureau.

Serious injury rates climb

Value to Self

Although many people learn first aid in order to help others, the training primarily helps oneself. It enables a person to give proper immediate care to one's own injuries and sudden illness. If victims are too seriously injured to help themselves, they may be able to direct others toward proper care.

First aid training also helps develop safety awareness. Discussing injuries sharpens the desire for injury prevention and shows how injuries occur.

Value to Others

Those with first aid training are more likely to properly assist family members if they are stricken. While the main benefits are to the trained individual and family, they extend further, usually to co-workers, acquaintances, and strangers.

Table 1-1: Health Problems Reported by Adults during the Previous Year

Problem	Percentage of Adults Reporting the Problem	
	Study 1	Study 2
Bruises	32	—
Cuts and scratches (minor)	46	57
Insect stings and bites	30	37
Sunburn	25	—

Source: American Pharmaceutical Association, *Handbook of Nonprescription Drugs,* 9th ed. (Washington, DC: American Pharmaceutical Association, 1990).

Value in Remote Locations

Should injuries or sudden illness require medical care, consideration must be given to time, distance, and availability. For most victims who are severely injured or suddenly ill, the EMS can reach them within 10 to 20 minutes. However, some victims are long distances from medical care. Although most people relate long distances and lack of medical care to wilderness settings involving outdoor recreational activities (e.g., hiking, camping, hunting, snowmobiling), other situations demand people be prepared to give first aid over an extended time:

- urban areas after a natural or manmade disaster that destroys or overwhelms the EMS
- remote occupations (e.g., farming, ranching, commercial fishing, forestry)
- remote communities
- developing countries

First aid needed in remote locations is similar to that needed in urban settings, but extra skills are sometimes needed. See Chapter 22 for wilderness first aid information.

What Is First Aid?

First aid is the immediate care given to an injured or suddenly ill person. First aid does *not* take the place of proper medical treatment. It consists only of furnishing temporary assistance until competent medical care, if needed, is obtained or until the chance for recovery without medical care is assured. Most injuries and illnesses do not require medical care.

Properly applied, first aid may mean the difference between life and death, rapid recovery and long hospitalization, or temporary disability and permanent injury. First aid involves more than doing things for others; it also includes the things that people can do for themselves.

The ability to recognize a serious medical emergency and knowledge of how to get help may mean the difference between life and death. The problem is that recognition can be delayed because neither the victim nor bystanders know basic symptoms (e.g., a heart attack victim may wait hours after the onset of symptoms before seeking help). Moreover, most people do not know first aid; even if they do, they may panic in an emergency.

Legal Considerations

Legal and ethical issues concern all first aiders. Is a first aider required to stop and give care at an automobile crash? Can a child with a broken arm be treated even when the parents cannot be contacted for their consent? These and many other legal and ethical questions confront first aiders.

Consent

Before giving first aid, a first aider must gain consent from a victim. Touching another person without his or her permission or consent is unlawful (known as battery) and could be grounds for a lawsuit. Likewise, giving first aid without the victim's consent is unlawful.

Expressed Consent

Consent must be obtained from every conscious, mentally competent (i.e., able to make a rational decision) adult (i.e., a person of legal age). Tell the victim your name and that you have first aid training and explain what you will be doing. Permission from the victim may be expressed either verbally or with a nod of the head.

Implied Consent

Implied consent involves an unconscious victim and a life-threatening condition. It is assumed or implied that an unresponsive victim would consent to lifesaving interventions. Consent also is implied

when the first aider begins care and the victim does not resist.

Children and Mentally Incompetent Adults

Consent must be obtained from a parent or guardian of a child victim, as legally defined by the state. The same is true for an adult who is mentally incompetent. When life-threatening situations exist and the parent or legal guardian is not available for consent, first aid should be given based on implied consent. Do not withhold first aid from a minor just to obtain parental or guardian permission.

Psychiatric emergencies present difficult problems of consent. Under most conditions, a police officer is the only person with the authority to restrain and transport a person against that person's will. A first aider should not intervene unless directed to do so by a police officer or unless it is obvious that the victim is about to do life-threatening harm to himself or herself or to others.

Refusing Help

Although it seldom happens, a person may refuse assistance for countless reasons, such as religious grounds, avoidance of possible pain, or the desire to be examined by a physician rather than by a first aider. Whatever the reason for refusing medical care, or even if no reason is given, the conscious and mentally competent adult can reject help. One exception to that rule is when a victim refuses to be moved, but relocating the person is necessary for the public good, such as movement of traffic.

Generally, the wisest approach is to inform the victim of his or her medical condition, what you propose to do, and why the help is necessary. If the victim understands the consequences and still refuses treatment, there is little else you can do. Call the emergency medical service (EMS) and, while awaiting their arrival:

- Try again to persuade the victim to accept care and encourage others at the scene to persuade the victim. A victim may have a change of mind after a short period of time.

- Make certain you have witnesses. All too often a victim will refuse consent and then deny having done so.

- Consider calling for law enforcement assistance. In most locations, the police can place a person in protective custody and require him or her to go to a hospital.

Table 1-2: Estimated Injuries Related to Selected Consumer Products, 1992

Product	Injuries*	Product	Injuries*
Home Maintenance		**Home Furnishings, Fixtures, and Accessories**	
Noncaustic cleaning equip., detergents	26,654		
Cleaning agents (except soaps)	43,758	Bathtub, shower structures	166,327
Miscellaneous household chemicals	24,679	Beds, mattresses, pillows	400,732
Paints, solvents, lubricants	23,383	Carpets, rugs	112,763
Drain, oven cleaners, caustics	10,319	Chairs, sofas, sofa beds	413,759
		Desks, cabinets, shelves, racks	228,676
Home Workshop Equipment		Electric fixtures, lamps, equipment	54,097
Batteries, all types	14,060	Ladders, stools	189,210
Hoists, lifts, jacks, etc.	16,562	Mirrors, mirror glass	24,928
Miscellaneous workshop equipment	46,407	Other misc. furniture, accessories	57,555
Power home tools, except saws	31,742	Sinks, toilets	61,281
Power home workshop saws, all	97,606	Tables, all types	345,271
Welding, soldering, cutting tools	20,686		
Wires, cords, not specified	12,789	**Home Structures and Construction Materials**	
Workshop manual tools	125,780		
		Cabinets or door hardware	24,876
Packaging and Containers, Household		Ceilings, walls, panels (inside)	262,572
		Counters, counter tops	36,888
Cans, other containers	239,521	Fences	123,014
Glass bottles, jars	63,170	Glass doors, windows, panels	216,193
Paper, cardboard, plastic products	47,495	Handrails, railings, banisters	42,965
		Miscellaneous construction materials	95,147
Housewares		Nails, carpet tacks, etc.	239,711
Cookware, pots, pans	36,700	Nonglass doors, panels	357,149
Cutlery, knives, unpowered	468,587	Porches, open side floors, etc.	129,152
Drinking glasses	130,200	Stairs, ramps, landings, floors	1,879,029
Miscellaneous housewares	61,201	Windows, door sills, frames	60,147
Scissors	34,602		
Small kitchen appliances	43,453	**General Household Appliances**	
Tableware and accessories	120,940	Cooking ranges, ovens, etc.	53,401
		Irons, clothes steamers (not toys)	17,266
		Miscellaneous household appliances	34,941
		Refrigerators, freezers	35,895
		Washers, dryers	22,590

Table 1-2: continued

Product	Injuries*	Product	Injuries*
Heating, Cooling, and Ventilating Equipment		**Yard and Garden Equipment**	
Radiators, all	15,771	Chain saws	38,692
Chimneys, fireplaces	26,664	Hand garden tools	36,374
Fans (except stove exhaust fans)	17,050	Hatchets, axes	16,760
Heating stoves, space heaters	37,805	Lawn, garden care equipment	51,324
Pipes, heating and plumbing	23,216	Lawn mowers, all types	85,202
		Trimmers, small power garden tools	14,635
Home Communication, Entertainment, and Hobby Equipment		Other power lawn equipment	21,598
Miscellaneous hobby equipment	15,785	**Sports and Recreation Equipment**	
Pet supplies, equipment	26,703	All-terrain vehicles, mopeds, minibikes	132,271
Sound recording, reproducing equipment	46,022	Barbecue grills, stoves, equipment	16,087
Television sets, stands	42,000	Bicycles, accessories	649,536
		Exercise equipment	95,127
Personal Use Items		Nonpowder guns, BBs, pellets	34,552
Cigarettes, lighters, fuel	23,547	Playground equipment	290,382
Clothing, all	142,457	Skateboards	44,068
Grooming devices	31,991	Toboggans, sleds, snow disks, etc.	43,273
Holders for personal items	16,529	Trampolines	43,665
Jewelry	55,142		
Paper money, coins	30,274	**Miscellaneous Products**	
Pencils, pens, other desk supplies	49,226	Dollies, carts	45,257
Razors, shavers, razor blades	43,365	Elevators, other lifts	14,457
Sewing equipment	29,814	Gasoline and diesel fuels	19,205
		Fireworks	13,263
		Nursery equipment	117,732
		Toys	177,061

*Estimated number of product-related injuries in the United States and territories that were treated in hospital emergency departments in 1992. Not all product categories are shown.
Source: Consumer Product Safety Commission, National Electronic Injury Surveillance System.

Table 1-3: Sports Injuries

Sport	Participants	Injuries
Archery	5,800,000	4,940
Badminton	(a)	2,612
Baseball, softball	34,600,000	437,207
Basketball	29,600,000	761,000
Bicycle riding	63,000,000[b]	604,066
Billiards, pool	29,400,000	5,194
Bowling	41,300,000	23,814
Boxing	700,000	7,537
Exercising with equipment[c]	34,900,000	91,359
Fishing	51,200,000	75,959
Football	14,700,000	409,296
Golf[d]	22,600,000	37,998
Gymnastics[e]	(a)	46,858
Handball	(a)	2,391
Horseback riding	(a)	68,517
Ice hockey	1,700,000	61,264
Ice skating	6,900,000	36,379
Racquetball	5,400,000	15,399[f]
Roller skating[g]	27,700,000	128,392
Skateboarding	5,600,000	27,718
Snowmobiling	(a)	14,729
Soccer	10,300,000	146,409
Surfboarding	(a)	2,424
Swimming	61,400,000	145,576
Table tennis	(a)	2,101
Tennis	14,200,000	30,532
Volleyball	20,500,000	112,120
Waterskiing	8,100,000	15,337
Wrestling	(a)	44,809

[a]Data not available.
[b]Includes on- and off-road mountain biking.
[c]Includes weight lifting.
[d]Excludes golf carts (6,372 injuries).
[e]Excludes trampolines (46,215 injuries).
[f]Includes squash and paddleball.
[g]Includes 2x2 (91,406 injuries) and in-line (36,986 injuries).
Source: Participants—National Sporting Goods Association (1993); figures include those who participate more than one time per year except for bicycle riding and swimming, which include those who participate more than six times per year. Injuries—Consumer Product Safety Commission (1993); figures include only injuries treated in hospital emergency rooms.

Abandonment

Abandonment means terminating the care of a victim without ensuring continued care at the same level or higher. Once you have responded to an emergency, you must not leave a victim who needs continuing first aid until another competent and trained person takes responsibility for the victim. This may seem obvious, but there have been cases in which critically ill or injured victims were left unattended and then died. Thus, a first aider must stay with the victim until another equally or better trained person takes over.

Negligence

Negligence means deviating from accepted standards of care that results in further injury to the victim. Factors involved in negligence include

1. duty to act
2. breach of duty (substandard care)
3. injury and damages inflicted

Duty to Act

No one is required to render first aid when no legal duty exists. For example, a physician could ignore a stranger suffering a heart attack or a fractured bone. While moral obligations may exist, they are not always the same as a legal obligation to help. Duty to act may occur in the following situations:

- *When employment requires it.* If your employer designates you as responsible for rendering first aid to meet OSHA (Occupational Safety and Health Administration) requirements and you are called to an accident scene, you have a duty to act. Other examples of occupations involving the giving of first aid include law enforcement officers, park rangers, athletic trainers, lifeguards, and teachers, all of whose job descriptions designate them to give first aid.

- *When a preexisting responsibility exists.* You may have a preexisting relationship with other persons that demands you be responsible for them, which means you must give first aid should they need it. Examples include a parent for a child, a driver for a passenger.

Duty to act means following guidelines for standards of care. Standards of care ensure quality care and protection for injured or suddenly ill victims. The elements that make up standards of care include the following:

- *The type of rescuer.* A first aider should provide the level and type of care expected of a reasonable person with the same amount of training and in similar circumstances. Different standards of care apply to physicians, nurses, emergency medical technicians (EMTs), and first aiders.

- *Published recommendations.* Emergency care–related organizations and societies publish recommended first aid procedures. For example, the American Heart Association publishes guidelines for giving cardiopulmonary resuscitation (CPR), and the Wilderness Medical Society publishes guidelines for assisting victims who are more than one hour from medical care.

Breach of Duty

Generally, a first aider breaches (i.e., "breaks") his or her duty to a victim by failing to provide the type of care as would a person having the same or similar training. There are two ways to breach one's duty: acts of omission and acts of commission. An *act of omission* is the failure to do what a reasonably prudent person with the same or similar training would do in the same or similar circumstances. An *act of commission* is doing something that a reasonably prudent person would *not* do under the same or similar circumstances. Forgetting to put on a dressing is an act of omission; cutting a snakebite site is an act of commission.

Injury and Damages Inflicted

Other than physical damage, injury and damage can include physical pain and suffering, mental anguish, medical expenses, and sometimes loss of earnings and earning capacity.

Confidentiality

First aiders may become privy to information that would be embarrassing to the victim or the victim's family if it were publicly revealed. It is important that you be extremely cautious about revealing information you learn while caring for someone. The law recognizes that people have the right to privacy.

Do not discuss what you know with anyone other than those who have a medical need to know. Some state laws do, however, require the reporting of certain incidents, such as rape, abuse, and gunshot wounds.

Hero Citation

Jose Gomez rescued Amelia J. Robitaille from burning, Lansing, Michigan, August 21, 1992. Amelia, 4, was inside her family's one-story house when fire erupted in a bedroom. Gomez, 31, who lived in the neighborhood, was alerted to the fire and went to the scene, where he learned that Amelia was still inside the burning house. Gomez entered the house through its front door; as dense smoke precluded visibility, he lay on the floor and crawled deeper into the house through a hall, which was adjacent to the burning bedroom. He found Amelia standing in the living room, then turned and took her outside to safety. Amelia required hospital treatment for smoke inhalation, and she sustained a minor burn to one foot. She recovered.

Good Samaritan Laws

Starting in the early 1960s, a number of states (California was the first, in 1959) enacted laws designed to protect physicians and other medical personnel from legal actions that may arise from emergency treatment they give while not in the line of duty. These laws, known as Good Samaritan laws, encourage people to assist others in distress by granting them immunity against lawsuits. While the laws vary from state to state, Good Samaritan immunity generally applies only when the rescuer is (1) acting during an emergency, (2) acting in good faith, which means he or she has good intentions, (3) acting without compensation, and (4) not guilty of any malicious misconduct or gross negligence toward the victim (deviating from all rational first aid guidelines).

Many legal experts believe that the main effect of Good Samaritan legislation has been to create a false sense of security in the minds of rescuers who erroneously believe that the law protects them from lawsuits regardless of their actions. Good Samaritan laws are easy to get around and should not be looked on as a substitute for competent first aid and keeping within the scope of your training.

While Good Samaritan laws primarily cover medical personnel, several states have expanded them to include laypersons serving as first aiders. In fact, some states have several Good Samaritan laws that cover different types of people in various situations (e.g., California has 15, New York 8, and Florida 4 different Good Samaritan laws).

Fear of lawsuits has made some people wary of getting involved in emergency situations. First aiders, however, are rarely sued; for those who are, the courts usually rule in their favor.

Rescue Doctrine

The *rescue doctrine* is an unfamiliar concept to most rescuers. The rescue doctrine says that a person who is injured while performing a rescue may, unless he or she has acted rashly or recklessly, recover from the person whose negligence created the peril that necessitated the rescue in the first place. In other words, in some cases an injured rescuer has the right to recover for injuries sustained while attempting to assist others who caused the dangerous rescue.

NOTES

C H A P T E R

2

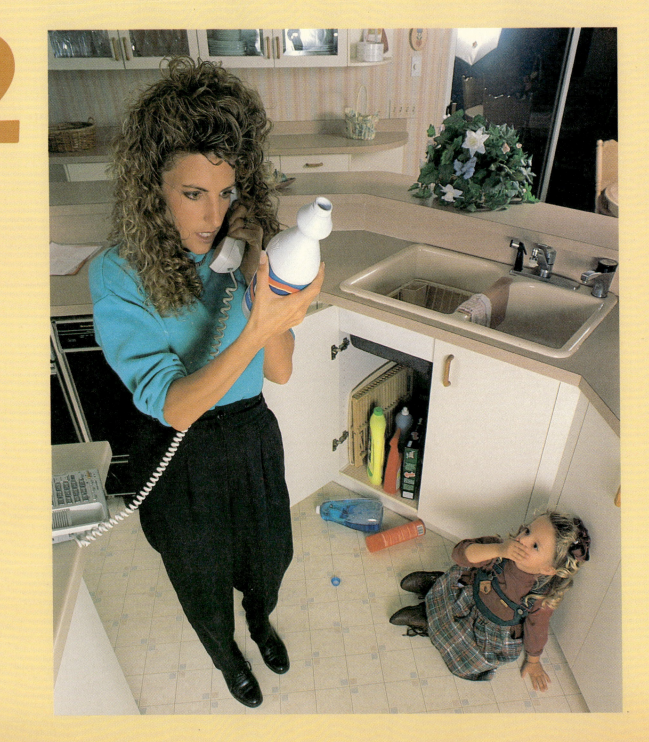

ACTION AT AN EMERGENCY

Bystander Intervention

The bystander is a vital link between the emergency medical service (EMS) and the victim. Typically it is a bystander who recognizes a situation as an emergency and decides to intervene to help the victim. A bystander must perform the following actions quickly and reliably:

1. recognize the emergency
2. decide to help
3. contact the EMS, if needed
4. assess the victim
5. provide first aid

Compared with health care professionals, laypersons are significantly less likely to offer help in emergencies that occur in public places. Several factors account for this fact:

- ignorance
- confusion about what is an emergency
- characteristics of the emergency (e.g., unpleasant physical characteristics of the victim, the presence of other bystanders)

Ignorance and Helping Behavior

The average layperson is ignorant of many aspects of emergency care and has difficulty recognizing common medical emergencies and deciding to call an ambulance.

Also, a person who does not feel competent to deal with an emergency is not likely to offer even minimal help. The person who does not feel competent may escape this uncomfortable feeling by failing to acknowledge the situation as an emergency. The implication is that bystanders who are uncertain of their ability to deal with a seriously injured victim may be more likely to assume that the victims are not seriously injured.

Confusion about What Is an Emergency

In general, laypersons have a great deal of difficulty deciding when an emergency exists. This difficulty can lead to delays in contacting the EMS and to inappropriate decisions to transport victims with life-threatening problems by private vehicles rather than to contact the EMS. For example, motor vehicle crashes may be easier for laypersons to recognize as emergencies when compared with other types of emergencies such as heart attacks.

Other Factors That Influence Whether a Bystander Helps

In addition to ignorance, bystanders encounter other barriers that can slow or prevent action in an emergency. Potential rescuers tend to be put off by unpleasant physical characteristics such as blood, vomit, or alcohol on the breath. Reluctance to help may reflect an unwillingness to approach or touch a bloody victim. Current public attention to HIV and AIDS may make this problem more difficult.

Another factor involved in helping behavior is the bystander's time of arrival. A bystander who has seen the emergency happen is more likely to help than a bystander who arrives after the event.

Quality of Help Provided by Bystanders

Some evidence suggests that much first aid treatment by bystanders is inadequate or potentially dangerous. Neglecting to keep the airway open and the decision to bypass the EMS and transport the victim in a private vehicle are two examples. One study concluded that 9 percent of the emergency victims who died would have had a greater chance for survival if they had received better care from laypersons and professionals. An Australian study examined 13 deaths from head and spinal injuries. For several of those deaths, inadequate first aid rendered by a layperson and the decision to transport the victim in a private vehicle were cited as potential contributing factors for the deaths.

What Should Be Done?

As stated at the beginning of this chapter, victims would benefit if bystanders were able to accomplish the following actions more often and more quickly:

1. recognize the emergency
2. decide to help
3. contact the EMS, if needed
4. assess the victim
5. provide first aid

Recognize the Emergency

To help in an emergency, the bystander first has to notice that something is wrong. Noticing that something is wrong is related to four factors:

- *Severity*. Severe, catastrophic emergencies (e.g., a traffic collision involving an overturned car or several vehicles) attract bystanders' attention.
- *Physical distance*. The closer a bystander is to an emergency situation, the more likely he or she will notice it.
- *Relationship*. Knowing the victim increases the likelihood of noticing an emergency. For example, your child's injuries would gain your attention more than a total stranger having the same injuries.
- *Time exposed*. Evidence indicates that the longer a bystander is aware of the emergency, the more likely he or she will notice it.

Decide to Help

Everyone will at some time have to make a decision whether to help another person. Unless the decision to act in an emergency is considered well in advance of encountering an emergency, the many obstacles that make it difficult or unpleasant for a bystander to help a stranger are almost certain to impede action. One important strategy that people use to avoid action is to refuse (consciously or unconsciously) to acknowledge the emergency. Many emergencies do not look like the ones portrayed on television, and the uncertainty of the real event can make it easier for the bystander to avoid acknowledging the emergency.

> *I shall pass through this life but once.*
> *Any good, therefore, that I can do*
> *Or any kindness I can show to any fellow creature*
> *Let me do it now.*
> *Let me not defer or neglect it,*
> *For I shall not pass this way again.*
>
> Etienne de Grellet

Making a quick decision to get involved at the time of an emergency is unlikely to occur unless the bystander has considered, in advance, the possibility of helping. Thus, the most important time to make the decision to help is *before* you ever encounter an emergency.

Deciding to help is an attitude about emergencies and about one's ability to deal with emergencies. It is an attitude that takes time to develop and is affected by a number of factors.

> *A hero is no braver than an ordinary man, but he is brave five minutes longer.*
>
> Emerson

Developing such an attitude means that you must:

- appreciate the importance of bystander help to an injured or suddenly ill person
- feel confident enough about helping someone who is seriously injured or suddenly ill to offer help even if someone else is present
- be willing to take the time to help
- be able to put the potential risks of helping in perspective
- feel comfortable about taking charge at an emergency scene
- feel comfortable about seeing or touching a victim who may be bleeding or vomiting or who may appear dead

Deciding Not to Help   Emergency situations exist in which a bystander uses excuses for not helping. The following excuses are possible reasons for why people fail to aid others.

- It would be harmful. Bystanders have lost their lives or been severely injured while attempting to rescue others. One example is Oklahoma teacher Ronnie Darden, who lost his left leg and part of his right foot when he tripped over a power line while attempting to help passengers in a car that had crashed. Another example is Joe Delaney, a star halfback for the Kansas City Chiefs, who died while trying to rescue three drowning boys in Louisiana. The fear of a lawsuit or of contracting a disease (e.g., HIV, tuberculosis) can also act as a deterrent. And some would-be rescuers are attacked by dogs protecting their disabled owners.
- "Helping doesn't matter." Some bystanders may feel that the victim is getting what he or she deserves. A negative image of the victim (e.g., if the victim is drunk or homeless) repulses some bystanders. Rewards, if any, are not high for rescuers, possibly consisting of a newspaper write-

up or a small cash prize. Often the rescuer gets nothing more than a hurried "Thanks," and in some cases rescuers are never known.

- Obstacles may prevent helping. Many bystanders do not know how to help. They cannot swim, do not know how to control bleeding or perform CPR, or do not have other necessary rescue and first aid skills. Also, the more bystanders there are, the less likely it is that one of them will respond.

Some would-be rescuers are adversely affected by the sight of blood, vomit, and other appalling conditions sometimes found at emergency scenes.

Contact the EMS, If Needed

Laypersons frequently make inappropriate decisions concerning the EMS. They delay contacting the EMS until they are absolutely sure that an emergency exists, or they elect to bypass the EMS and transport the victim to medical care in a private vehicle. These actions present significant dangers to victims.

Assess the Victim

The bystander must decide if life-threatening conditions exist and what kind of help a victim needs immediately.

Provide First Aid

Often the most critical life-support measures are effective only if started immediately by the nearest available person. That person usually will be a layperson—a bystander.

Rescuer Reactions

The sight of blood and the cries of victims can be very upsetting to persons attempting to rescue and assist the injured. Grotesque sights such as amputations, being splattered with vomitus or blood, and disagreeable odors from urine and feces can be quite unnerving. More than one rescuer has felt nauseated and weak, vomited, or fainted when helping injured victims. Even the toughest of physicians and EMTs have difficult moments when exposed to certain situations.

It is essential that rescuers stay conscious and working at an injury scene. A rescuer who collapses while aiding the injured detracts attention from the original victim, whose condition is usually more serious. All the knowledge and skills a rescuer has are useless if he or she collapses or has to leave the scene because of weakness or fainting.

There are those in the emergency care field who seem to have "ice in their veins." They always appear calm and unaffected by even the worst injuries. Such people may seem callous, but the proper psychological term is *desensitized*. A specialty within psychology deals with desensitization and suggests ways of overcoming anxieties caused by unpleasant sights and sounds. Desensitization is a deconditioning or a counterconditioning process that can be effective in eliminating fears and anxieties. The idea is to weaken an undesirable response (e.g., fainting) by strengthening an incompatible response. When responses are incompatible (e.g., calmness versus anxiety), the occurrence of either one prevents the occurrence of the other. By desensitizing, you learn to associate relaxation with situations that elicit anxiety so that eventually you do not experience anxiety. But first you need to learn how to invoke relaxation and then gradually expose yourself to anxiety situations (such as the sight of blood).

There are some simple ways to desensitize (calm) yourself while helping another person:

- Close your eyes for a moment and take several long, deep breaths. Let your mind go blank and just say the number "one" as you breathe out. Do not count—just repeat the number "one" at the end of each exhalation.

- Change your thought patterns from the unpleasant to the pleasant by singing a favorite song to yourself (not out loud, of course, for the obvious reason of how you might appear to the victim or observers).

Once you have learned a relaxation response technique, you can start gradual exposure by viewing videos, slides, or pictures of injuries in medical journals. Another step in the process of conditioning yourself might be to volunteer at a hospital emergency department.

In a number of cases, a fainting rescuer had failed to eat breakfast. It is strongly recommended that everyone maintain an adequate blood sugar level through proper eating habits.

Post-Care Reactions

After giving first aid for severe injuries, rescuers often feel an emotional "letdown," which is frequently overlooked. Discussing your feelings, fears, and reactions within 24 to 72 hours of helping at a traumatic injury scene helps prevent later emotional problems. Such discussion may be with a trusted

friend, a mental health professional, or a member of the clergy. Bringing out your feelings quickly helps to relieve personal anxieties and stress.

Scene Survey

If you are at the scene of an emergency situation, do a 10-second survey that includes looking for three things: (1) hazards that could be dangerous to you, the victim(s), or bystanders; (2) the mechanism or cause of the injury or injuries; and (3) the number of victims.

As you approach an emergency scene, scan the area for immediate dangers to yourself or to the victim. For example, if an automobile accident has left the involved vehicle in the roadway obstructing traffic, you have to consider whether you can safely go to that vehicle to help the victim. Or you might notice that gasoline is dripping from the gas tank and that the battery has shorted out and is sparking—the car could explode at any moment. In such circumstances you should withdraw and get help before proceeding. You are not being cowardly, merely realistic. Never attempt a rescue that you have not been specifically trained to do. You cannot help another if you also become a victim. Always ask yourself: Is the scene safe to enter? (For details about hazards at an emergency scene, refer to Chapter 23.)

The second thing to do in the first 10 seconds is to determine the cause of the injury. For example, if the emergency department physician knows that a victim was thrown against a steering wheel, he or she will check for liver, spleen, and cardiac injuries. Be sure to tell the EMS personnel about that, so the physician may initially be able to fully recognize the extent of the injuries.

Determine how many people are injured. There may be more than one victim, so look around and ask about others involved.

When to Call the EMS

Generally you will know when an emergency happens. You can tell by the type of injuries or by how the victim looks that it is time to call for help. Call the EMS whenever a situation is more than you can handle. In the following instances, calling the EMS is definitely the right thing to do:

- severe bleeding
- drowning

Do a 10-second scene survey by looking for three things:

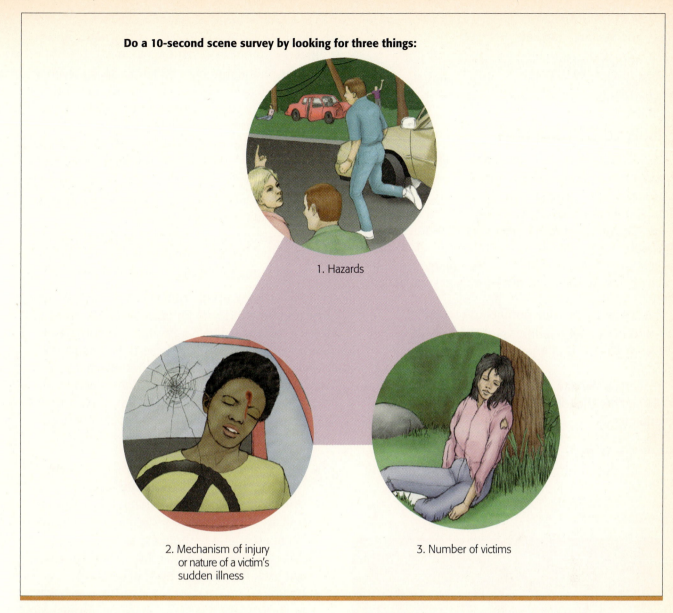

1. Hazards

2. Mechanism of injury or nature of a victim's sudden illness

3. Number of victims

Scene Survey

- electrocution
- possible heart attack
- breathing difficulty or no breathing
- choking
- altered mental status
- poisoning
- attempted suicide
- some seizure cases (most do not require EMS assistance)
- critical burns
- paralysis
- spine injury
- imminent childbirth

When a serious situation occurs, call the EMS (911 in most communities) *first*. Do *not* call your doctor, the hospital, a friend, relatives, or neighbors for help before you call the EMS. Calling anyone else first only wastes time.

Calling the EMS has several advantages:

- Many victims should not be moved except by trained personnel.
- The emergency medical technicians (EMTs) who arrive with the ambulance know what to do. In addition, they are in radio contact with hospital physicians.
- Care provided by EMTs at the scene and on the way to the hospital can increase a victim's chances of survival and rate of recovery.

- An EMS ambulance usually can get a victim to the hospital quicker.

If the situation is not an emergency, call your doctor. However, if you are in *any* doubt as to whether the situation is an emergency, call the EMS.

How to Call the EMS

To receive emergency assistance of every kind in most communities, you simply phone 911. Check to see if this is true in your community. Emergency telephone numbers usually are listed on the inside front cover of all telephone directories. Keep these numbers near or on every telephone. Call "O" (the operator) if you do not know the emergency number. A community 911 number has several benefits:

- There is only one number to remember.
- Calls are received by specially trained persons.
- Response time is reduced.

If you have to call the EMS, be ready to give the dispatcher the following information. Speak slowly and clearly.

1. The victim's location. Give the address, names of intersecting roads, and other landmarks, if

possible. This information is the most important you can give. Also, tell the specific location of the victim (e.g., "in the basement").

2. Your phone number and name. This prevents false calls and allows a dispatch center without the enhanced 911 system to call back for additional information, if needed.

3. What happened. State the nature of the emergency (e.g., "My husband fell off a ladder and is not moving").

4. Number of persons needing help and any special conditions.

5. Victim's condition (e.g., "My husband's head is bleeding") and any first aid you have tried (such as pressing on the site of the bleeding).

Do *not* hang up the phone unless the dispatcher instructs you to do so. Enhanced 911 systems can track a call, but some communities lack this technology or are still using a seven-digit emergency number. Also, the EMS dispatcher may tell you how to best care for the victim. If you send someone else to call, have the person report back to you so you can be sure the call was made. Other tips include:

- Teach children what 911 is for and how and when to call. Refer to "nine-one-one," not "nine-eleven," because children may expect to find an 11 on the dial or on the push buttons.
- Do not hang up without explanation if 911 is called by mistake, or the dispatcher will have to call back to see if you need help.
- If your area does not have a 911 system, add EMS, fire, and police numbers to a list by your phones. During an emergency, you may not have the time or presence of mind to find a number in a directory.

Disease Precautions

First aiders must be aware of the risks associated with emergency medical care. One such risk comes from infectious diseases, which can range in severity from mild to life threatening. First aiders should know how to reduce the risk of contamination to themselves and to others. This section stresses the importance of precautionary measures that help to protect against infection from disease agents such as viruses and bacteria.

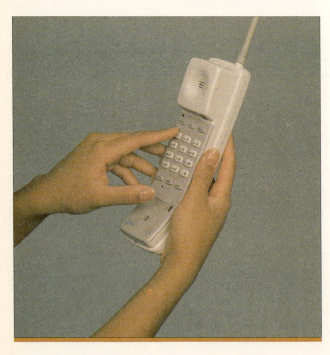

For help, phone 911 or the local emergency number

Bloodborne Disease

Some diseases are caused by microorganisms that are "borne" (carried) in a person's bloodstream. Contact with blood infected with such microorganisms may cause infection. Of the many bloodborne pathogens, three pose significant health threats to first aiders: hepatitis B virus (HBV), hepatitis C virus, and human immunodeficiency virus (HIV).

Hepatitis B

Each year, as many as 12,000 people come down with hepatitis B, the most common form of hepatitis. Hepatitis is a viral infection of the liver. Types A, B, and C are seen most often. Each is caused by a different virus.

A vaccine for hepatitis B is available and is recommended for all infants and for adults who may have contact with carriers of the disease or with blood. Medical and laboratory workers, police, intravenous drug users, people with multiple sexual partners, and those living with someone who has lifelong infection are at high risk of hepatitis B (and hepatitis C as well). Vaccination is the best defense against HBV. There is no chance of developing hepatitis B from the vaccine. Federal laws require employers to offer a series of three vaccine injections free to all employees who may be at risk of exposure.

Without vaccination shots, exposure to hepatitis B may produce symptoms within two weeks to six months following exposure. People with hepatitis B infection may be symptom free, but that does *not* mean they are not contagious. These people may infect others through exposure to their blood. Symptoms of hepatitis B resemble those of the flu and include fatigue, nausea, loss of appetite, stomach pain, and perhaps a yellowing of the skin.

Hepatitis B starts as an inflammation of the liver and usually lasts one to two months. In a few people, the infection is very serious, and in some, mild infection continues for life. The virus may stay in the liver and can lead to severe damage (cirrhosis) and liver cancer. Medical treatment that begins immediately after exposure may prevent infection from developing.

Hepatitis C

Hepatitis C, first identified in the 1980s, is caused by a different virus from HBV, but both diseases have a great deal in common. Like hepatitis B,

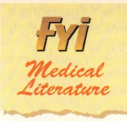

What Is the Risk of HIV Transmission from Contacting Blood? In professional football, there are almost four bleeding injuries per game, yet researchers estimate the risk of HIV transmission in an NFL game to be less than one in one million.

Source: L. S. Brown et al., "Bleeding Injuries in Professional Football: Estimating the Risk for HIV Transmission," *Annals of Internal Medicine* 122:271–74 (1995).

hepatitis C affects the liver and can lead to long-term liver disease and liver cancer. Hepatitis C varies in severity and may even cause no symptoms at the time of infection. Currently, there is no vaccine or effective treatment for hepatitis C.

HIV

Estimates are that over 1.5 million people in the United States are infected with HIV but have no symptoms. A person infected with HIV can infect others, and HIV-infected persons almost always develop acquired immunodeficiency syndrome (AIDS), which interferes with the body's ability to fight off other diseases. No vaccine is available to prevent HIV infection, which eventually proves fatal. Since 1981, more than 250,000 Americans have died of AIDS-related illnesses. It is predicted that by the year 2000, the majority of those afflicted with HIV will be females and children. The best defense against AIDS is to avoid becoming infected.

How Bloodborne Pathogens Are Transmitted

HIV and HBV are usually transmitted (passed on) when disease organisms in body fluids enter the body through mucous membranes or through breaks in the skin. The most common forms of transmission are:

- sexual contact with an infected person
- from an infected mother to her unborn child
- sharing needles with infected intravenous drug users

A first aider may be exposed through an open sore or wound that comes in contact with a victim's

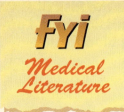

FYi
Medical Literature

Facts about the Human Immunodeficiency Virus and Its Transmission

Research has revealed a great deal of valuable information about the human immunodeficiency virus (HIV) and acquired immunodeficiency syndrome (AIDS). The ways in which HIV can be transmitted have been clearly identified.

HIV is spread by sexual contact with an infected person, by needle-sharing among injecting drug users, or, less commonly (and now very rarely in countries where blood is screened for HIV antibodies), through transfusions of infected blood or blood clotting factors. Babies born to HIV-infected women may become infected before or during birth, or through breast-feeding after birth.

In the health-care setting, workers have been infected with HIV after being stuck with needles containing HIV-infected blood or, less frequently, after infected blood gets into the worker's bloodstream through an open cut or splashes into a mucous membrane (e.g., eyes or inside of the nose).

Some people fear that HIV might be transmitted in other ways; however, no scientific evidence to support any of these fears has been found. The Centers for Disease Control and Prevention (CDC) reports:

1. Since HIV does not survive well outside its living host it does not spread or maintain infectiousness outside its host.

2. Although HIV has been transmitted between family members in a household setting, this type of transmission is very rare. These transmissions are believed to have resulted from contact between skin or mucous membranes and infected blood or body fluids.

3. Closed-mouth or "social" kissing is not a risk for HIV transmission. Because of the theoretical potential for contact with blood during "French" or open-mouthed kissing, the CDC recommends against engaging in this activity with an infected person. However, no case of AIDS reported to the CDC can be attributed to transmission through any kind of kissing.

4. HIV has been found in saliva and tears in only minute quantities from some AIDS patients. HIV has not been recovered from the sweat of HIV-infected persons. Contact with saliva, tears, or sweat has never been shown to result in HIV transmission.

5. No evidence of HIV transmission through biting or blood-sucking insects even in areas where there are many cases of AIDS and large populations of mosquitoes exist. When an insect bites a person, it does not inject its own or a previous victim's blood into the new victim. Rather, it injects saliva (yellow fever and malaria are transmitted through the saliva of certain mosquito species).

6. No transmission has occurred involving rescue breathing during CPR manikin practice or actual resuscitation attempts.

CDC National AIDS Hotline:
1-800-342-AIDS (2437)
Spanish: 1-800-344-7432
Deaf: 1-800-243-7889

Source: Adapted from the Centers for Disease Control and Prevention.

---

infectious blood or other body fluids that contain blood or when the first aider is not wearing the proper personal protective equipment (PPE) to protect against contact with infectious material.

Protection

In most cases, you can control the risk of exposure to bloodborne pathogens by wearing the proper PPE and by following some simple procedures.

Personal Protective Equipment (PPE)

This equipment blocks entry of an organism into the body. The most common type of protection is gloves. The Food and Drug Administration (FDA),

the Centers for Disease Control and Prevention (CDC), and the Occupational Safety and Health Administration (OSHA) have stated that vinyl and latex gloves are equally protective. Research indicates that latex has fewer micropores (very small holes) and thus offers the most protection. However, latex tends to break down faster over time (several years) while they may be in a first aid kit, waiting to be used. All first aid kits should have several pairs of gloves.

Protective eyewear and a standard surgical mask may be necessary at some emergencies; first aiders ordinarily will not have or need such equipment.

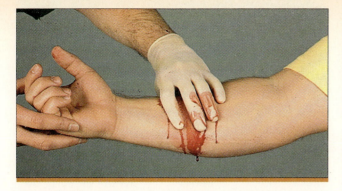

Whenever possible, use gloves as a barrier.

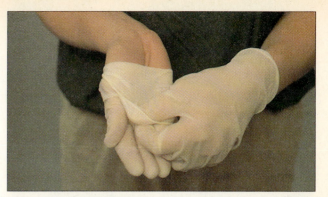

Glove Removal

Proper glove removal is as important as wearing gloves to protect against infection. Follow this procedure:

1. Grip one glove near the cuff and peel it down until it comes off inside out. Cup it in the palm of your gloved hand.
2. Place two fingers of your bare hand inside the cuff of the remaining glove.
3. Peel that glove down so it also comes off inside out and over the first glove.
4. Properly dispose of the gloves.
5. Wash your hands with soap and water.

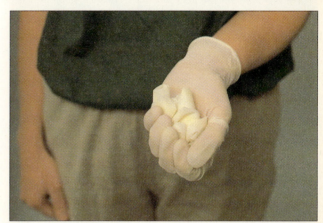

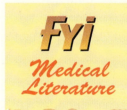

Do Gloves Really Protect? A study tested the effectiveness of vinyl and latex gloves as barriers to hand contamination. Gloves were checked according to the American Society for Testing and Materials and leaks occurred with 43 percent of vinyl gloves and 9 percent of latex gloves. The researchers concluded that latex gloves, and to a lesser extent vinyl gloves, provide substantial protection during hand contact with moist body substances, functioning as a barrier even when leaks are present. Since leaks are not always detected by the wearer, hand washing should routinely follow the use of disposable gloves.

Source: R. J. Olsen et al., "Examination Gloves as Barriers to Hand Contamination in Clinical Practice," *Journal of the American Medical Association,* 270:350–53, (1993).

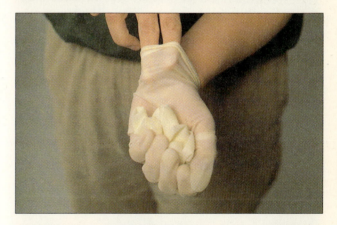

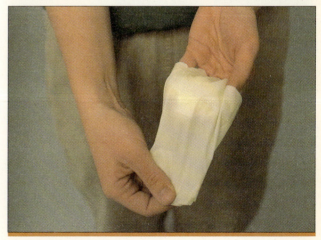

Glove removal

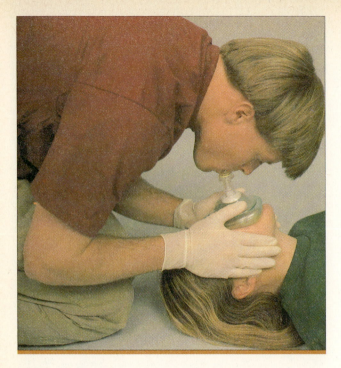

Pocket face mask, one-way valve

Mouth-to-barrier devices are recommended for rescue breathing and CPR. No case of disease transmission to a rescuer as a result of performing unprotected CPR on an infected victim has been

Handwashing

Wearing PPE is the best method for personal protection, and handwashing is the second best. If you have been exposed to blood or body fluids, follow these steps:

1. Remove your gloves and wash your hands and contaminated body area immediately with soap and water. Rub your hands together vigorously for at least 10 to 15 seconds (work up a lather), then rinse your hands and dry them with a paper towel.

2. Use a paper towel to turn off the faucet so you do not recontaminate yourself or others.

3. If you cannot wash immediately with soap and water, use antiseptic towelettes and wash with soap and water as soon as possible.

4. Flush your eyes, nose, and other mucous membranes with water if they have been exposed.

documented. Nevertheless, a mouth-to-barrier device should be used whenever possible.

Universal Precautions or Body Substance Isolation?

Individuals infected with HBV or HIV may not show symptoms and may not even know they are infectious. For that reason, all human blood and body fluids should be considered infectious, and precautions should be taken to avoid contact. The *body substance isolation* (BSI) technique assumes that *all* body fluids are a possible risk. EMS personnel routinely follow BSI procedures, even if blood or body fluids are not visible.

OSHA requires any company with employees who are expected to give first aid in an emergency to follow *universal precautions,* which assume that *all* blood and *certain* body fluids pose a risk for transmission of HBV and HIV. OSHA considers an employee who assists another with a nosebleed or a cut to fall under the definition of "Good Samaritan." Such acts, however, are not considered occupational exposure unless the employee who provides the assistance is a member of a first aid team or is designated or expected to render first aid as part of his or her job. In essence, OSHA's requirement excludes unassigned employees who perform unanticipated first aid.

Whenever there is a chance you could be exposed to bloodborne pathogens, your employer must provide appropriate PPE, which might include eye protection, gloves, gowns, and masks. The PPE must be accessible, and your employer must provide training to help you choose the right PPE for your work.

While EMS personnel follow BSI procedures and OSHA requires designated worksite first aiders to follow universal precautions, what should a typical first aider do? It makes sense for first aiders to follow BSI procedures and assume that *all* blood and body fluids are infectious and follow appropriate protective measures.

Coping with Emergencies

When an injury occurs, first aiders can protect themselves and others against bloodborne pathogens by following these steps:

1. Wear appropriate PPE, such as gloves.
2. If you have been trained in the correct proce-

dures, use absorbent barriers to soak up blood or other infectious materials.

3. Clean the spill area with an appropriate disinfecting solution, such as diluted bleach.

4. Discard contaminated materials in an appropriate waste disposal container.

If you have been exposed to blood or body fluids:

1. Use soap and water to wash the parts of your body that have been contaminated.

2. If the exposure happens while at work, report the incident to your supervisor. Otherwise, contact your personal physician. Early action can prevent the development of hepatitis B and enable affected workers to track potential HIV infection.

The best protection against bloodborne disease is using the safeguards described here. By following these guidelines, first aiders can decrease their chance of contracting bloodborne illness.

Airborne Disease

Infective organisms (e.g., bacteria, viruses) that are introduced into the air by coughing or sneezing are said to be "airborne." Droplets of mucus that carry those bacteria or viruses can then be inhaled by other individuals. The rate of tuberculosis (TB) has increased recently and is receiving much attention. TB, caused by bacteria, sometimes settles in the lungs and can be fatal. In most cases, a first aider will not know that a victim has TB. Assume that any person with a cough, especially one who is in a nursing home or a shelter, may have TB. Other symptoms include fatigue, weight loss, chest pain, and coughing up blood. If a surgical mask is available, wear it or wrap a handkerchief over your nose and mouth.

Death

The Dying Victim

A dying person presents a difficult situation. To assist such a victim:

- Avoid negative statements about the victim's condition. Even a semiconscious person can hear what is being said.

- Assure the victim that you will locate and in-

form his or her family of what has happened. Attempt to have family members present—they can provide great comfort to the victim.

- Allow some hope. Don't tell the victim that he or she is dying. Instead, say something like, "I don't know for sure. I won't give up on you, so don't give up on yourself. Keep trying."

- Do not volunteer information about the victim or others who may also be injured. However, if the victim asks a question about a family member, tell the truth. Provide simple, honest, clear information if it is requested and repeat it as often as necessary.

- Use a gentle tone of voice.

- Use a reassuring touch, if appropriate.

- Let the person know that everything that can be done to help will be done.

The Stages of Grieving

Both the dying and the surviving go through a grieving process that has been described as having the following five stages:

1. Denial ("Not me"). This is an attempt to create a buffer against the shock of dying and dealing with the illness or injury.

2. Anger ("Why me?"). Bystanders may be the target of the anger. Do not take the anger or insults personally. Be tolerant, use good listening skills, and be empathetic.

3. Bargaining ("OK, but first let me . . ."). In the victim's mind, an agreement will postpone the death for a short time.

4. Depression ("OK, but I haven't . . ."). This stage is characterized by sadness and despair. The person is usually silent and retreats into his or her own world.

5. Acceptance ("OK, I am not afraid"). This does not mean the person is happy about dying. The family often requires more support during this stage than does the victim.

Survivors of the Dead

Deal with the family members of a dead or dying victim as follows:

- Do not pronounce death; leave the confirmation of death to a physician.

- Allow survivors to grieve in whatever way seems right to them (anger, rage, crying).
- Provide simple, honest, clear information as it is requested, and repeat it as often as necessary. The survivors should not be told everything at once.

- Offer as much support and comfort as possible, by your presence as well as by your words. Do not leave an individual survivor alone, but do respect that person's right to privacy.
- Use a gentle tone of voice.
- Use a reassuring touch, if appropriate.

NOTES

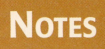

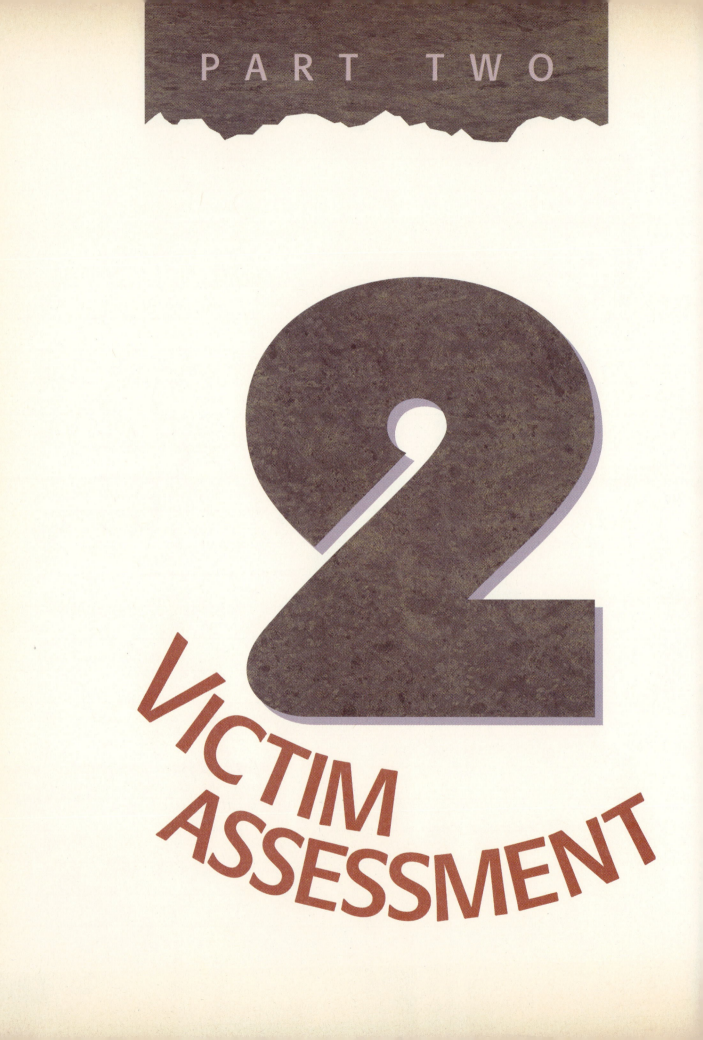

2

VICTIM ASSESSMENT

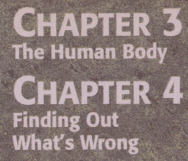

CHAPTER

3

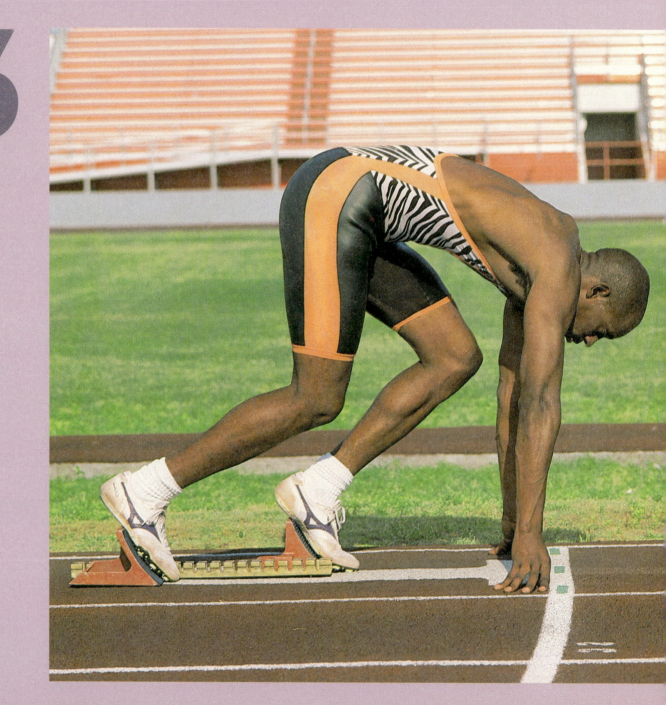

THE HUMAN BODY

To adequately assess a victim's condition and to give effective first aid, a first aider must be familiar with the anatomy and physiology of the human body. Such knowledge is a solid cornerstone on which a first aider can build the essentials of quality victim assessment and emergency first aid.

In injuries and illnesses, the respiratory, circulatory, and nervous systems can have conditions that are the most life-threatening. These three body systems include the most important and most sensitive organs: the lungs, the heart, the brain, and the spinal cord.

The other body systems are also important, and a good victim assessment can locate injury and/or sudden illnesses affecting them. The major body systems described in this chapter are respiratory, circulatory, nervous, skeletal, and muscular systems, and the skin. The other body systems—the endocrine, gastrointestinal, and genitourinary systems—are not discussed.

The Respiratory System

The body can store food to last several weeks and water to last several days, but it can store enough oxygen for only a few minutes. Ordinarily this does not matter because we have only to inhale air to get the oxygen we need. If the oxygen supply of the body is cut off, as in drowning, choking, or smothering, death will come in about four to six minutes unless oxygen intake is restored. Oxygen from air is made available to the blood through the respiratory system and then to the body cells by the circulatory system.

Nose

Air normally enters the body through the nostrils. It is warmed, moistened, and filtered as it flows over the damp, sticky lining (mucous membrane) of the nose. When a person breathes through the mouth instead of the nose, there is less filtration and warming. Breath passing through the nasal passages enters the nasal portion of the pharynx.

Pharynx and Trachea

From the back of the nose or the mouth, the air enters the throat (**pharynx**). The pharynx is a common passageway for food and air. At its lower end, the pharynx divides into two passageways, one for food and the other for air. Food is routed by muscular control in the back of the throat to the food tube (**esophagus**), which leads to the stomach; air is routed from the pharynx to the windpipe (**trachea**), which leads to the lungs. The trachea and the esophagus are separated by a small flap of tissue (**epiglottis**), which acts as a kind of valve that closes the trachea while food is being swallowed. At other times, the trachea remains open to permit breathing. Usually this diversion works automatically to keep food out of the trachea and air from going into the esophagus. When the epiglottis fails to close, however, food or liquid can enter the trachea instead of the esophagus.

During unconsciousness, normal swallowing controls do not operate. *If liquid is poured into the mouth of an unconscious person in an attempt to revive him or her, it may get into the windpipe and cause suffocation.* Foreign objects, such as false teeth or a piece of food, may lodge in the throat or windpipe and cut off the passage of air.

In the upper two inches of the trachea, just below the epiglottis, is the voice box (**larynx**), which contains the vocal cords. The larynx can be felt in the front of the throat (Adam's apple).

Lungs

The trachea branches into two main tubes (bronchial tubes or bronchi), one for each lung. Each bronchus divides and subdivides somewhat like the branches of a tree. The smallest bronchi end in thousands of tiny pouches (air sacs), just as the twigs of a tree end in leaves. Each air sac is enclosed in a network of capillaries. The adjoining walls of the air sacs and the walls of the capillaries are very thin. Through those walls, oxygen combines with hemoglobin in red blood cells to form oxyhemoglobin, which is carried to all parts of the body. Carbon dioxide and certain other waste gases in the blood move across the capillary walls into the air sacs and are exhaled from the body. The lungs occupy most of the chest cavity.

Mechanics of Breathing

The passage of air into and out of the lungs is called **respiration.** Breathing in is called **inhalation;** breathing out is **exhalation.**

Respiration is a mechanical process brought about by alternately increasing and decreasing the size of the chest cavity. When the diaphragm (dome-shaped muscle dividing the chest from the abdomen) moves down, the chest moves out, drawing air into the lungs (inhalation). An exchange of oxygen and carbon dioxide takes place in the lungs. When the diaphragm moves up, it causes air to flow out of the lungs (exhalation).

Infants and children differ from adults. Their respiratory structures are smaller and more easily obstructed than those of adults. Infants' and children's tongues take up proportionally more space in the mouth than do adults'. The trachea is more flexible in infants and children. The primary cause of cardiac arrest in infants and children is an uncorrected respiratory problem.

The average rate of breathing in an adult at rest is 12 to 20 complete respirations per minute. Normal rates for children are from 15 to 30 times per minute; infants' rates will be between 25 and 50 times per minute. Normally the rate is less when a person is lying down, faster during vigorous exer-

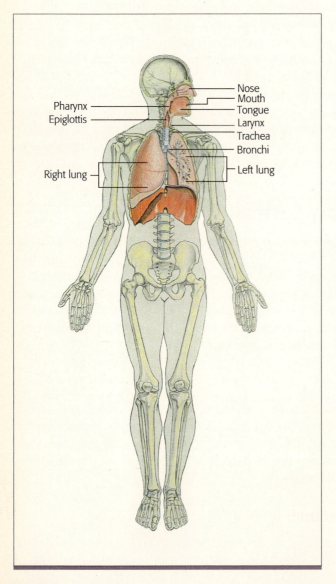

Pharynx
Epiglottis
Right lung

Nose
Mouth
Tongue
Larynx
Trachea
Bronchi
Left lung

Respiratory System

Table 3-1: Normal Respiration Rate Ranges	
Breaths per Minute*	
Adults	12 to 20
Children	15 to 30
Infants	25 to 50

*To obtain the breathing rate in a person, count the number of breaths in a 30-second period and multiply by 2. Avoid letting the person know you are counting to prevent influencing the rate.

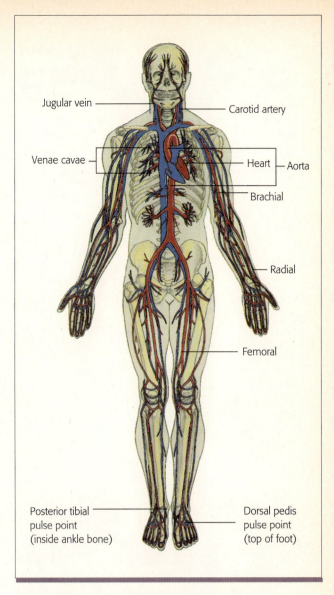

Circulatory System (principal arteries and major veins)

cise. The rate of breathing is controlled by a nerve center in the brain (the respiratory center).

Signs of inadequate breathing include a rate of breathing outside normal ranges, skin that is pale or cyanotic (blue-gray) and cool and **clammy**, and nasal flaring, especially in children.

When a person performs hard muscular work, the lungs cannot get rid of carbon dioxide or take in oxygen fast enough at the normal rate. As carbon dioxide increases in the blood and tissues, the respiratory center sends impulses along its nerves to cause deeper and more rapid respirations. At the same time, the heart rate increases. A greater supply of oxygen becomes available to the blood and lungs, because more blood moves through the lungs as a result of the increased heart rate.

The Circulatory System

The circulatory system is made up of the blood, the heart, and the blood vessels. Blood is the great common carrier to cells throughout the body. It carries nutrients and other products from the digestive tract in its plasma and oxygen from the lungs in its hemoglobin. It also transports wastes produced by the cells to the lungs, kidneys, and other excretory organs for removal from the body.

Heart

The human circulatory system is a completely closed circuit of tubelike vessels through which blood flows. The heart, by contracting and relaxing, pumps blood through the vessels. It is a powerful, hollow, muscular organ about as big as a man's clenched fist, shaped like a pear, and located in the left center of the chest, behind the sternum. The heart is divided by a wall in the middle. Right and left compartments are divided into two chambers, atrium above, ventricle below. A check valve is located between each atrium and its corresponding ventricle and at the exit of the major arteries leading out of each ventricle. The opening and shutting of these valves at just the right time in the heartbeat keeps the blood from backing up.

At each beat, or contraction, the heart pumps blood rich in carbon dioxide and low in oxygen from the right ventricle to the lungs and back to the left atrium of the heart. Blood rich in oxygen freshly obtained from the lungs is pumped from the left ventricle to the rest of the body and back to the right atrium. At each relaxation of the heart, blood flows into the left atrium from the lungs and into the right atrium from the rest of the body.

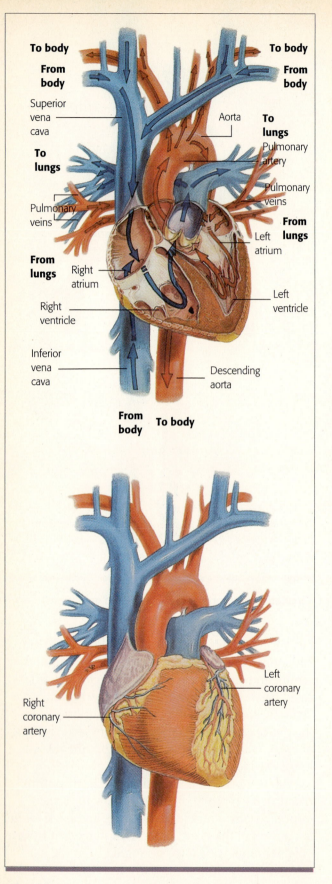

Top: The heart in cross section showing circulation. Arrows indicate direction of blood flow. **Bottom:** Exterior view of the heart showing the coronary arteries.

Table 3-2: Normal Heart Rates

Beats per Minute*	
Adults	60 to 100
Children	80 to 100
Toddlers	100 to 120
Newborns	120 to 140

*To obtain a heart rate in most people, count the number of beats over a 30-second period and multiply by 2.

Blood Vessels

The **arteries** are elastic, muscular tubes that carry blood away from the heart. They begin at the heart as two large tubes: the pulmonary artery, which carries blood to the lungs for the carbon dioxide–oxygen exchange, and the aorta, which carries blood to all the other parts of the body. The aorta divides and subdivides until it ends in networks of extremely fine vessels (**capillaries**) smaller than hairs. Through the thin walls of the capillaries, oxygen and food pass out of the bloodstream into the stationary cells of the body. Into the capillaries, the body cells discharge their waste products. In the capillaries of the lungs, carbon dioxide is released and oxygen is absorbed. Capillaries, having reached their limit of subdivision, begin to join together again into **veins.** The veins become larger and larger and finally form major trunks that empty blood returning from the body into the right atrium and blood from the lungs into the left atrium.

It is impossible to prick normal skin anywhere without puncturing capillaries. Because the flow of blood through the capillaries is relatively slow and under little pressure, blood merely oozes from a

FYI
Did You Know?

Arteries received their name (from the Greek for *windpipe*) because the Greek physician Praxagoras thought they carried air. (In corpses they are usually empty and that was probably where his observations were made.)

Source: Skinner, Henry A., *The Origin of Medical Terms,* 2nd edition (Baltimore: Williams and Wilkins).

punctured capillary and usually has time to clot, promptly plugging the leak.

Each time the heart contracts, the surge of blood can be felt as a pulse at any point where an artery lies close to the surface of the body. When an artery is cut, blood spurts out. There is no pulse in a vein because the pulse is lost by the time the blood has passed through the capillaries. Hence, blood from a cut vein flows out in a steady stream. It has much less pressure behind it than blood from a cut artery.

A pulse can be felt anywhere an artery passes near the skin surface and over a bone. Major locations for feeling pulses include the following:

- **Carotid:** the major artery of the neck, which supplies the head with blood. Pulsations can be palpated (felt) on either side of the neck (do not try to feel both at the same time). Use the carotid to check an unconscious person's pulse.
- **Femoral:** the major artery of the thigh supplying the lower extremities with blood. Pulsations can be palpated in the groin area (the crease between the abdomen and thigh).
- **Radial:** the major artery of the lower arm. Pulsations can be palpated at the palm side of the wrist on the thumb side. Use the radial to check a conscious person's pulse.
- **Brachial:** an artery of the upper arm. Pulsations can be palpated on the inside of the arm between the elbow and the armpit. Use the brachial to determine a pulse in an infant.
- **Posterior tibial:** located behind the inside ankle knob. Pulsations can be palpated on the posterior surface of the medial malleolus.
- **Dorsalis pedis:** Pulsations can be palpated on the top surface of the foot (pulsations felt in only 20 percent of the population).

Blood Pressure

Blood pressure is a measure of the pressure exerted by the blood on the walls of the flexible arteries. Blood pressure may be high or low according to the resistance offered by the walls to the passage of blood. This difference in resistance may be due to several causes. For example, if blood does not fill the system, as following hemorrhage, the pressure will be low (**hypotension**). High blood pressure (**hypertension**) may be present when the arterial walls have become hard and cannot expand readily.

Blood

Blood has liquid and solid portions. The liquid portion is called *plasma.* The solid portion, which is transported by the plasma, includes disk-like red blood cells; slightly larger, irregularly shaped white blood cells; and an immense number of smaller bodies called platelets.

Plasma, the liquid part of the blood, is about 90 percent water, in which minerals, sugar, and other materials are dissolved. Plasma carries food materials picked up from the digestive tract and transports them to the body cells. It also carries waste materials produced by cells to the kidneys, digestive tract, sweat glands, and lungs for elimination (excretion) in urine, feces, sweat, and expired breath.

The red blood cells, which give the blood its color, carry oxygen to the organs. The white blood cells are part of the body's defense against bacteria. The cells can go wherever they are needed in the body to fight infection, for example, a wound in the skin or other tissue that is diseased or injured. Pus, a sign of wound infection, gets its yellowish-white color from the innumerable white blood cells that are fighting the invading bacteria.

Platelets are essential for the formation of blood clots. If blood plasma did not clot at the site of a wound, the slightest cut or abrasion would produce death from bleeding. Clots plug the openings through which blood escapes from punctured blood vessels. Bleeding from a large blood vessel may be too rapid to permit the formation of a clot. **Hemorrhage** is the term for profuse bleeding.

Inadequate circulation is known as **shock** (hypoperfusion). Shock is a state of profound depression of the vital processes of the body, characterized by the following signs and symptoms: pale, cyanotic, cool, clammy skin; rapid pulse; rapid breathing; restlessness, anxiety, or mental dullness; nausea and vomiting; reduction in total blood volume; low or decreasing blood pressure; and subnormal temperature.

Perfusion refers to the circulation of blood through an organ or a structure. **Hypoperfusion** is the inadequate circulation of blood through an organ or a structure. The average-size adult male has about six quarts (12 pints) of blood.

The Nervous System

The nervous system is a complex collection of nerve cells (neurons), which coordinate the work of all parts of the human body and keep the individual in touch with the outside world. Neurons receive stimuli from the environment and transmit impulses to nerve centers in the brain and spinal cord. Then, by a complicated process of thinking (reasoning) plus reflex and automatic reactions, they produce nerve impulses that regulate and coordinate all bodily movements and functions and govern behavior and consciousness.

Once nerve cells have been destroyed, the body cannot regenerate them. Some limited nerve repair is possible, however, as long as the vital cell body is intact. If a nerve fiber is cut or injured, the section attached to the cell body remains alive, but the part beyond the injury withers away.

The nervous system can be classified in different ways. From a structural standpoint, there is (1) the central nervous system, which includes the brain and the spinal cord, and (2) the peripheral nervous system, a network of nerve cells that originates in the brain and spinal cord and extends to all parts of the body, including the muscles, the surface of the skin, and the special sense organs, such as the eyes and the ears. The peripheral nervous system is further subdivided into the voluntary and the autonomic (involuntary) nervous systems.

Central Nervous System

The central nervous system (CNS) consists of the brain, which is enclosed within the skull, and the spinal cord, which is housed in a semiflexible bony column of vertebrae. The CNS serves as the controlling organ of the body. The brain enables us to think, judge, and act. The spinal cord is a major communication pathway between the brain and the rest of the body.

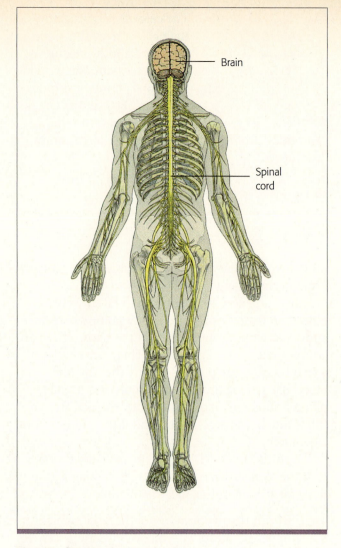

Nervous System (major nerves)

Brain

The brain, which is the headquarters of the human nervous system, is probably the most highly specialized organ in the body. It weighs about three pounds in the average adult, is richly supplied with blood vessels, and requires considerable oxygen to perform effectively.

The brain has three main subdivisions: the cerebrum (large brain), which occupies nearly all (75%) of the cranial cavity; the cerebellum (small brain), and the brain stem. The cerebrum is divided into two hemispheres by a deep cleft. The outer surface of the cerebrum, the cerebral cortex, is about one-eighth of an inch thick, is composed mainly of cell bodies of nerve cells and is often referred to as "gray matter."

Certain sections of the cerebrum are localized to control specific body functions such as sensation,

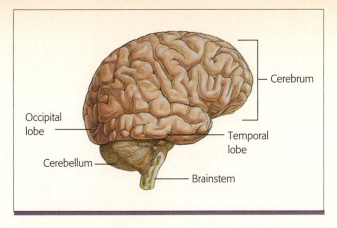

Surface View of the Brain

thought, and associative memory, which allows us to store, recall, and make use of past experiences. The sight center of the brain is located in the back part of the cerebrum, called the occipital lobe. The temporal lobes, at the sides of the head, deal with smell and hearing.

The cerebellum is located at the back of the cranium and below the cerebrum. Its main function is to coordinate muscular activity.

The third major area of the brain is the brain stem, which extends from the base of the cerebrum to the foramen magnum (a large opening at the base of the skull).

Small cavities in the brain contain the **cerebrospinal fluid** (CSF), which is a clear, watery solution similar to blood plasma. Circulating throughout the brain and the spinal cord, CSF serves as a protective cushion and exchanges food and waste materials. The total quantity of CSF in the brain–spinal cord system is 100–150 ml, although up to several liters may be produced daily. It is constantly being produced and reabsorbed.

Knowledge of nerve structure and function enables physicians to locate brain sections that are diseased. It is known that nerves from one side of the body eventually connect with the opposite side of the brain. Thus, a person whose left arm is paralyzed after a stroke is known to have suffered damage to the right side of the brain.

Spinal Cord

The spinal cord is a soft column of nerve tissue continuous with the lower part of the brain that is enclosed in the bony vertebral column. The spinal cord exits through the foramen magnum. Thirty-one pairs of spinal nerves branch from the spinal cord. These nerves are large trunks similar to telephone cables because they house many nerve fibers. Some fibers carry impulses into the spinal cord; others carry impulses away from it. Spinal nerves at different levels of the cord regulate activities of various parts of the body.

The closeness of the spinal cord to the bony walls of the vertebra, especially in the cervical and thoracic regions, makes it particularly vulnerable to injury. Damage to the cord is almost irreversible. An injury to the lumbar spine causes paralysis and loss of sensation in the legs; an injury to the cervical cord causes paralysis and loss of sensation in the arms as well as in the legs.

Peripheral Nervous System

At each vertebral level on each side of the spinal cord a spinal nerve exits the spinal cord and passes through an opening in the bony canal. These nerves make up the peripheral nervous system.

The peripheral nervous system consists of the sensory and motor nerves. The sensory nerves carry sensations such as smell, touch, heat, and sound from the body to the brain and the spinal cord. The motor nerves carry information from the brain and the spinal cord to the body.

Autonomic Nervous System

The autonomic nervous system consists of a group of nerves that control heart rate, digestion, sweating, and other automatic body processes. These processes are not controlled by the conscious mind, but they can be influenced by the CNS to a limited extent.

If a nerve is cut or seriously damaged, the area of the brain and the body that the nerve connects will not be able to work. For example, if the motor nerve going to the right leg is cut, the leg will be unable to move. This may be a permanent loss. Injuries to the nerves in the spinal cord can be very serious.

Fortunately, the CNS is well protected against injury. The brain is enclosed in the cranial cavity of the skull. The spinal cord is contained in a hollow space inside the vertebrae. The brain and the spinal cord are also protected by three layers of tissue known as the meninges. The space between the layers of the meninges is filled with CSF, which protects the brain and spinal cord from injury.

The Skeletal System

The human body is shaped by its bony framework. Without its bones, the body would collapse. The adult skeleton has 206 bones. Bones are composed of living cells that are surrounded by hard deposits of calcium. The bone cells are well supplied by blood vessels and nerves. The calcium deposits give bones their strength and rigidity. Broken bones are repaired by bone-building cells lying in the bone and its covering sheath, the periosteum. New bone is formed at the site of the break, much as two pieces of steel are welded together.

Skull

The skull rests at the top of the spinal column. It contains the brain, certain special-purpose glands (such as the pituitary and the pineal), and the centers of special senses—sight, hearing, taste, and smell. The skull has two parts, the brain case (cranium) and the face.

Blood vessels and nerve trunks pass to and from the brain through openings in the skull, mostly at the base. The largest opening, through which the brain and the spinal cord are joined, is the foramen magnum. The brain, which fits snugly in the cranium, is covered by the meninges membranes. The very narrow spaces between the membranes are filled with CSF.

Although the skull is very tough, a blow may fracture it. Even if there is no fracture, a sudden impact may tear or bruise the brain and cause it to swell, as any soft tissue will swell following an injury or bruise. Because the skull does not "give," injury to the brain is magnified by the contained pressure. Unconsciousness or even death may result from swelling (**edema**), tearing wound (**laceration**), bleeding, or other damage to the brain.

The face extends from the eyebrows to the chin and forms the eyes, nose, cheeks, mouth, and lower jaw (mandible).

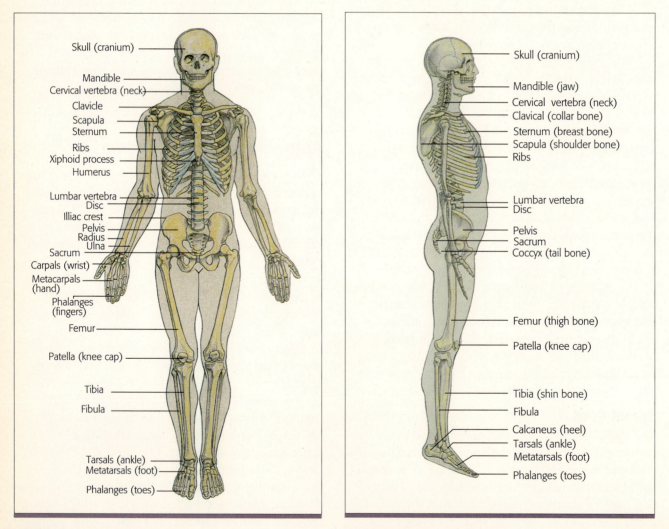

Skeletal System (front view)

Skeletal System (side view)

Spinal Column

The spinal column is made up of irregularly shaped bones called **vertebrae** (singular is *vertebra*). Lying one on top of the other to form a strong flexible column, the vertebrae are bound firmly together by strong ligaments. Between each two vertebrae is an intervertebral disk, which is a pad of tough elastic cartilage that acts as a shock absorber.

The spinal column can be damaged by disease or by injury. If any of the vertebrae is crushed or displaced, the spinal cord at that point may be squeezed, stretched, torn, or severed. Movement of the disabled part by the injured person or careless handling by well-meaning but uninformed persons can result in displacement of sections of the spinal column, causing further injury to the cord and possibly resulting in permanent paralysis. For that reason, a person with a back or neck injury must be handled with extreme care.

Thorax

The thorax (rib cage) is made up of ribs and the sternum (breastbone). The sternum is a flat, narrow bone in the middle of the front wall of the chest. The collar bones and certain ribs are attached to the sternum.

The 24 ribs are semiflexible arches of bone. There are 12 on each side of the chest. The back ends of the 12 pairs of ribs are attached to the 12 thoracic vertebrae. Strong ligaments bind the back ends of the ribs to the backbone but allow slight gliding or tilting movements. The front ends of the top 10 pairs are attached in the front to the sternum by means of cartilage. The front ends of the last two pairs (pairs 11 and 12) hang free; they are called floating ribs.

Fracture of the sternum or the ribs usually results from crushing or squeezing the chest. A fall, blow, or penetration of the chest wall by an object may have the same effect. The chief danger from such injuries is that the lungs or heart may be punctured by the sharp ends of broken ribs.

The lowest portion of the sternum is the **xiphoid process**, which is used as the landmark for determining the hand position for chest compressions given in CPR.

Pelvis

The two hipbones and the sacrum form the pelvic girdle (pelvis). Muscles help attach the pelvic

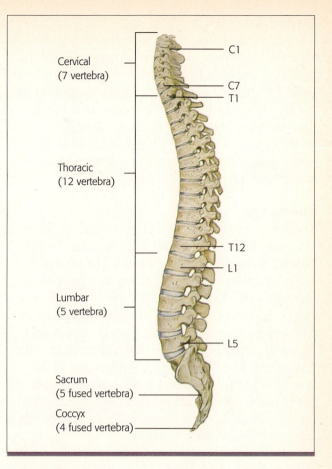

Spinal Column

bones, the trunk, the thighs, and the legs. The pelvis forms the floor of the abdominal cavity. The lower part of the cavity, sometimes called the pelvic cavity, holds the bladder, rectum, and internal parts of the reproductive organs. The floor of the pelvic cavity helps to support the intestines.

Leg Bones

Upper Leg (Thigh)

At the outer side of each hipbone is a deep socket into which the round head of the thighbone (**femur**) fits, forming a ball-and-socket joint. The lower end of the femur is flat and has two knobs. These knobs articulate with the shinbone (**tibia**) at the knee joint. Although the femur is the longest and strongest bone in the skeleton, its fracture is common. A fractured femur is always serious because of the difficulties in getting a good position for union between the broken or splintered ends of this large, strong bone. Because of the force required to break the femur, laceration of the surrounding tissues, pain, and blood loss may be extensive.

Knee

The knee joint is the largest joint in the body and is a strong hinge joint. The joint is protected and stabilized in the front by the kneecap (**patella**). The patella is a small triangular-shaped bone in front of the knee joint and within the tendon of the large muscle of the front of the thigh. Because the patella usually receives the force of falls or blows to the knee, it frequently is bruised or dislocated and sometimes fractured.

Lower Leg

The lower leg pertains to that portion of the lower extremity between the knee and the ankle. Its two bones are the **tibia** and the **fibula.** The tibia is at the front and inner side of the leg. It is palpable throughout its length. Its broad upper surface receives the end of the femur to form the knee joint. The lower end, much smaller than the upper end, forms the inner rounded knob of the ankle (medial malleolus). The fibula, which is not a part of the true knee joint, is attached at the top to the tibia. Its lower end forms the ankle knob (lateral malleolus) on the outside of the ankle. The fibula is more often fractured alone than is the tibia.

Ankle, Feet, and Toes

The ends of the tibia and fibula form the socket of the ankle joint. Both ankle knobs are easily palpated. The seven ankle bones (**tarsals**) are bound firmly together by tough ligaments. The heel bone (calcaneus) transmits the weight of the body to the ground and in walking forms a base for the muscles of the calf of the leg.

The sole and the instep of the foot are formed by the five long **metatarsals.** These articulate with the tarsals and with the front row of toe bones (phalanges).

Shoulder

The collar bone (**clavicle**) and the shoulder blade (**scapula**) form each shoulder girdle. Each clavicle—a long, slightly double-curved bone—is attached to the breastbone at its inner end and to the shoulder blade at its outer end. Each clavicle is palpable throughout its length. Fracture is common because the clavicle lies close to the surface and must absorb blows.

Each scapula—a large, flat, triangular bone—is located over the upper ribs at the back of the thorax.

Arm Bones

Upper Arm

The bone of the upper arm, the **humerus,** is the arm's largest bone. Its upper end (the head) is round; its lower end, flat. The round head fits into a shallow cup in the shoulder blade, forming a ball-and-socket joint. This is the most freely movable joint in the body and is easily dislocated. Dislocation may tear the capsule of the joint (synovial membrane) and cause damage. Improper manipulation during attempts to reduce or "set" the dislocation may add to the damage. Therefore, it is important to treat dislocation of the shoulder with gentle care.

Forearm

The two bones of the forearm (**radius** and **ulna**) lie side by side. The larger of the two, the ulna, is on the little finger side, and part of it forms the elbow. The flat, curved lower end of the humerus fits into a big notch at the upper end of the ulna to form the elbow joint. This hinge joint permits movement in one direction only. The radius, shorter and smaller than the ulna, is on the thumb side of the forearm.

Wrist, Hand, and Fingers

The wrist is composed of eight small, irregularly shaped bones (**carpals**) united by ligaments. Tendons extending from the muscles of the forearm to the bones of the hand and fingers pass down the front and the back of the wrist close the surface. Wrist lacerations may result in the cutting of these tendons, yielding total or partial immobility of the fingers.

The palm of the hand has five long bones (**metacarpals**). The 14 bones of the fingers (phalanges) give the hand its great flexibility. The thumb is the most important digit. A good thumb and one or two fingers make a far more useful hand than four fingers minus the thumb.

Joints

A joint is where two or more bones meet or join. Some joints, such as those in the cranium, allow little, if any, movement of the bones. Other joints, such as the hip and the shoulder, allow a wide range of motion. In a typical joint, the layer of cartilage (gristle), which is softer than bone, acts as a pad or buffer. The bones of such a joint are held in place by firmly attached ligaments, which are bands of very dense, tough, but flexible connective tissue.

Joints are enclosed in a capsule, a layer of thin tough material, strengthened by the ligaments. The inner side of the capsule (synovial membrane) secretes a thick fluid (**synovial fluid**) that lubricates and protects the joint.

Muscular System

When the body moves itself, it is due to work performed by muscles. Examples are walking, breathing, the beating of the heart, and the movements of the stomach and the intestines. What enables muscle tissue to perform work is its ability to contract—that is, to become shorter and thicker—when stimulated by a nerve impulse. The cells of a muscle, usually long and threadlike, are called *fibers*. Each muscle has countless bundles of closely packed, overlapping fibers bound together by connective tissue. The three different kinds of muscles

are skeletal muscle (voluntary), smooth muscle (involuntary), and cardiac muscle (heart). They differ in appearance and the specific jobs they do.

Skeletal Muscles

The skeletal muscles, which are under the control of a person's will, make possible all deliberate acts: walking, chewing, swallowing, smiling, frowning, talking, moving the eyeballs. Most voluntary muscles are attached by one or both ends to the skeleton by tendons. However, some muscles are attached to skin, cartilage, and special organs, such as the eyeball, or to other muscles, such as the tongue.

Muscles help to shape the body and to form its walls. Most skeletal muscles end in tough, whitish cords (**tendons**) by which they are attached to the bones they move. Tendons continue into the fascia, which covers the skeletal muscles. The fascia is

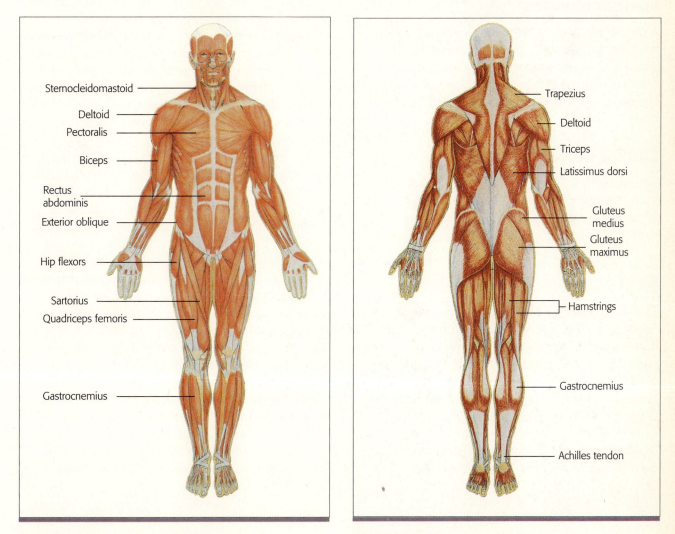

Muscular System (major muscles—front view)

Muscular System (major muscles—back view)

much like the skin of a sausage in that it surrounds the muscle tissue. At either end of the muscle, the fascia extends beyond the muscle to attach to a bone. That area is lined with a synovial membrane, which secretes a lubricating substance, the synovial fluid. This makes it easier for the tendon to move when the muscle contracts or relaxes. Muscular contraction pulls the bone in the direction permitted by a joint.

When not working, muscles become comparatively slack. But they are never completely relaxed; some fibers are contracting all the time. They always have some tension (muscle tone).

Muscles can be injured in many ways. Overexerting a muscle can break fibers. Muscles can be bruised, crushed, cut, torn, or otherwise injured, with or without breaking the skin. Muscles injured in any of those ways are likely to become swollen, tender, painful, or weak.

Smooth Muscles

A person has little or no control over the smooth muscles and usually is not conscious of them. Smooth muscles are in the walls of tubelike structures such as the gastrointestinal tract, the urinary system, the blood vessels, and the bronchi of the lungs.

Cardiac Muscles

Cardiac muscle is a specialized form of muscle found only in the heart. A continuous oxygen supply and glucose are needed for cardiac muscle to work properly.

Skin

The skin covers the entire body, protecting the deep tissues from injury, drying out, and invasion by bacteria and other foreign bodies. The skin helps to regulate body temperature, by aiding in the elimination of water and various salts. The skin senses heat, cold, touch, pressure, and pain and transmits that information to the brain and the spinal cord.

The skin consists of two layers: the outer layer (**epidermis**) and the inner layer (**dermis**). The epidermis varies in thickness in different parts of the

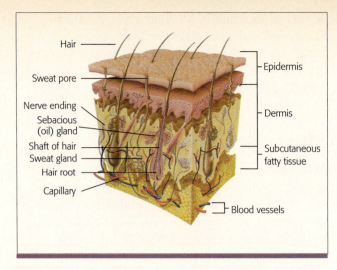

Skin

body, being thickest on the palms and the soles, and its dead cells are constantly worn off. The dermis has a rich supply of blood vessels and nerve endings. Hair grows from the dermis through openings in the skin called hair follicles. Sweat glands and oil glands in the dermis empty onto the surface of the epidermis through pores in the skin. Beneath the dermis is the subcutaneous ("under the skin") layer, which is well supplied with fat cells and blood vessels.

Sweat, or perspiration, glands occur in nearly all parts of the skin. Sweat contains essentially the same minerals as blood plasma and urine, but it is more dilute. Normally, only traces of the waste products excreted in urine are in sweat. But when sweating is profuse or when the kidneys are diseased, the amounts of such wastes excreted in the sweat may be considerable. Several mineral salts are removed from the body in sweat. Chief among those in quantity is sodium chloride (the same mineral as common table salt).

A general knowledge of the human body, similar to that given in this chapter, should help in understanding the other chapters in this book. Even though you will not be making a medical diagnosis, you will be able to suspect what is wrong with a victim and provide proper first aid. You will also be able to communicate to medical personnel correct information with the least possible confusion.

STUDY QUESTIONS 3

Name _____   Course _____   Date _____

Activities

Activity 1

Mark each statement as true (T) or false (F).

T   F   1. Conditions involving the respiratory, nervous, and skeletal systems can threaten life.

T   F   2. Cerebrospinal fluid (CSF) is blood found on the surfaces of the brain and spinal cord.

T   F   3. The brain can swell and press against the skull.

T   F   4. Floating ribs are the bottom two pairs of ribs hanging free.

T   F   5. The longest and strongest bone in the body is the sternum.

T   F   6. Normal swallowing controls do not work in an unconscious person.

T   F   7. The malleolus in the ankle are the lower ends of the tibia and fibula bones.

T   F   8. Of the two bones in the forearm, the ulna is on the thumb side.

T   F   9. The epiglottis closes when food is being swallowed.

T   F   10. The Adam's apple is a common term for the front of the larynx.

T   F   11. The heart is about the size of a clenched fist and shaped like a pear.

T   F   12. A pulse happens where a vein passes near the skin's surface and over a bone.

T   F   13. Hemorrhage is the term for profuse bleeding.

Activity 2

Choose the best answer.

_____ 1. How many quarts of blood are in the body of an average sized adult?
   a. 4 quarts
   b. 6 quarts
   c. 8 quarts
   d. 10 quarts

_____ 2. The bone between the shoulder and elbow is the
   a. femur
   b. humerus
   c. scapula
   d. radius
   e. tibia

_____ 3. The _____ is the pulse point used in unconscious victims.
   a. carotid
   b. aorta
   c. brachial
   d. femoral

_____ 4. The collarbone is known as the
   a. ulna
   b. metacarpal
   c. tarsal
   d. clavicle

_____ 5. The major artery that leaves the left side of the heart and carries freshly oxygenated blood to the body is referred to as
   a. vena cava
   b. carotid artery
   c. aorta
   d. pulmonary vein

Match the following:

_____ 6. prevents food and liquid from entering the lungs

_____ 7. part of the larynx that can be felt in front of the throat

_____ 8. outer layer of skin

_____ 9. attaches muscle to bone

_____ 10. kneecap

   a. tendon
   b. patella
   c. epiglottis
   d. Adam's apple
   e. epidermis

_____ 11. The trachea is the
    a. passageway leading to the stomach
    b. passageway leading to the lungs
    c. opening from the stomach to the small intestines
    d. opening between the esophagus and stomach

Which structure(s) are located in the upper arm?

_____ 12. scapula

_____ 13. humerus

_____ 14. sciatic nerve

_____ 15. radial pulse

_____ 16. The bones of the upper extremity include which of the following?
    a. occipital
    b. femur
    c. ulna
    d. patella

What is the average rate of breathing for

17. _____ adults

18. _____ children

19. _____ infants

What is the average rate of pulse for

20. _____ adults

21. _____ children

22. _____ toddlers

23. _____ newborns

Name the major locations for feeling each of the following pulses.

Name	Location
24. Carotid	_____
25. Radial	_____
26. Brachial	_____
27. Posterior tibial	_____
28. Dorsalis pedis	_____

Which of the following statements are true?

_____ 29. The heart receives its nutrients and oxygen via the coronary veins.

_____ 30. The heart is cone-shaped and about the size of a golf ball.

_____ 31. The right ventricle pumps blood to the body.

_____ 32. The heart has four chambers.

Match the following elements of blood with their corresponding definition(s).
    a. red blood cells
    b. white blood cells
    c. plasma
    d. platelets

_____ 33. tiny, disk-shaped elements that, when ruptured, release chemical factors needed to form blood clots

_____ 34. carry oxygen to and carbon dioxide away from the tissues

_____ 35. involved in destroying germs and producing antibodies that help the body resist infection

_____ 36. watery, salty fluid that makes up more than half the blood's volume

37. List the three types of blood vessels:
    a. _____
    b. _____
    c. _____

38. List the three most important body systems sustaining life:
    a. _____
    b. _____
    c. _____

C H A P T E R

4

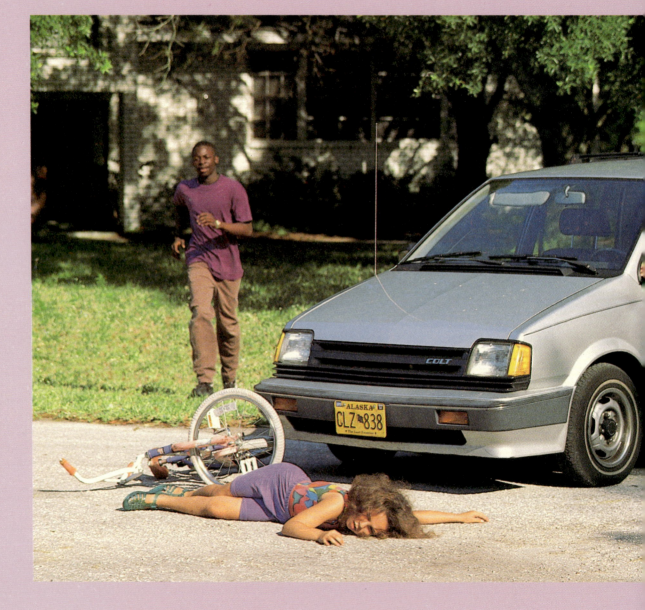

FINDING OUT WHAT'S WRONG

Chances are you will treat someone who has been injured. In fact, almost everyone will, at some time, witness at least one life-threatening injury. During emergency situations, when panic is likely to exist, knowing what to do and what *not* to do can be vital. Effective first aid depends on effective assessment—you need to find what is wrong before you can treat it.

The saying "first things first" may seem obvious in most emergency situations, but it is not always obvious which injuries take precedence. What should be done first, for instance, when an unconscious victim with a leg at an odd angle, which suggests a fracture, is also bleeding profusely from several facial wounds? A logical, systematic format known as **victim assessment** will help you evaluate the situation. Victim assessment is divided into three steps:

1. the primary survey to determine any life-threatening conditions
2. the physical exam to evaluate nonemergency conditions
3. the victim's history (*For a suddenly ill person you may want to complete the victim's history before conducting the physical exam.*)

After you have determined that the situation is safe (see page 20), you can perform the primary survey. Make all assessments while kneeling close to the victim.

If two or more people are injured, attend to the quiet one first. A quiet victim may not have an open airway or a pulse. A victim who is talking, crying, or yelling obviously has an open airway.

Most injured or ill victims do not require a complete victim assessment. The circumstances of the same type of injury usually will determine if a complete assessment is necessary. For example, a victim who cut a finger while peeling a potato won't require a complete assessment, but a victim with a cut finger from a bicycle collision will because other injuries may be present.

The Primary Survey

The respiratory, circulatory, and nervous systems include the most important organs in the body. A serious problem in any of those three body systems generally produces a serious threat to life. And if any one of those systems stops functioning, death occurs within minutes.

The goal of the primary survey is to quickly assess the three most important body systems. The heart, lungs, brain, and spinal cord are essential to life.

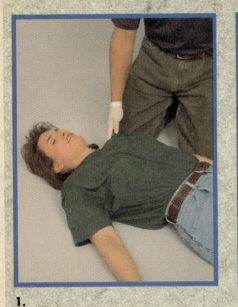

1.

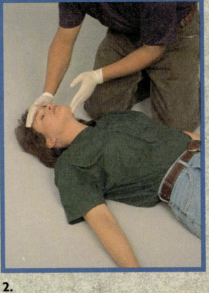

2.

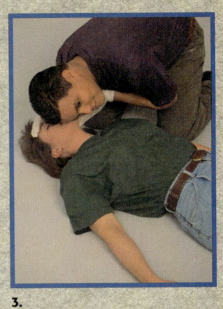

3.

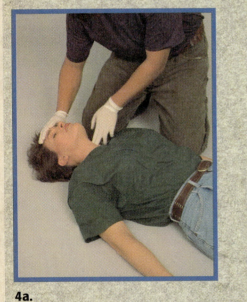

4a.

1. Responsive? Victim's mental status—use AVPU scale

2. A = Airway open?

3. B = Breathing?

4. C = Circulation

    a. Carotid pulse?

    b. Hemorrhage/severe bleeding?

    c. Condition of skin? (not shown)

      • color

      • temperature

      • moisture

5. D = Disability

      • spinal cord response

      • mental status (AVPU scale)

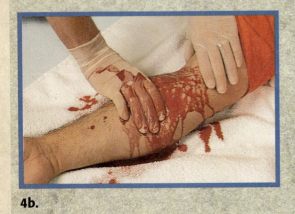

4b.

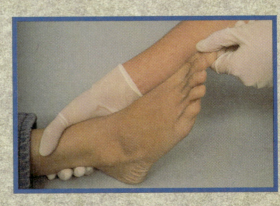

5.

Any life-threatening condition, such as an obstructed airway or massive bleeding, found during the primary survey, must be corrected before you continue the victim assessment. Since most injured victims won't have life-threatening conditions, most primary surveys will be completed quickly.

"You can observe a lot just by watchin'.

Yogi Berra (former New York Yankee catcher)

The first step in caring for any victim is to find the most life-threatening conditions. Always assess and care for the three most important body systems in the ABCD order of importance:

- Respiratory system
  A: **A**irway open?
  B: **B**reathing?
- Circulatory system
  C: **C**irculation (Pulse? Hemorrhage? Skin condition?)
- Nervous system
  D: **D**isability (Spinal cord response? Level of responsiveness?)

Give priority to caring for the ABCDs for life- and limb-saving first aid. (You may need to remove some of a victim's clothing to complete the assessment. This step, sometimes called **E**xpose, is why you may hear references to "ABCDE.")

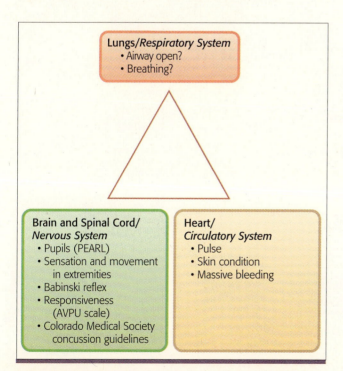

How to assess the three most important body systems

First, form a general impression of the victim based on an immediate assessment of the scene and the victim's chief complaint. Look at the surroundings and the mechanisms of injury (MOI). Then assess the victim's responsiveness or mental status. Begin by asking if he or she is okay. State your name, tell the victim you are a first aider, and explain that you are there to help. Then gain consent by asking if you can help. If you suspect a spine injury, stabilize the spine against moving.

A victim's level of responsiveness or mental status can be described according to the following **AVPU** scale. The V, P, and U levels can help determine damage from decreased oxygen to the brain, drug or alcohol overdose, central nervous system (CNS) injury, or metabolic derangement from diabetes, a seizure, or a heart condition.

> **A**: **A**lert. The victim's eyes are open, and he or she can answer questions clearly. A victim who knows the date (*time*), where he or she is (*place*), and his or her own name (*person*) is said to be alert.
>
> **V**: Responsive to **V**erbal stimulus. The victim may not be oriented to time, place, and person but does respond in some meaningful way when spoken to.
>
> **P**: Responsive only to **P**ainful stimulus. The eyes do not open, and the victim does not respond to questions. The victim does respond to your pinching of the skin over the collarbone.
>
> **U**: **U**nresponsive to any stimulus. The eyes do not open, and the victim does not respond to pinching of the skin.

A: Open the Airway

If the victim is talking or responsive, the airway is open. For an unresponsive victim, open the airway with the head-tilt/chin-lift method unless you suspect a neck injury (see pages 70 and 73).

B: Assess Breathing

Responsive victims are breathing. Note any breathing difficulties or unusual breathing sounds such as wheezing, crowing, gurgling, or snoring. If the victim is unresponsive, keep the airway open and look for the chest to rise and fall, listen for breathing, and feel for air coming out of the victim's nose and mouth. If there is no breathing, give two breaths. (Refer to page 73 for details.) If an unresponsive victim is breathing, place the victim on his or her left side (**recovery position**, see page 72).

PRIMARY SURVEY

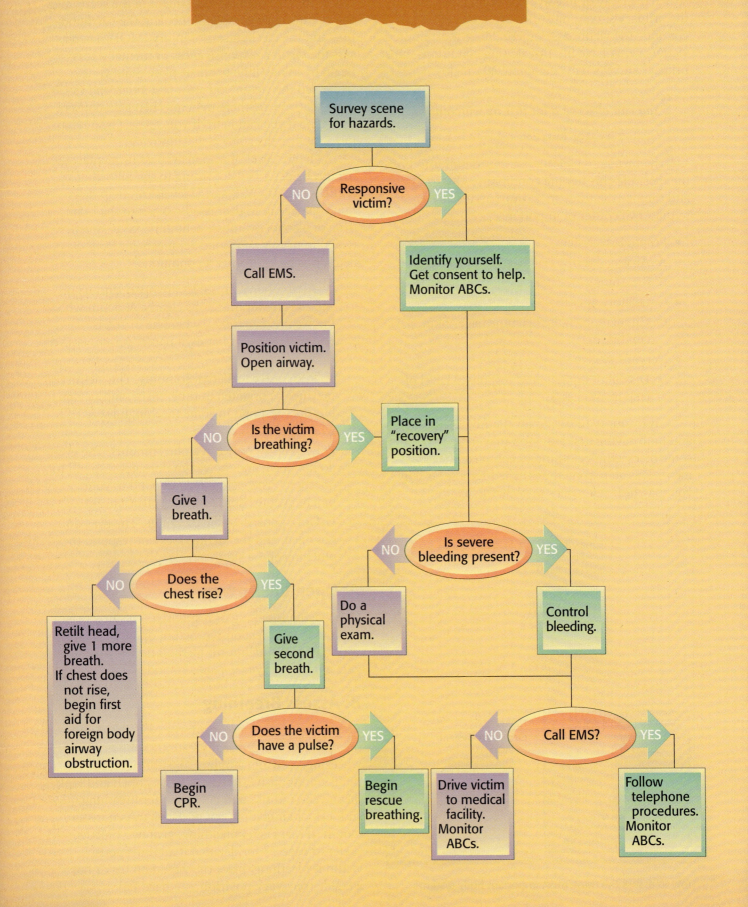

Survey scene for hazards.

Responsive victim?

NO → Call EMS. → Position victim. Open airway. → Is the victim breathing?

YES → Identify yourself. Get consent to help. Monitor ABCs.

Is the victim breathing?
NO → Give 1 breath. → Does the chest rise?
YES → Place in "recovery" position.

Does the chest rise?
NO → Retilt head, give 1 more breath. If chest does not rise, begin first aid for foreign body airway obstruction.
YES → Give second breath. → Does the victim have a pulse?

Is severe bleeding present?
NO → Do a physical exam.
YES → Control bleeding.

Does the victim have a pulse?
NO → Begin CPR.
YES → Begin rescue breathing.

Call EMS?
NO → Drive victim to medical facility. Monitor ABCs.
YES → Follow telephone procedures. Monitor ABCs.

C: Assess Circulation

First, check an unresponsive victim's pulse by feeling at the side of the neck (carotid artery) or, for an infant, at the upper arm (brachial artery). If a pulse is absent, cardiopulmonary resuscitation (CPR) is required. If a pulse is present, but there is no breathing, give rescue breathing. Refer to page 75 for details.

Second, check for major bleeding by looking over the victim's entire body for blood (blood-soaked clothing or blood pooling on the floor or the ground). Bleeding requires the application of direct pressure or a pressure bandage. Avoid contact with the victim's blood, if possible, by using latex gloves or extra layers of cloth or dressings. Control any bleeding as described on pages 112–114.

Finally, check the victim's skin condition (color, temperature, and moisture). Skin color, especially in light-skinned people, reflects the circulation un-

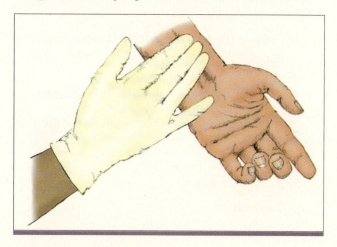

Palpating (feeling) the radial pulse

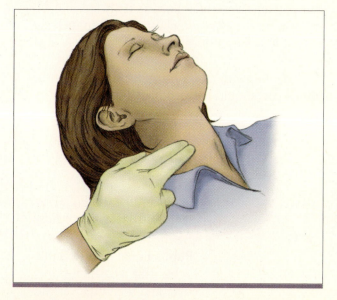

Palpating (feeling) the carotid pulse

der the skin as well as oxygen status. In darkly pigmented people, changes may not be readily apparent but can be assessed by the appearance of the nail beds, the inside of the mouth, and the inner eyelids. When the skin's blood vessels constrict or the pulse slows, the skin becomes cool and pale or cyanotic (blue-gray color). When the skin's blood vessels dilate or blood flow increases, the skin becomes warm and pink.

You can get a rough idea of temperature by putting the back of your hand or wrist on the victim's forehead and your other hand on your own forehead or that of another healthy person. If the victim has a fever, you should feel the difference. Abnormal skin temperature will feel hot, cool, cold, or clammy (cool and moist).

Notice if the skin seems dry (normal) or moist or wet (abnormal).

D: Assess Disability

Check for a spine injury especially if the victim has been injured in a fall, a motor vehicle crash, or other incident that could produce a spine injury. Assume that a victim with a head injury has a spine injury until it is proved otherwise. To assess a victim for a spine injury: (1) check sensation by squeezing the victim's fingers and toes; (2) check movement by having the victim wiggle his or her fingers and toes; and (3) have the victim perform a hand squeeze and a foot push. See page 203 for details. Another test for a possible spine injury is the Babinski test; refer to page 204 for details.

If you suspect a spine injury, do not move the victim's head or neck. See page 205 for the best way to stabilize a neck at the accident scene.

Next, check the victim's level of responsiveness. Avoid using confusing terms such as "semiconscious" and "in and out" to describe the victim's responsiveness. Instead, use one of four levels on the AVPU scale (see page 53).

E: Expose the Injury

Clothing can hide an injury. How much clothing you should remove varies, depending on the victim's condition and injuries. The general rule is to remove as much clothing as necessary to determine the presence or absence of a condition or an injury. Keep in mind that most injured victims are susceptible to hypothermia. If the removal of certain items of clothing may prove embarrassing to the victim or to bystanders, explain what you intend to do and why.

The Physical Exam

After you have completed the primary survey and attended to any life-threatening conditions, next make a systematic **physical exam.** The physical exam will uncover injuries or illnesses that, while not posing an immediate threat to life, may do so if they remain uncorrected. Even minor injuries need treatment, but first they must be found. If there are two or more victims, complete the primary survey on each before checking either with a physical exam.

Carry out a physical exam while kneeling close to the victim. Standing over someone lying on the ground sends the signal to the victim and to others that you want to keep your clothes clean or that you do not really want to help.

By now, you will have a good idea whether the victim's condition involves an injury or a sudden illness. The physical exam of a victim with a sudden illness focuses on a particular complaint. The physical exam of an injured victim may focus on a specific part of the body. Make sure you tell the victim what you are doing and why.

CAUTION: DO NOT

- aggravate injuries or contaminate wounds.
- move a victim with a possible spine injury.

Systematically start a "looking and feeling" exam at the victim's head and proceed down the body to the feet. With children, start at their feet, since it is less frightening to them. The mnemonic **LAF** can remind you how to examine an area:

L: Look at the area for deformity, open wounds, and swelling.

A: And

F: Feel for deformity, tenderness, and swelling.

Use the mnemonic **DOTS** to remember the signs of injury:

D: Deformity

O: Open wounds

T: Tenderness

S: Swelling

Use the LAF method to briefly inspect (look at) and palpate (feel) the following body areas in a logical manner: head, neck, chest, abdomen, pelvis, and all four extremities. Use DOTS to locate any injuries.

The following checklist indicates some of the things you should look and feel for:

- Head   Deformity?

                     Open wounds?

                     Tenderness?

                     Swelling?

                     Cerebrospinal fluid (CSF, a clear fluid) from ear or nose?

- Eyes   Use the mnemonic **PEARL** (**P**upils **E**qual **A**nd **R**eact to **L**ight). Use a flashlight or cover and then uncover the victim's eyes with your hand to

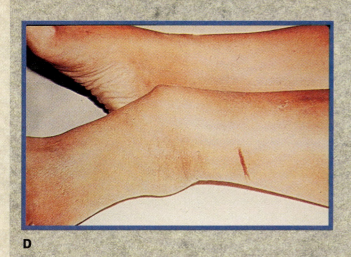

D

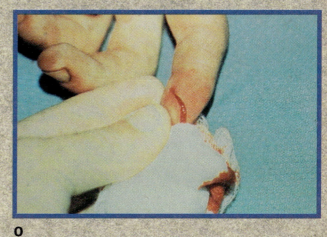

O

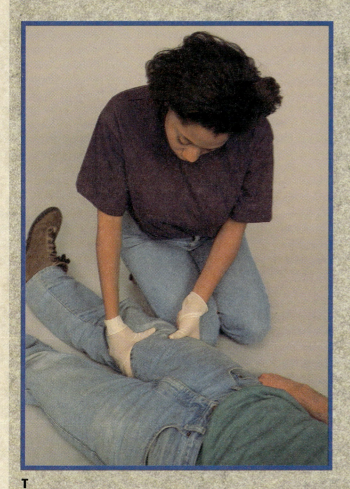

T

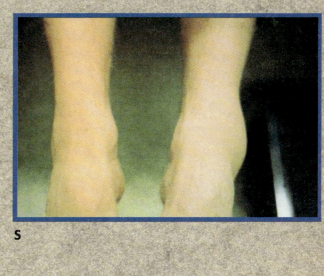

S

Examine an area by looking and feeling (LAF) for deformity, open wounds, tenderness, and swelling (DOTS).

D = Deformity
O = Open wounds
T = Tenderness
S = Swelling

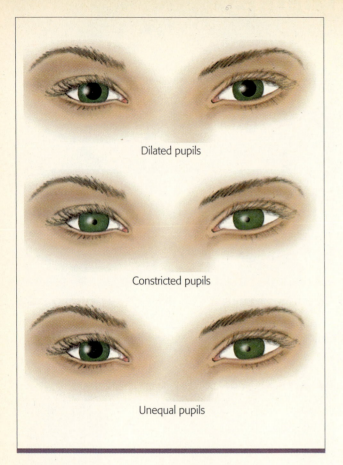

Dilated pupils

Constricted pupils

Unequal pupils

Changes in pupil size can have medical significance.

Open wounds?
Tenderness? (Gently press downward and squeeze inward.)
Swelling?

- Extremities   Deformity?
  Open wounds?
  Tenderness?
  Swelling?
  Circulation, **S**ensation, and **M**ovement (**CSM**)
  (See page 225.)

The Victim's History

The interview usually involves the victim, but it may include the family and bystanders if the victim is unresponsive or a young child.

Ask the victim about his or her condition. Those with chronic health problems can often tell you what is best for them. For example, an asthmatic will tell you that he or she needs to stand or sit up and cannot tolerate lying flat. Well-meaning emergency medical personnel have been known to

determine if the pupils are reactive (i.e., they constrict in response to light). Unequal pupils occur normally in 2 to 4 percent of the population but should be of equal size when the brain is not injured.

- Neck   Deformity?
  Open wounds?
  Tenderness?
  Swelling?
- Chest   Deformity?
  Open wounds?
  Tenderness? (Squeeze or compress the sides for rib pain.)
  Swelling?
- Abdomen   Deformity?
  Open wounds?
  Tenderness? (Gently press the four abdominal quadrants for firmness and softness.)
  Swelling?
- Pelvis   Deformity?

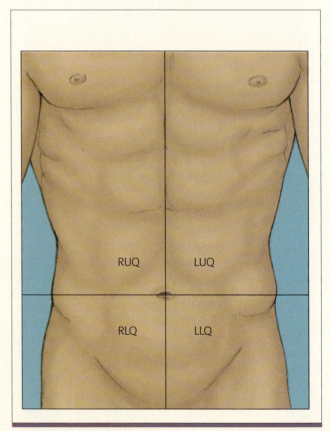

Gently press the four quadrants for firmness and softness.

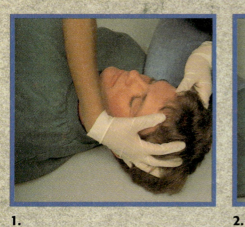

1.

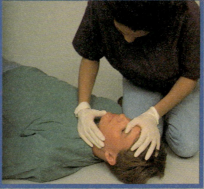

2.

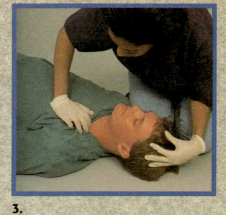

3.

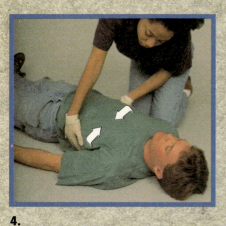

4.

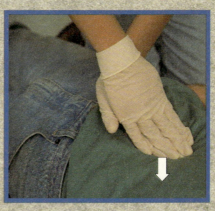

5.

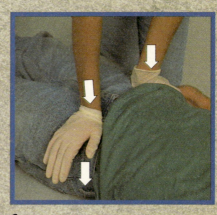

6a.

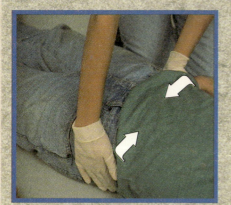

6b.

Briefly inspect by looking and feeling:

1. Head: DOTS; cerebrospinal fluid
2. Eyes: PEARL—Pupils are Equal And React to Light
3. Neck: DOTS
4. Chest: DOTS; squeeze chest
5. Abdomen: DOTS; gently press four quadrants
6. Pelvis: a. Gently press downward
        b. Gently squeeze inward
7. Extremities: DOTS arms and legs; check CSM—Circulation, Sensation, Movement

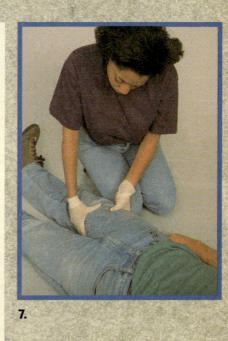

7.

insist that an asthmatic victim lie down despite the victim's protests and increasing shortness of breath.

Question the victim or the victim's family, if time permits, to learn the victim's relevant medical history. The information gained may indicate what is wrong or what needs to be passed along to medical personnel. Ask the victim about his or her chief complaint; often it is obvious (e.g., a twisted ankle). Most chief complaints are characterized by pain or an abnormal function. Use the mnemonic **SAMPLE** to help you collect the victim's history.

Note: For suddenly ill victims, you may want to collect the SAMPLE history before you conduct the physical exam.

> **S**: **S**igns and symptoms. A **sign** is any condition or injury *displayed* by the victim and identifiable by the first aider (e.g., bleeding, skin temperature). A **symptom** is any condition *described* by the victim (e.g., headache, stomachache). As you locate signs and symptoms of illness or injury, there may be specific questions that you as a first aider should ask (described in later chapters on illness and injury).
>
> **A**: **A**llergies. "Are you allergic to anything?" The answer may give a clue as to the problem. Always look for a medical-alert tag.
>
> **M**: **M**edications. "Do you take any prescription or over-the-counter medicine?" The answer may give a clue as to the problem and help prevent the administration of contraindicated medication.
>
> **P**: **P**ertinent past illnesses. "Are you seeing a doctor for anything?" (relating to the present problem)
>
> **L**: **L**ast oral intake. "When was the last time you had anything to eat or drink? How much? Was it solid or liquid?" The answers are important in case surgery is necessary or food poisoning is suspected.
>
> **E**: **E**vents leading to the injury or illness. "What were you doing when this happened?"

Medical Identification Tags

Look for medical identification tags, which may be beneficial in identifying allergies, medications, or medical history. A medical-alert tag, worn as a necklace or as a bracelet, contains the wearer's medical problem(s) and a 24-hour telephone number that offers, in case of an emergency, access to the

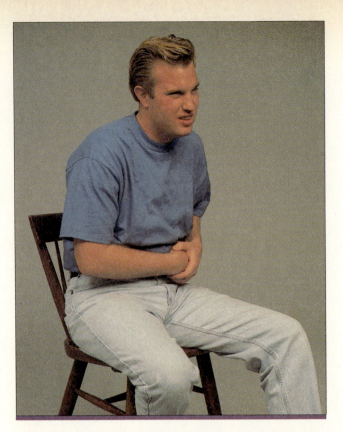

Symptom: condition described by victim, such as abdominal pain

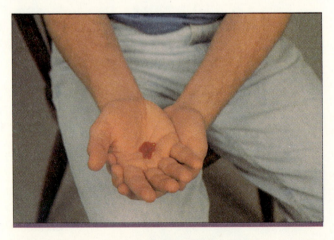

Sign: condition or injury displayed, such as blood

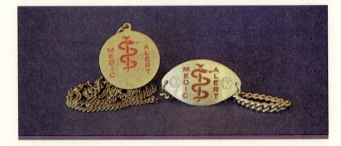

Medical-alert tag

during those hectic, panicky, emergency situations when you may be wondering what to do first.

While you are waiting for an ambulance, continue to check the victim. Ongoing assessment allows you to calm and reassure the victim and at the same time to reassess the ABCs. Repeat the primary assessment every 15 minutes for a responsive victim and every 5 minutes for an unresponsive victim. Use the AVPU scale to check the victim's mental status. Check any first aid that has been given, including bandages and splints.

When the ambulance arrives, report to the emergency medical personnel the following information:

Hero CITATION

Ronald Miracle saved Darlene F. Musselman from burning, Mesa, Arizona, September 29, 1989. Miss Musselman, 35, was semi-conscious in the front seat of a burning car after a fatal, three-vehicle accident. After witnessing the accident from nearby, Miracle, 41, ran to the driver's door of Miss Musselman's car and opened it. Despite growing flames on the wreckage and heavy smoke, Miracle entered the car, seized Miss Musselman, and pulled her out. As he dragged her to safety, flames engulfed the interior of the car. Miss Musselman required hospital treatment for her injuries, and Miracle was treated for smoke inhalation, from which he recovered.

victim's medical history plus names of doctors and close relatives. Necklaces and bracelets are durable, instantly recognizable, and less likely than cards to be separated from the victim in an emergency.

Putting It All Together

The victim assessment will be influenced by whether the victim is suffering from a sudden illness or from an injury, whether the victim is responsive or unresponsive, and whether life-threatening conditions are present. Be sure to conduct a primary survey and correct any life-threatening problem *before* going on to the physical exam and the victim's history.

Medical personnel at all levels follow a systematic method of assessing an injured person. The assessment methods may vary, but all share a similar format. The method presented here can help you

1. victim's chief complaint
2. responsiveness (AVPU scale)
3. ABCD (airway, breathing, circulation, disability) status
4. physical exam findings
5. SAMPLE history
6. any first aid that has been provided

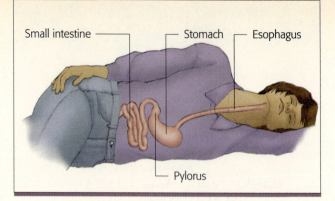

Stomach placement of person in left-side position.

Advantages of the Left-Side Position

Left-side positioning is referred to by several terms: recovery position, left lateral recumbent position, left lateral decubitus position, and stable-side position. Positioning a person on his or her left side has several advantages:

- It keeps the airway open in an unresponsive breathing victim without a spine injury.

- It protects the lungs from aspiration should vomiting occur.

- It delays vomiting by placing the esophagus above the stomach.

- It delays a poison's effects by retaining the poison in the stomach (the pyloric sphincter is kept straight up). A poison can be better dealt with in the stomach than in the small intestines.

- It relieves pressure on a pregnant woman's vena cava (the body's largest vein). Many pregnant women will pass out or at least feel dizzy if they lie supine (on their backs), because of the reduced blood flow.

NOTES

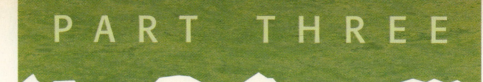

PART THREE

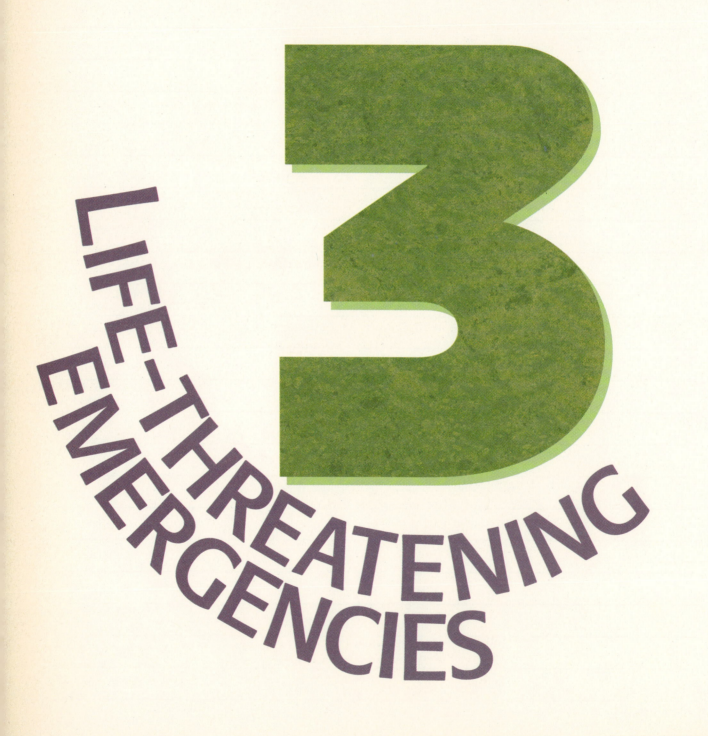

LIFE-THREATENING
EMERGENCIES

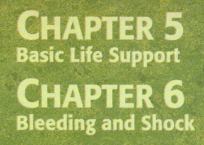

CHAPTER 5
Basic Life Support

CHAPTER 6
Bleeding and Shock

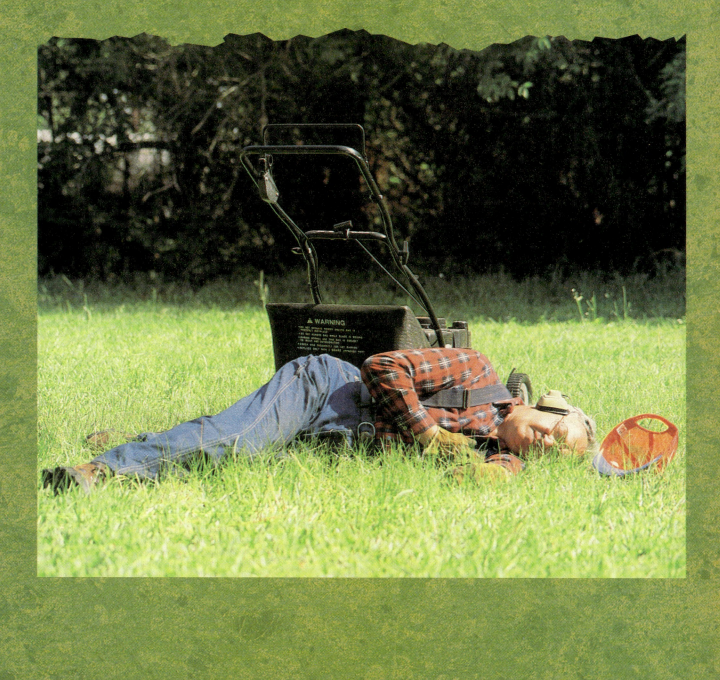

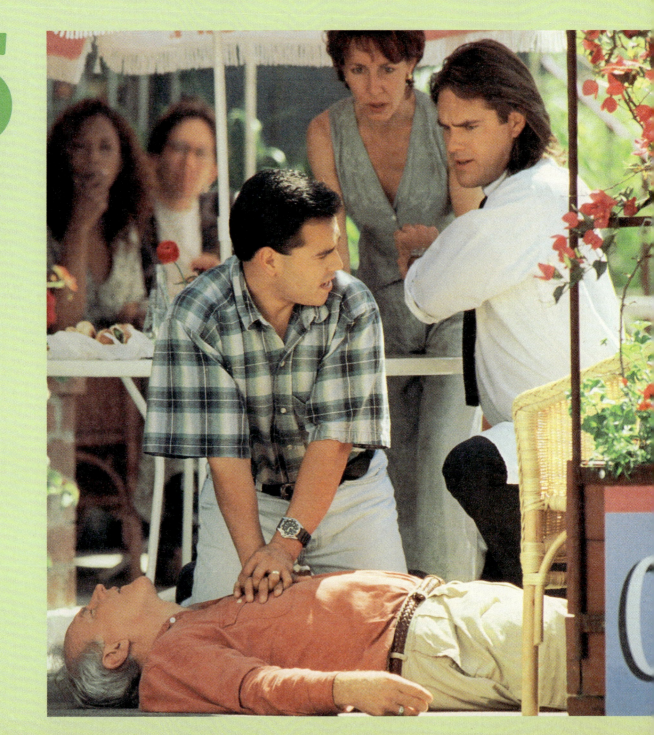

BASIC LIFE SUPPORT*

The American Heart Association reports that nearly 500,000 yearly deaths are due to heart attacks in the United States. Heart attacks are the most prominent medical emergency in North America. In addition, drownings, suffocations, electrocutions, and drug intoxication cause cardiac arrest. Many deaths could be prevented if the victims got prompt help—if someone trained in CPR provided proper life-saving measures until trained EMS professionals could take over.

Adult Basic Life Support

For the nonbreathing victim, rescue breathing must be started immediately. This is one of the most important procedures that you as a first aider will be called on to do. For best results, you must understand the process so well that you can proceed automatically. Every second you do not have to spend trying to recall the proper procedure is a precious second you can use to resuscitate a victim.

Essentially, there are eight steps for performing adult basic life support:

1. Check victim's responsiveness.
2. Activate the Emergency Medical Service (EMS).
3. Position the unresponsive victim.
4. Open the victim's airway.
5. Check for breathing.
6. Give 2 slow breaths.
7. Check for a pulse.
8. Perform rescue procedures based on findings: either rescue breathing or CPR.

Check Responsiveness

The first step is to recognize that a person is unresponsive. The simplest method to determine unresponsiveness is to tap the victim's shoulder and shout, "Are you okay?" Do not forcefully shake the victim, since he or she may have a spine injury.

*Based on the American Heart Association, Guidelines for Cardiopulmonary Resuscitation and Emergency Cardiac Care, *JAMA*, 268: 2172 (1992).

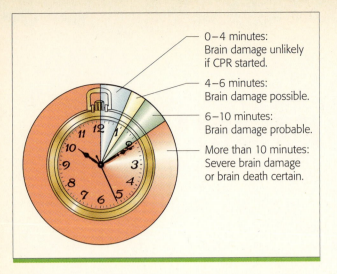

0–4 minutes:
Brain damage unlikely
if CPR started.

4–6 minutes:
Brain damage possible.

6–10 minutes:
Brain damage probable.

More than 10 minutes:
Severe brain damage
or brain death certain.

Start resuscitation efforts at once. Brain damage occurs without oxygen.

Activate EMS

If the victim is unresponsive, activate the EMS *immediately,* to avoid unnecessary loss of time in acquiring advanced cardiac life support. Direct a bystander to activate the EMS (usually by telephoning 911). If no bystanders are present, activate the EMS yourself.

Position the Unresponsive Victim

An unresponsive victim lying facedown must be turned over so CPR can be given, if necessary. If you must turn the victim over, keep the head, neck, and shoulders aligned to avoid any twisting of the body. To turn an unresponsive victim, see page 71.

Open the Airway

The most important maneuver in performing rescue breathing is opening the victim's airway. The most common cause of airway obstruction in an unconscious person is blockage by the tongue. When a victim's airway is opened, the lower jaw is moved forward, bringing the base of the tongue (which is attached to the lower jaw) forward also and away from the back of the throat. The easiest way to open an injured person's airway is by tilting the head and lifting the chin.

To perform the head-tilt/chin-lift, place one hand, palm down, on the victim's forehead and push downward so the head tilts back. Then place the index and middle fingers of your other hand under the lower edge of the chin to lift the jaw. Simply opening the victim's airway sometimes results in restoration of breathing.

If you suspect a spine injury, first try to open the airway by lifting the chin without tilting the head back. If the airway remains blocked, tilt the head slowly and gently until the airway is open enough to allow breaths to go in. Another technique for a victim with a possible spine injury is to use a jaw thrust without a head tilt. While stabilizing the head, place the fingers of each hand behind the angles of the victim's lower jaw on each side of the head and move the lower jaw forward without tilting the head backward. If the airway does not open, it may be necessary to tilt the head slightly.

Check for Breathing

After determining unresponsiveness and opening the airway, the next step is to look, listen, and feel for breathing. *Look* to see whether there is any visible movement of the victim's chest, *listen* for air by placing your ear next to the victim's mouth and nose, and *feel* for air by placing your cheek next to the victim's mouth and nose. If breathing is present, you will see the victim's chest rise and fall, hear air coming from the victim's mouth and nose, and feel air against your cheek. This process should take only three to five seconds. Place a breathing unconscious victim in the recovery position (see Chapter 4).

Perform Rescue Breathing

If a victim is not breathing, perform rescue breathing by using one of the following methods: mouth

Definitions

Cardiopulmonary resuscitation (CPR) combines rescue breathing (also known as mouth-to-mouth breathing) and external chest compressions. *Cardio* refers to the heart, and *pulmonary* refers to the lungs. *Resuscitation* means "to revive." Proper and prompt CPR serves as a holding action by providing oxygen to the brain and heart until advanced cardiac life support can be provided.

Basic life support (BLS) refers to lifesaving procedures that focus on the victim's airway, breathing, and circulation. BLS includes rescue breathing, CPR, and obstructed airway management.

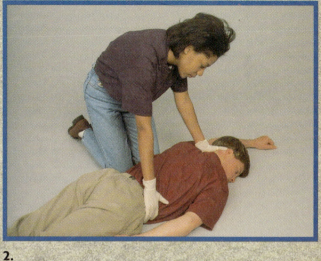

1.

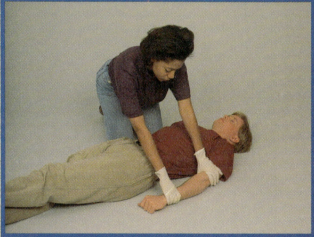

2.

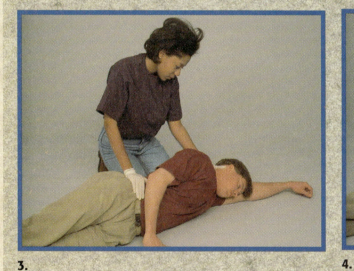

3.

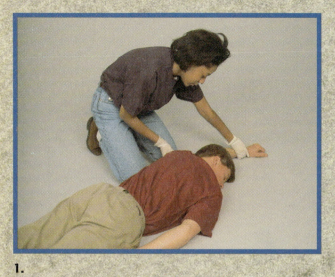

4.

1. Kneel at victim's side. Raise victim's arm closest to you. Adjust victim's legs so they are nearly straight (crossing ankles helps).
2. Support head and neck with one hand. Reach over to victim's outside hip and grasp clothing or edge of hip with your other hand.
3. Turn victim as a complete unit, pulling steadily and evenly to roll him or her toward you.
4. Reposition the extended arm next to body.

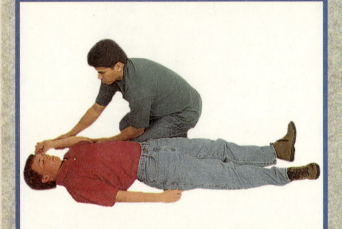

1.

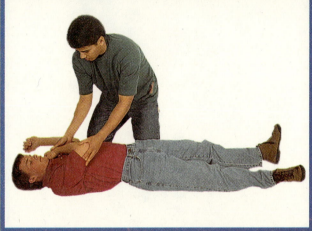

2.

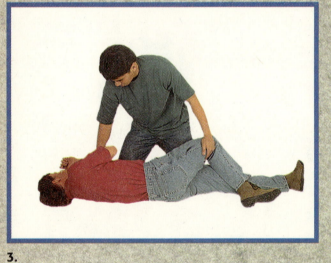

3.

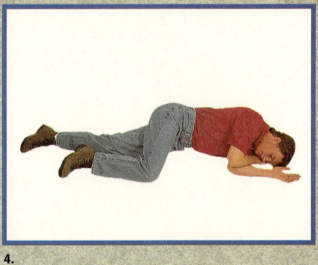

4.

1. Bend arm. Keep legs straight.
2. Place back of victim's hand against cheek and hold there.
3. Hold victim's hand against cheek to support head. Pull bent leg and roll victim toward you.
4. Hand supports head. Bent knee prevents rolling. Bent arm gives stability. Front view of recovery position.

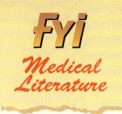

FYI *Medical Literature*

Chain of Survival The National Safety Council advocates the Chain of Survival model of emergency cardiac care. The Chain of Survival includes four links: (1) early access; (2) early cardiopulmonary resuscitation (CPR); (3) early defibrillation; and (4) early advanced care. Bystanders are a vital part of the first two links—activation of the EMS and CPR. Skilled EMS personnel provide the other two links—defibrillation and advanced care. A weak or missing link decreases the chance of survival.

1. **Early access.** Early access of the emergency medical service (EMS) enables defibrillation-trained and equipped personnel to arrive at the victim's side more rapidly and enables trained emergency dispatchers to coach bystanders in the provision of CPR until help arrives. The bystander must recognize the emergency, be willing to help, and be able to notify the local EMS.

2. **Early CPR.** Early CPR, which provides rescue breathing and chest compressions, serves as a holding action providing blood and oxygen to vital organs for a few extra minutes until defibrillation and advanced care can be provided. It takes more than CPR to save a life when the heart stops.

   CPR, as we do it today, was first described in 1960. Since then, the technique has changed very little. The earlier it is used, the better. Bystander CPR improves a victim's likelihood of survival. CPR alone has a minimal effect if early defibrillation cannot be provided. Experts claim that poorly performed CPR may be no more effective than no CPR at all.

3. **Early defibrillation.** In most cases of adult cardiac arrest, the heart is in an abnormal rhythm called ventricular fibrillation that can only be reversed by delivering an electrical shock with a machine known as a defibrillator. Each minute delayed for attempted defibrillation reduces the likelihood of survival.

4. **Early advanced care.** Early advanced care includes the three above links plus special care (e.g., intravenous medications) to help stabilize the victim and prevent recurrence of cardiac arrest.

to mouth, mouth to nose, mouth to barrier device, or mouth to stoma.

Mouth-to-Mouth Method

The mouth-to-mouth method of rescue breathing is the simplest, quickest, and most effective method for an emergency situation.

During rest, the normal adult breathing rate is about 12 times per minute, and the volume is 0.5 to 1.0 liter per breath. Mouth-to-mouth rescue breathing provides 0.8 to 1.2 liters of exhaled air per breath. Exhaled air is about 16 percent oxygen (which is enough to sustain life) in comparison to room air, which is 21 percent.

Mouth-to-mouth breathing is preferred over mouth-to-nose breathing, especially if there is nasal bleeding, injury, or blockage. To perform mouth-to-mouth rescue breathing, follow these steps:

1. Make sure the victim's head is positioned with the neck extended and the head tilted backward to open the airway.
2. Pinch the victim's nose closed to prevent air from escaping, using the same hand that is on the victim's forehead to keep the neck extended.
3. Take a deep breath.
4. Make a tight seal with your mouth around the victim's mouth.
5. Slowly blow air into the victim's mouth until you see the chest rise.
6. Remove your mouth to allow the air to come out and turn your head away as you take another breath.
7. Repeat one more breath.

If the first breath does not go in, retilt the victim's head and try a second breath. If the second breath does not go in, use the procedure to aid an unconscious choking victim described later in this chapter (page 86).

Do not remove a victim's dentures unless they interfere with rescue breathing. Even loose dentures give form and shape to the victim's mouth.

Mouth-to-Nose Method

Although mouth-to-mouth breathing is successful in the majority of cases, certain complications necessitate mouth-to-nose rescue breathing: the victim's mouth cannot be opened, a good seal cannot be made around the victim's mouth, the victim's mouth is severely injured, or the victim's mouth is too large or has no teeth.

The mouth-to-nose technique is performed like

mouth-to-mouth breathing, except that you force your exhaled breath through the victim's nose while holding his or her mouth closed with one hand pushing up on the chin. The victim's mouth then must be held open so any nasal obstruction does not impede exhalation of air from the victim's lungs.

Mouth-to-Stoma Method

Cancer and other diseases of the vocal cords often make surgical removal of the larynx necessary. This operation is called a *laryngectomy,* and an individual who has had the larynx removed is called a *laryngectomee.* Laryngectomees do not have a connection between the upper airway and the lungs. They breathe through a small permanent opening called a *stoma,* which is surgically made in the lower part of the neck and joined to the trachea. Some laryngectomees have a tracheostomy tube temporarily inserted inside their surgically created airway until the surrounding tissues mature. A person with a tracheostomy tube can be recognized by the tube that projects out of the front of the neck.

In mouth-to-stoma rescue breathing, the victim's mouth and nose must be closed during the delivery of breaths because the air can flow upward into the upper airway through the larynx as well as downward into the lungs. You can close the victim's mouth and nose with one hand. Determine breathing by looking, listening, and feeling at the stoma. Keep the victim's head and neck level.

Mouth-to-Barrier Device

A mouth-to-barrier device is an apparatus that is placed over a victim's face as a safety precaution for the rescuer during rescue breathing. There are two types of mouth-to-barrier devices:

- *Face masks.* Face masks cover the victim's mouth and nose. Most have a one-way valve so exhaled air from the victim does not enter the rescuer's mouth. According to the American Heart Association, face masks are more effective than face shields.
- *Face shields.* These clear plastic devices have a mouthpiece through which the rescuer breathes. Some models have a short airway that is inserted into the victim's mouth over the tongue. They are smaller and less expensive than face masks, but air can leak around the shield. Also, they cover only the victim's mouth, so the nose must be pinched. The American Heart Association recommends replacing face shields with face masks as soon as possible.

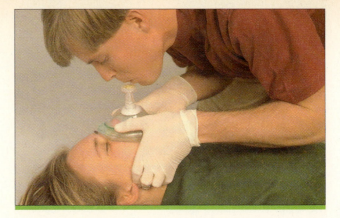

Mouth-to-barrier device

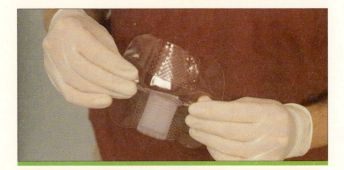

Face shield

Use of a barrier device requires the victim's neck to be hyperextended and the chin lifted. After the mask is in place, the rescuer breathes through the device. The technique is performed like mouth-to-mouth breathing.

Check for a Pulse

After you have given the first two breaths, locate the victim's pulse to see if the heart is beating. To find the pulse, maintain the head-tilt position with one hand pushing backward on the victim's forehead and use the tips of the index and the middle fingers of your other hand to locate the victim's Adam's apple (larynx or voice box). Then slide the two fingers into the groove between the Adam's apple and the muscle at the side of the neck for the carotid pulse.

Feel for the carotid artery on the side of the victim's neck closer to you. You should not feel for the carotid artery on the far side of the victim's neck for two reasons: (1) there is a greater tendency to apply unnecessary pressure on the trachea, which can obstruct the airway, and (2) there is a greater tendency to feel for the pulse by using your thumb and feeling both sides of the neck simultaneously. Feeling with the thumb, which has its own pulse, can give a false indication of a pulse in the victim.

The reasons for feeling the carotid pulse are that it is immediately accessible and you are already positioned at the victim's head and neck. Also, a felt carotid pulse will persist when other pulses (e.g., radial pulse) cannot be detected. Locating the carotid pulse is easily learned.

Feel for the carotid artery gently and without undue pressure. It should take five to ten seconds to feel for the pulse, except in cases of hypothermia, when 30 to 45 seconds should be taken.

If the victim has no pulse, CPR must be started immediately.

If the victim has a pulse but is not breathing, continue rescue breathing at a rate of one breath every five seconds, or 12 times per minute. Between breaths, remove your mouth to take a breath and to permit air to flow out of the victim's lungs. As you remove your mouth, turn your head toward the victim's feet to see whether the victim's chest falls after each breath. A method for timing the breaths for every five seconds is to breathe into the victim for about two seconds, count "one–one thousand, two–one thousand," then take a breath for yourself on the fifth second. After 12 breaths, recheck the victim's pulse and breathing.

Perform External Chest Compressions

External chest compressions are required only if a pulse is not present. After each minute of rescue breathing, you should feel for a pulse. If a pulse cannot be felt, external chest compressions must be given.

If there is no pulse initially, external chest compressions must be given in addition to rescue breathing. This procedure is known as **cardiopulmonary resuscitation (CPR)**. External chest compressions require a smooth application of pressure over the lower half of the sternum. External pressure applied to the sternum causes pressure in the chest (intrathoracic) to increase, thus producing blood movement to the brain. Compressions must not be sharp or jabbing or applied over the tip of the sternum (xiphoid process). Proper hand position and placement on the victim's chest are necessary to avoid internal injury such as bruising of the heart, laceration of the liver, or rupture of the spleen.

Blood flow in the carotid arteries as a result of external chest compressions is only one-fourth to one-third the normal flow, but it is adequate until advanced life support can be given. Because the blood circulates oxygen, chest compressions must be accompanied by rescue breathing.

Follow these steps to accomplish effective chest compression:

1. Place the victim on his or her back on a firm, level surface. The lower extremities may be raised to promote the return of venous blood.

2. Locate the lower part of the victim's sternum by sliding your middle and index fingers along the margin of the victim's rib cage until the notch is located in the center of the lower chest where the ribs and the sternum meet. Keep the middle finger on the center of the notch and place your index finger on the lower end of the victim's sternum, next to your middle finger.

3. Place the heel of your hand nearest the victim's head next to your index finger. Place the heel of the other hand on the back of the first hand. Your fingers should be pointing away from you. Interlock or extend your fingers but keep them off the victim's chest wall to avoid rib fractures and other internal injuries. The heel of the hand that is in direct contact with the sternum must remain in contact with the chest during both the compression and the release to prevent bouncing or jerking movements. If you have arthritic hands or wrists, grasp the wrist of the hand touching the sternum, instead of placing one hand on top of the other.

4. Lean forward so your shoulders are directly over your hands. Keeping your arms straight, press straight downward on the sternum 1½ to 2 inches, using the weight of the upper part of your body, then relax pressure on the sternum completely. The pressure and relaxation phases of each chest compression should be of equal duration; do not pause between each phase. Be sure to give each compression straight downward. Pushing at an angle is less effective and creates pressure over the ends of the ribs where they attach to the sternum, resulting in injury to the victim.

5. Give 15 chest compressions at a rate slightly faster than one every second. Perform each series of 15 compressions while counting aloud, "One and, two and, three and, four and, five and, six and, seven and, eight and, nine and, ten and, eleven and, twelve and, thirteen and, fourteen and, fifteen and," to achieve the rate of 80 to 100 compressions per minute.

6. After 15 compressions, immediately give two slow breaths (take a breath between them).

Basic Life Support Procedures and Techniques

Adult and Child Rescue Breathing and CPR

If you see a motionless person . . .

1

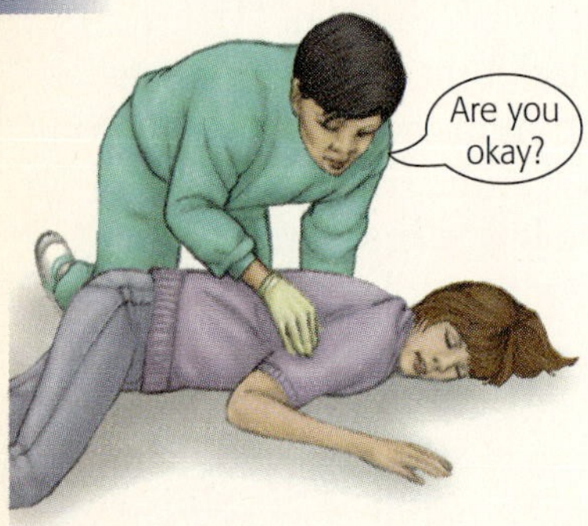

Are you okay?

Check responsiveness
- If spine injury is suspected, move victim only if absolutely necessary.
- Tap victim's shoulder.
- Shout near victim's ear, "Are you okay?"

2

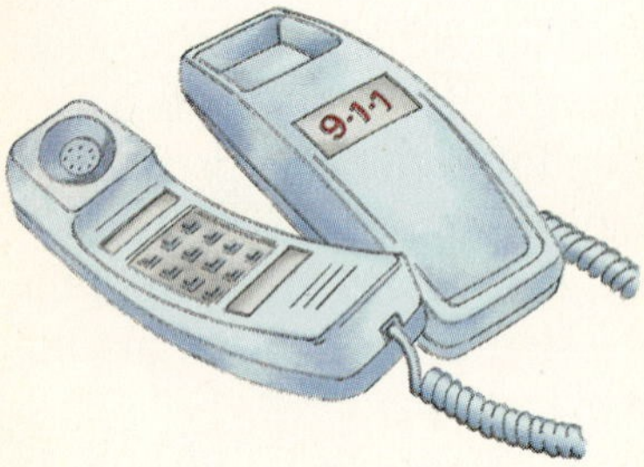

9-1-1

Activate the EMS for help
- Ask a bystander to call the local emergency telephone number, usually 911.
- If you are alone, shout for help. If no one comes quickly, call the local emergency telephone number. If someone does come quickly, ask him or her to call.

For a child (1–8 years)
- If you are alone, call the EMS after 1 minute of resuscitation unless a nearby bystander can be sent.

3

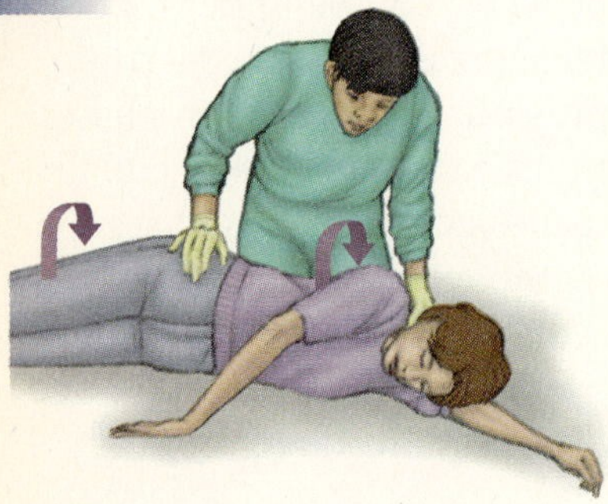

Roll person onto back
- Gently roll victim's head, body, and legs over at the same time. Do this without further injuring the victim.

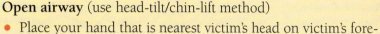

4

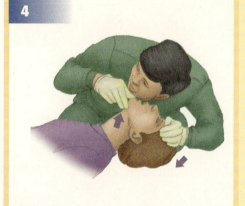

Open airway (use head-tilt/chin-lift method)

- Place your hand that is nearest victim's head on victim's forehead and apply backward pressure to tilt head back.
- Place fingers of your other hand under bony part of jaw near chin and lift. Avoid pressing on soft tissues under jaw.
- Tilt head backward without closing victim's mouth.
- Do *not* use your thumb to lift the chin.

If you suspect a spine injury

Do *not* move victim's head or neck. First try lifting chin without tilting head back. If breaths do not go in, slowly and gently bend the head back until breaths go in.

5

Check for breathing (take 3–5 seconds)

- Place your ear over victim's mouth and nose while keeping airway open.
- *Look* at victim's chest to check for rise and fall; *listen* and *feel* for breathing.

6

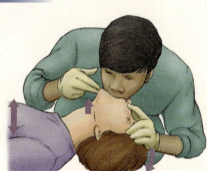

Give 2 slow breaths

- Keep head tilted back with head-tilt/chin-lift to keep airway open.
- Pinch nose shut.
- Take a deep breath and seal your lips tightly around victim's mouth.
- Give 2 slow breaths, each lasting 1½ to 2 seconds (you should take a breath after each breath given to victim).
- Watch chest rise to see if your breaths go in.
- Allow for chest deflation after each breath.

If first breath did not go in

Retilt the head and try another breath. If second breath is unsuccessful, suspect choking, also known as foreign body airway obstruction (use *Unconscious Adult and Child Foreign Body Airway Obstruction* procedures, described later in this chapter).

7

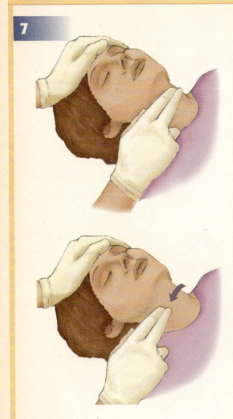

Check for pulse (take 5–10 seconds)

- Maintain head tilt with your hand nearest the victim's head on forehead.
- Locate Adam's apple with 2 or 3 fingers of hand nearer victim's feet.
- Slide your fingers down into groove of neck on side closest to you (do not use your thumb because you may feel your own pulse).
- Feel for carotid pulse (take 5–10 seconds). Carotid artery is used because it lies close to the heart and is accessible.

8

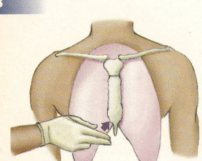

Perform rescue procedures based on what you found:

If there is a pulse but no breathing

Give one rescue breath every 5 to 6 seconds. Use the same techniques for rescue breathing given in Step 6 but give only one. Every minute (10 to 12 breaths) stop and check the pulse to make sure there is a pulse. For a child: give 1 breath every 3 seconds lasting 1 to 1½ seconds. Check the pulse every 20 breaths. Continue until:

- Victim starts breathing on his or her own.

OR

- Trained help, such as emergency medical technicians (EMTs), arrives and relieves you.

OR

- You are completely exhausted.

If there is no pulse, give CPR

- Find hand position:

    1. Slide the fingers of your hand nearest the victim's feet up rib cage edge nearer to you to notch at the end of sternum.

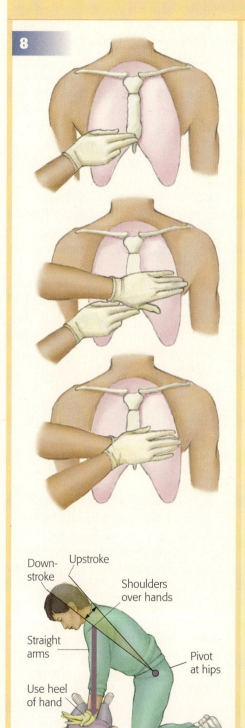

Downstroke
Upstroke
Shoulders over hands
Straight arms
Pivot at hips
Use heel of hand

2. Place your middle finger on or in the notch and the index finger next to it.

3. Put heel of other hand (one closer to victim's head) on sternum next to index finger.

4. Remove hand from notch and put it on top of hand on chest.

5. Interlace, hold, or extend fingers up.

- Do 15 compressions.

1. Place your shoulders directly over your hands on the chest.

2. Keep arms straight and elbows locked.

3. Push sternum straight down 1½ to 2 inches.

4. Do 15 compressions at a rate of 80 per minute. Count as you push down: "One and, two and, three and, four and, five and, six and, seven and, . . . , fifteen and."

5. Push smoothly; do not jerk or jab; do not stop at the top or at the bottom of the compression action.

6. When pushing, bend from your hips, not knees.

7. Keep fingers pointing across victim's chest, away from you.

- Give 2 slow breaths.

- Complete 3 more cycles of 15 compressions and 2 breaths (takes about 1 minute), then check the pulse. *If there is no pulse,* restart CPR with chest compressions. Recheck the pulse every few minutes. *If there is a pulse,* give rescue breathing.

- Continue CPR until:

  Victim revives.

OR

  Trained help, such as emergency medical technicians (EMTs), arrives and relieves you.

OR

  You are completely exhausted.

For a child

- Compress sternum with 1 hand with other hand on child's forehead.

- Compression rate to 100 times per minute. Count as you push down, "one, two, three, four, five."

- Compress 1 to 1½ inches.

- Give 1 breath after every 5 chest compressions.

After the two breaths, quickly reassess your hand location and position, then begin another cycle of 15 compressions and two breaths.

7. After you have completed four cycles (which should take about one minute), check the victim's pulse. If you cannot feel a pulse, continue CPR starting with 15 compressions. Check the pulse every few minutes.

Two-Rescuer CPR

CPR given by two rescuers (training usually reserved for professional rescuers and other health care providers) is more advantageous than one-rescuer CPR for the following reasons:

■ It increases the frequency of rescue breaths per minute (from 8 to 12).
■ It is less fatiguing to the rescuers and provides more effective resuscitation.

■ It allows one of the rescuers to evaluate the chest compressions by checking for a pulse.

In two-rescuer CPR, the compression rate is 80 to 100 times per minute, which is sufficient to maintain adequate blood flow. The ratio of compressions to breathing in two-rescuer CPR is 5 to 1. Preferably, the two rescuers should work on opposite sides of the victim so that if they later decide to switch functions, they can do so smoothly and without interfering with each other.

A second rescuer should tell the first rescuer that he or she can help, has activated the EMS, and has had CPR training. Then, while the first rescuer is giving chest compressions, the second rescuer checks for five seconds for a carotid pulse produced by each compression to evaluate the compressions being given.

The first rescuer completes the CPR cycle of 15 compressions and two breaths, then checks the victim's pulse. If there is no pulse, the first rescuer tells the second rescuer to begin chest compressions. The second rescuer gives five compressions, then pauses for the first rescuer to give one slow breath. Chest compressions are given at a rate of 80 to 100 per minute to the count of "one and, two and, three and, four and, five and." Counting out loud helps time the compressions and also lets the rescuer giving breaths know when to do so.

While the compressions are being given, the rescuer giving the breaths should frequently feel for the carotid pulse to check the effectiveness of the compressions.

Switching Functions

Two rescuers giving CPR should switch functions before one of them becomes fatigued. The switch should be done quickly with minimal interruption of CPR. The rescuer giving chest compressions initiates the switch by saying aloud, "Change and, two and, three and, four and, five and." Immediately following completion of the fifth compression, the other rescuer breathes into the victim once, then moves to the victim's chest. The rescuer who was compressing the chest moves to the victim's head and checks the pulse for five seconds. If the pulse is absent, that rescuer says aloud, "No pulse." The other rescuer then gives five more compressions. If a pulse is found during the check, the rescuer who found the pulse says aloud, "There is a pulse—I'll give rescue breathing," and begins rescue breathing at a rate of one breath every five seconds, or 12 times per minute.

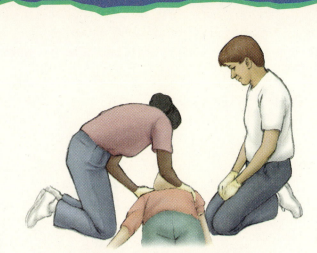

1. First rescuer checks responsiveness.

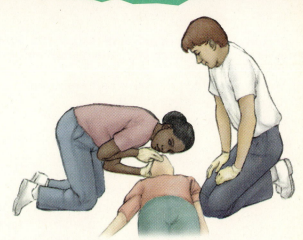

2. First rescuer opens airway and checks breathing.

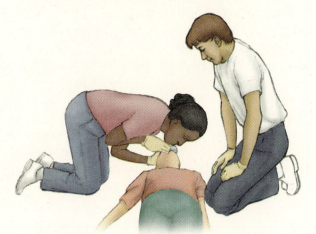

3. First rescuer gives 2 slow breaths.

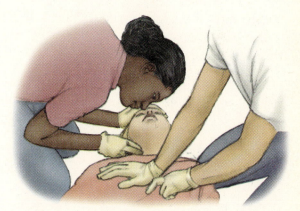

4. First rescuer checks pulse. Second rescuer locates proper hand placement.

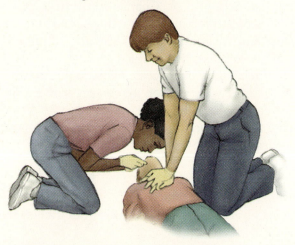

5. Second rescuer gives 5 chest compressions.

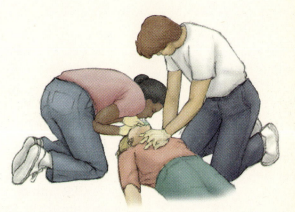

6. First rescuer gives 1 slow breath. Two rescuers repeat cycles of CPR.

After about 1 minute of CPR and then every few minutes thereafter, the first rescuer checks pulse. If there is still no pulse, both rescuers continue CPR, beginning with compressions.

Two-Rescuer CPR Procedures

(Laypersons should learn only one-rescuer CPR. Professional rescuers such as EMTs and other health care professionals should learn both one-rescuer and two-rescuer CPR.)

Entry of second rescuer when one-person CPR is in progress	#1 is performing one-rescuer CPR
	#2 says:
	   • "I know CPR."
	   • "EMS has been activated."
	   • "Can I help?"
	#1 • completes CPR cycle (15 compressions and ends on 2 breaths)
	   • says, "Take over compressions."
	   • checks pulse and breathing (5 seconds)
	   • if pulse absent, says, "No pulse, continue CPR."
	#2 • gives 5 compressions (at rate of 80–100 per minute)
	   • after every 5th compression, pauses for #1 rescuer to give 1 full breath
	#1 • monitors victim while #2 performs compressions:
	     (a) watches chest rise during breaths
	     (b) feels carotid pulse during compressions
	   • gives 1 full breath after every 5th compression given by #2 rescuer

Two rescuers starting CPR at the same time	#1 (ventilator) • assesses victim; if no breaths, gives 2 slow breaths; if no pulse, tells #2 to start compressions
	                 • gives 1 full breath after every 5th compression given by #2
	#2 (compressor) • finds hand position and gets ready to give compressions
	                 • gives 5 compressions after #1 says to start them
	                 • pauses after every 5th compression for #1 to give 1 full breath

Switching during two-rescuer CPR	#2 (compressor) • signals when to change by saying, "Change and, two and, three and, four and, five" or "Change on the next breath."
	                 • after #1 gives breath, #2 moves to victim's head and completes pulse and breathing check (5 seconds); if pulse is absent, says, "No pulse, begin CPR."
	                 • gives a full breath after every cycle of 5 compressions
	#1 (ventilator) • gives 1 full breath at the end of 5th compression and moves to victim's chest
	                 • finds hand position and gets ready to give compressions
	                 • begins cycles of 5 compressions after every breath

How an untrained rescuer can help	• goes for help • monitors pulse and breathing, with some direction • gives CPR with directions (can learn compressions easier with trained rescuer giving breaths)

Airway Obstruction (Choking) —Adult

Recognizing Choking

Choking victims vary as to whether the victim (1) is conscious and has a partial airway obstruction, (2) is conscious and has a complete airway obstruction, (3) becomes unconscious as a result of complete airway obstruction, or (4) is found unconscious with complete airway obstruction.

A foreign body lodged in the airway may cause partial or complete airway obstruction. When a foreign body partially blocks the airway, either good or poor air exchange may result. When good air exchange is present, the victim is able to make forceful coughing efforts in an attempt to relieve the obstruction. The victim should be permitted and encouraged to cough. Sometimes, a good air exchange may progress to a poor air exchange.

A choking victim who has poor air exchange has weak and ineffective coughs, and breathing becomes more difficult. The skin, the fingernail beds, and the inside of the mouth may appear bluish-gray in color (indicating cyanosis). Each attempt to inhale is usually accompanied by a high-pitched noise. A partial airway obstruction with poor air ex-

Types of Upper Airway Obstruction

- *Tongue.* Unconsciousness produces relaxation of soft tissues, and the tongue can fall into the airway. "Swallowing one's tongue" is impossible, but the widespread belief that that can happen is explained by slippage of the relaxed tongue into the airway. The tongue is the most common cause of airway obstruction.
- *Foreign body.* The National Safety Council reports that 3,000 deaths occur in the United States each year because of foreign body airway obstruction. People, especially children, inhale all kinds of objects. Foods such as hot dogs, candy, peanuts, and grapes are major offenders because of their shapes and consistencies. Meat is the main cause of choking in adults. Balloons are the top cause of nonfood choking deaths in children, followed by balls, marbles, toys, and coins. Unconscious victims' airways also can be obstructed by a foreign body (e.g., vomit, teeth).
- *Swelling.* Severe allergic reactions (anaphylaxis) and irritants (e.g., smoke, chemicals) can cause swelling. Even a nonallergic person who is stung inside the throat by a bee, yellow jacket, or flying insect can experience swelling in the airway.
- *Spasm.* Water that is suddenly inhaled can cause a spasm in the throat. This happens in about 10 percent of all drownings. When such a spasm does not allow the lungs to fill with water, it is known as a "dry drowning."
- *Vomit.* Most people vomit when they are at or near death. Therefore, always expect vomit during CPR.

Causes of Choking

There are many reasons why people choke on objects, including:

- They try to swallow large pieces of food.
- Drunkenness contributes to choking for several reasons:
  - Alcohol can deaden sensations in the mouth and interfere with swallowing.
  - An excessive amount of alcohol can affect one's judgment as to proper chewing and swallowing of food.
  - Before-dinner drinking extends the start of eating, so the hungry eater may attempt to swallow large chunks of food without proper chewing.
- Loose dentures (false teeth) inhibit the proper chewing of food.
- Eating too fast.
- Eating while talking or laughing.
- Walking, running, or playing with objects in the mouth.

change should be treated as if it were a complete airway blockage.

Complete airway obstruction in a conscious victim commonly occurs when the victim has been eating. The victim is unable to speak, breathe, or cough. When asked, "Can you speak?" the victim is unable to respond verbally. Choking victims with complete foreign body obstruction of the airway may instinctively reach up and clutch their necks to communicate that they are choking. This motion is known as the distress signal for choking. The victim becomes panicked and desperate and may appear pale in color. Because a complete obstruction prevents air from entering the lungs, oxygen deprivation occurs within a few minutes.

Abdominal Thrusts

Giving abdominal thrusts to a choking victim can dislodge the foreign body from the airway. To give abdominal thrusts to a choking victim who is sitting or standing, position yourself behind the victim. Place your arms around the victim's waist and form a fist with one hand. Place the thumb side of the fist with the knuckles up against the victim's abdomen slightly above the navel. With your other hand, grasp and hold your fist, then give up to five quick upward and inward thrusts to the victim's abdomen. If the victim is sitting in a chair, you probably will have to turn the victim, since reaching around the victim and the back of the chair usually is not practical.

To give abdominal thrusts to a victim who is lying down, kneel and straddle the victim's thighs. Place the heel of one hand against the victim's abdomen slightly above the navel. Place the other hand over the first hand. Point the fingers of the bottom hand toward the victim's head. Then give five quick inward, upward thrusts. Use this method, too, if you are unable to reach around the waist of a conscious victim.

A conscious choking victim who is alone can self-administer abdominal thrusts. The victim places the thumb side of a closed fist in the same position described above, covers the first with the other hand, then gives inward, upward thrusts. Also, if a firm object such as a chair or table is available, the victim can lean over the back of the chair or a corner of the table, pressing the abdomen upward and inward.

If the choking victim is extremely obese or in an advanced stage of pregnancy, give chest thrusts. Position yourself behind the victim and place the thumb side of a fist on the middle of the victim's sternum. Then thrust straight back for five thrusts. If the pregnant or obese victim is lying down, kneel at the victim's side and position your hands the same as for external chest compressions.

Finger Sweep of the Mouth

Use this maneuver only for an unconscious choking victim. First, open the victim's mouth by means of the tongue-jaw lift. With the victim's head up, place your thumb in the victim's mouth over the tongue. Then grasp the victim's tongue and lower jaw between your thumb and fingers and lift upward.

If you are unable to open the victim's mouth, use the crossed-finger technique. To perform that maneuver, cross your index finger and thumb and use them as a wedge to push the victim's teeth apart. Once the mouth is opened, insert a thumb for the tongue-jaw lift.

While keeping the victim's mouth open with the tongue-jaw lift, use the index finger of your other hand to sweep down along the inside of one cheek. This finger should probe deeply into the throat to the base of the tongue. Using a hooking action, try to dislodge the foreign body and maneuver it so it can be removed. Be careful not to force the object deeper into the airway.

Conscious Choking Victims

First determine if the victim has good or poor air exchange. A victim with good air exchange is able to speak, cough forcefully, and make effective breathing efforts. Encourage such a victim to cough; do not interfere with the victim's efforts to expel the object.

For a conscious victim with a partial airway obstruction who has poor air exchange, help the victim as for a complete obstruction. Poor air exchange is marked by ineffective, weak coughing, high-pitched noise, breathing difficulty, possible cyanosis, and inability to speak. To assist these victims:

1. Ask, "Can you speak?"
2. If the victim is unable to speak, give five abdominal thrusts (chest thrusts for extremely obese or pregnant victims).
3. Assess the victim and your technique.
4. Repeat the sequence of five thrusts and a reassessment until the airway is clear or the victim becomes unconscious.

Unconscious Choking Victims

To help an unconscious choking victim:

1. Determine the victim's responsiveness.
2. Call for help—either send someone or call yourself.
3. Open the victim's airway using the head-tilt/chin-lift method.
4. Determine if the victim is breathing by looking at the chest and listening for air coming out of the mouth and nose.
5. Give two slow breaths. If the first breath does not go in, retilt the victim's head and try a second breath. *The breaths not going in indicates choking.*

Conscious Adult and Child Foreign Body Airway Obstruction (Choking)

If person is conscious and cannot speak, breathe, or cough . . .

1

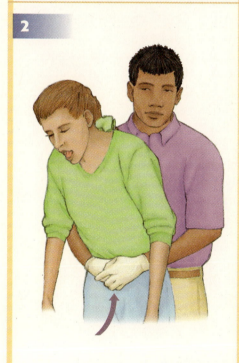

Give up to 5 abdominal thrusts (Heimlich maneuver)
- Stand behind the victim.
- Wrap your arms around victim's waist. (Do not allow your forearms to touch the ribs.)
- Make a fist with 1 hand and place the thumb side just above the victim's navel and well below the tip of the sternum.
- Grasp fist with your other hand.
- Press fist into victim's abdomen with 5 quick upward thrusts.
- Each thrust should be a separate and distinct effort to dislodge the object.

After every 5 abdominal thrusts, check the victim and your technique.

Note: If the victim is obese or in an advanced stage of pregnancy, consider using chest thrusts.

2

Repeat cycles of up to 5 abdominal thrusts until
- Victim coughs up object.

OR

- Victim starts to breathe or coughs forcefully.

OR

- Victim becomes unconscious (activate EMS and start methods for an unconscious victim with a finger sweep first).

OR

- You are relieved by EMS or other trained person. Reassess victim and your technique after every 5 thrusts.

If person is unconscious and breaths have not gone in . . .

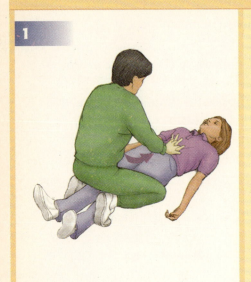

1

Give up to 5 abdominal thrusts (Heimlich maneuver)

- Straddle victim's thighs.
- Put heel of one hand against middle of victim's abdomen slightly above navel and well below sternum's notch (fingers of hand should point toward victim's head).
- Put other hand directly on top of first hand.
- Press inward and upward using both hands with up to 5 quick abdominal thrusts.
- Each thrust should be a separate and distinct effort to relieve the airway obstruction. Keep heel of hand in contact with abdomen between abdominal thrusts.

Note: If the victim is obese or in an advanced stage of pregnancy, consider using chest thrusts.

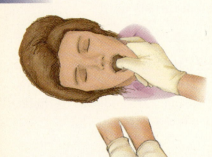

2

Perform finger sweep

- Use only on an unconscious victim. On a conscious victim, it may cause gagging or vomiting.
- Use your thumb and fingers to grasp victim's jaw and tongue and lift upward to pull tongue away from back of throat and away from foreign object.
- If you are unable to open mouth to perform the tongue-jaw lift, use the crossed-finger method by crossing the index finger and thumb and pushing the teeth apart.
- With index finger of your other hand, slide finger down along the inside of one cheek deeply into mouth and use a hooking action across to other cheek to dislodge foreign object.
- If foreign body comes within reach, grab and remove it. Do not force object deeper

For a child: Use finger sweep only if foreign object is seen.

3

If Steps 1 and 2 are unsuccessful

Cycle through the following steps in rapid sequence until the object is expelled or EMS arrives:

- Give 1 rescue breath.
- Do up to 5 abdominal thrusts.
- Do a finger sweep

S = self-check / P = partner check / I = instructor check

Adult Rescue Breathing

	S	P	I
1. Check responsiveness.	☐	☐	☐
2. Activate EMS.	☐	☐	☐
3. Roll victim onto back.	☐	☐	☐
4. Airway open.	☐	☐	☐
5. Breathing check.	☐	☐	☐
6. 2 slow breaths.	☐	☐	☐
7. Check pulse at carotid.	☐	☐	☐
8. Rescue breathing (1 every 5–6 seconds).	☐	☐	☐
9. Recheck pulse and breathing after first minute, then every few minutes.	☐	☐	☐

Adult One-Rescuer CPR

	S	P	I
1. Check responsiveness.	☐	☐	☐
2. Activate EMS.	☐	☐	☐
3. Roll victim onto back.	☐	☐	☐
4. Airway open.	☐	☐	☐
5. Breathing check.	☐	☐	☐
6. 2 slow breaths.	☐	☐	☐
7. Check pulse at carotid.	☐	☐	☐
8. Hand position.	☐	☐	☐
9. 15 compressions.	☐	☐	☐
10. 2 slow breaths.	☐	☐	☐
11. Continue CPR (3 more cycles, for total of 4).	☐	☐	☐
12. Recheck pulse.	☐	☐	☐
13. Continue CPR (start with compressions).	☐	☐	☐
14. Recheck pulse after first minute, then every few minutes.	☐	☐	☐

Conscious Adult Choking Management

	S	P	I
1. Recognize choking.	☐	☐	☐
2. Up to 5 abdominal thrusts.	☐	☐	☐
3. Reassess.	☐	☐	☐
4. Repeat cycles of up to 5 thrusts; reassess after each cycle.	☐	☐	☐

Unconscious Adult Choking Management

	S	P	I
1. Check responsiveness.	☐	☐	☐
2. Activate EMS.	☐	☐	☐
3. Roll victim onto back.	☐	☐	☐
4. Airway open.	☐	☐	☐
5. Breathing check.	☐	☐	☐
6. Try 2 slow breaths. (If first breath unsuccessful, retilt head and try 1 more breath.)	☐	☐	☐
7. Up to 5 abdominal thrusts.	☐	☐	☐
8. Finger sweep.	☐	☐	☐
9. Try 1 slow breath.	☐	☐	☐
10. Repeat sequence of 5 thrusts, sweep, 1 breath.	☐	☐	☐

Basic Life Support Steps for Adult Victims

R: Responsiveness of victim?
A: Activate EMS (usually call 911).
P: Position victim on back.

A: Airway open. Use head-tilt/chin-lift or jaw thrust.
B: Breathing check. Look, listen, and feel for 3–5 seconds.
- If victim is breathing and spine injury is not suspected, place victim in recovery position.
- If victim is not breathing, give 2 slow breaths; watch chest rise.
  - If 2 breaths go in, proceed to step C.
  - If first breath did not go in, retilt head and try 1 more breath.
  - If second breath did not go in, give 5 abdominal thrusts; perform tongue-jaw lift followed by a finger sweep; give 1 breath. Repeat sequence of 5 thrusts, sweep, 1 breath.

C: Circulation check (at carotid pulse for 5–10 seconds).
- If there is a pulse but no breathing, give rescue breathing (1 breath every 5–6 seconds).
- If there is no pulse, give CPR (cycles of 15 chest compressions followed by 2 breaths).

After 1 minute (4 cycles of CPR or 10–12 breaths of rescue breathing), check pulse.
- If no pulse, give CPR (cycles of 15 compressions and 2 breaths) starting with chest compressions.
- If there is a pulse but no breathing, give rescue breathing.

6. Give five abdominal thrusts.

7. Using one hand, open the victim's mouth with the tongue-jaw lift. With the index finger of the other hand, finger sweep the mouth and remove any reachable foreign body.

8. Reposition the victim in a head-tilt/chin-lift position and give one breath.

9. If unsuccessful, repeat the sequence of five thrusts, finger sweep, one breath until the airway is clear or until the victim becomes conscious.

Basic Life Support Steps for a Child or Infant Victim

E: Establish unresponsiveness.
S: Send bystander, if available, to activate EMS (usually call 911).
P: Position victim on back.

A: Airway open. Use head-tilt/chin-lift or jaw thrust.
B: Breathing check. Look, listen, and feel for 3–5 seconds.
- If victim is breathing and spine injury is not suspected, place victim in recovery position.
- If victim is not breathing, give 2 slow breaths; watch chest rise.
  - If 2 breaths go in, proceed to step C.
  - If first breath did not go in, retilt head and try 1 more breath.
  - If second breath did not go in, then . . .
  For a child: Give 5 abdominal thrusts; perform tongue-jaw lift and if object is seen perform a finger sweep; give 1 breath. Repeat sequence of 5 thrusts, mouth check, 1 breath.
  For an infant: Give 5 back blows and 5 chest thrusts; perform tongue-jaw lift and if object is seen perform a finger sweep; give 1 breath. Repeat sequence of 5 blows, 5 thrusts, mouth check, 1 breath.

C: Circulation check (for 5–10 seconds).
- *For a child:* Check carotid pulse.
- *For an infant:* Check brachial pulse.
- If there is a pulse but no breathing, give rescue breathing (1 breath every 3 seconds).
- If no pulse, give CPR (cycles of 5 chest compressions followed by 1 breath).

After 1 minute (20 cycles of CPR or 20 breaths of rescue breathing), check pulse.
- If you are alone, activate EMS.
- If there is no pulse, give CPR (cycles of 5 compressions and 1 breath) starting with chest compressions.
- If there is a pulse but no breathing, give rescue breathing.

Differences between Adult and Child (1–8 years) Basic Life Support

IF child . . .	THEN . . .
is *not* responsive and rescuer is alone	if alone, **activate EMS after 1 minute of resuscitation** (in adults, activate EMS immediately after determining unresponsiveness).
is *not* breathing but has a pulse	• give **1- to 1½-second breaths** (in adults give 1½- to 2-second breaths). • give **1 breath every 3 seconds** (in adults give 1 breath every 5 to 6 seconds).
does *not* have a pulse	• after locating the tip of the breastbone, lift your fingers off and put heel of the **same hand** on breastbone immediately above where index finger was (adult requires one hand to locate and the other hand placed next to it). • give **chest compressions with 1 hand** (nearest feet) while keeping other hand on child's forehead (adult requires 2 hands on victim's chest for compressions). • **compress breastbone 1 to 1½ inches** (adults require 1½ to 2 inches). • **compression rate is 100 times per minute;** with breaths, it becomes about 80 compressions per minute (adult rate is 80–100 per minute). • give **one breath after every 5 chest compressions** (one-rescuer adult CPR requires 2 breaths after every 15 compressions).
has a foreign body airway obstruction (choking), and after up to 5 abdominal thrusts (Heimlich maneuver), the airway still remains obstructed	look into mouth; **if foreign body is visible, use finger sweep to remove it—do not perform blind finger sweeps** (in an adult, you can perform blind finger sweeps).

Child Basic Life Support Proficiency Checklist

S = self-check / P = partner check / I = instructor check

Child Rescue Breathing

	S	P	I
1. Check responsiveness.	☐	☐	☐
2. Send a bystander, if available, to call EMS.	☐	☐	☐
3. Roll victim onto back.	☐	☐	☐
4. **A**irway open.	☐	☐	☐
5. **B**reathing check.	☐	☐	☐
6. 2 slow breaths.	☐	☐	☐
7. **C**heck pulse at carotid.	☐	☐	☐
8. Rescue breathing (1 every 3 seconds).	☐	☐	☐
9. If alone, call EMS after 1 minute.	☐	☐	☐
10. Recheck pulse and breathing after first minute, then every few minutes.	☐	☐	☐

Child One-Rescuer CPR

	S	P	I
1. Check responsiveness.	☐	☐	☐
2. Send a bystander, if available, to call EMS.	☐	☐	☐
3. Roll victim onto back.	☐	☐	☐
4. **A**irway open.	☐	☐	☐
5. **B**reathing check.	☐	☐	☐
6. 2 slow breaths.	☐	☐	☐
7. **C**heck pulse at carotid.	☐	☐	☐
8. Hand position using same hand used to locate tip of sternum.	☐	☐	☐
9. 5 compressions with only 1 hand.	☐	☐	☐
10. 1 slow breath.	☐	☐	☐
11. Continue CPR for 1 minute (19 more cycles, for total of 20).	☐	☐	☐

	S	P	I
12. If alone, call EMS after 1 minute.	☐	☐	☐
13. Recheck pulse.	☐	☐	☐
14. Continue CPR (start with compressions).	☐	☐	☐
15. Recheck pulse after first minute, then every few minutes.	☐	☐	☐

Conscious Child Choking Management

	S	P	I
1. Recognize choking.	☐	☐	☐
2. Up to 5 abdominal thrusts.	☐	☐	☐
3. Reassess.	☐	☐	☐
4. Repeat cycles of up to 5 thrusts; reassess after each cycle.	☐	☐	☐

Unconscious Child Choking Management

	S	P	I
1. Check responsiveness.	☐	☐	☐
2. Send a bystander, if available, to call EMS.	☐	☐	☐
3. Roll victim onto back.	☐	☐	☐
4. **A**irway open.	☐	☐	☐
5. **B**reathing check.	☐	☐	☐
6. Try 2 slow breaths. (If first breath unsuccessful, retilt head and try 1 more breath.)	☐	☐	☐
7. Up to 5 abdominal thrusts.	☐	☐	☐
8. Check mouth for foreign object (finger sweep only if object is visible).	☐	☐	☐
9. Try 1 slow breath.	☐	☐	☐
10. Repeat sequence of 5 thrusts, mouth check, 1 breath.	☐	☐	☐

Infant Basic Life Support

Basic life support techniques for an infant differ from those for an adult or child. Initially occurring cardiac arrest in infants is rare. Usually, infants have a respiratory arrest with cardiac arrest developing later because the heart muscle did not receive sufficient oxygen.

Infant Rescue Breathing and CPR

Check Responsiveness

The first priority in a cardiopulmonary emergency is to determine the victim's responsiveness. This is done by tapping the victim and speaking loudly. If basic life support is necessary, give resuscitation for one minute before activating the EMS. The rescuer should shout for help if alone.

Positioning an Unresponsive Infant

Properly position the victim so that if any resuscitation efforts are needed, they can be performed. If the victim is found lying facedown, turn the infant as a complete unit onto his or her back. The victim's head and neck should always be supported with one of your hands so that they remain aligned with the rest of the body and do not twist.

Opening the Airway

After unresponsiveness has been determined and the victim has been properly positioned, open the victim's airway by using the head-tilt/chin-lift method. To do this, place one hand to apply pressure on the victim's forehead to gently tilt the head backward. Do not overtilt the head backward because it can block the airway because of the pliability of the infant's tissues. To lift the chin, place the finger(s) of your other hand under the bony part of the jaw. Then lift your fingers to bring the chin up. The fingers should not press on the soft tissue under the victim's chin because it can interfere with the opening of the airway. While the chin is lifted, the hand on the forehead maintains the head-tilt position of the victim. Sometimes, opening the airway may be all that is necessary for the victim to breathe.

When a spine injury is suspected, open the airway using the chin-lift without tilting the head back. If the airway remains blocked, tilt the head slowly and gently until the airway is open. Another technique for a suspected spine-injured victim is using a jaw thrust without a head tilt. While stabi-lizing the head, place the fingers of each hand behind the angles of the victim's lower jaw on each side of the head and move the lower jaw forward without tilting the head backward; however, it may be necessary to tilt the head slightly if the airway cannot be opened.

Check for Breathing

After unresponsiveness has been determined and the airway has been opened, you should look, listen, and feel for breathing. You should (1) look to see whether there is any visible movement of the victim's chest, (2) listen for air by placing your ear next to the victim's mouth and nose, and (3) feel for air by placing your cheek next to the victim's mouth and nose. If breathing is present, you will see the victim's chest rise and fall, hear air coming from the victim's mouth and nose, and feel air against your own cheek.

Rescue Breathing

To give rescue breaths to an infant, place your mouth over the infant's nose and mouth, forming an airtight seal. Give two slow breaths, taking time to quickly breathe between them.

If both breaths went into the infant, check the victim's pulse. If the first breath did not go in, retilt the infant's head and try a second breath.

The breaths for an infant should be limited to the amount needed to raise the victim's chest. For infants, use shallow puffs of air.

To perform rescue breathing for an infant, follow these steps:

1. Make sure the victim's head is positioned with a moderate head-tilt/chin-lift to open the airway.
2. Form an airtight seal over the victim's nose and mouth.
3. Give two breaths using shallow puffs of air.
4. Watch to see if the victim's chest rises.
5. Remove your mouth to allow the air to come out and move your head away as you take another breath.

If the first breath did not go in, retilt the victim's head and try a second breath. If breaths do not go in, see the section on unconscious choking management on page 101.

If the breaths went in and the victim has a pulse, continue giving rescue breathing. Because infants breathe faster than adults, breathe into an infant once every three seconds or 20 times a minute. Between breaths, remove your mouth from

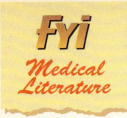

Facts about Sudden Infant Death Syndrome (SIDS) Many more children die of SIDS in a year than all who die of cancer, heart disease, pneumonia, child abuse, AIDS, cystic fibrosis, and muscular dystrophy combined . . .

What Is SIDS?

- Sudden Infant Death Syndrome (SIDS) is a medical term that describes the sudden death of an infant that remains unexplained after all known and possible causes have been carefully ruled out through autopsy, death scene investigation, and review of the medical history. SIDS is responsible for more deaths than any other cause in childhood for babies one month to one year of age, claiming 150,000 victims in the United States in this generation alone—7,000 babies each year—*nearly one baby every hour of every day*. It strikes families of all races, ethnic, and socioeconomic origins without warning; neither parent nor physician can predict that something is going wrong. In fact, most SIDS victims appear healthy prior to death.

What Causes SIDS?

- While there are still no adequate medical explanations for SIDS deaths, current theories include: (1) stress in a normal baby, caused by infection or other factors; (2) a birth defect; (3) failure to develop; and/or (4) a critical period when all babies are especially vulnerable, such as a time of rapid growth.

- Many new studies have been launched to learn how and why SIDS occurs. Scientists are exploring the development and function of the nervous system, the brain, the heart, breathing and sleep patterns, body chemical balances,

autopsy findings, and environmental factors. It is likely that SIDS, like many other medical disorders, will eventually have more than one explanation.

Can SIDS Be Prevented?

- No, not yet. But, some recent studies have begun to isolate several risk factors that, though not causes of SIDS in and of themselves, may play a role in some cases. (*It is important that, since the causes of SIDS remain unknown, SIDS parents refrain from concluding that their child care practices may have caused their baby's death.*)

Some Basic Facts about SIDS:

- SIDS is a definite medical entity and is the major cause of death in infants after the first month of life.
- SIDS claims the lives of over 7,000 American babies each year . . . *nearly one baby every hour of every day.*
- SIDS victims appear to be healthy prior to death.
- Currently, SIDS cannot be predicted or prevented, even by a physician.
- There appears to be no suffering; death occurs very rapidly, usually during sleep.

What SIDS Is Not:

- SIDS is **not** caused by external suffocation.
- SIDS is **not** caused by vomiting and choking.
- SIDS is **not** contagious.
- SIDS does **not** cause pain or suffering in the infant.
- SIDS can**not** be predicted.

Source: SIDS Network. Used with permission.

---

the victim's to allow air to flow out of the victim's lungs. As you remove your mouth, you should turn your head to the side to see if the victim's chest fell after each breath. For rescue breathing, breathe into the infant for the first second, count "one–one thousand," then take a breath yourself for the third second.

Gastric Distention Rescue breaths tend to cause stomach or gastric distention more often in infants than in adults. Minimize this problem by limiting the breaths to the amount needed to make the chest rise. Avoid overinflating the lungs. Gastric distention can cause regurgitation and aspiration of stomach contents.

Check for Pulse

After a nonbreathing infant has been given two breaths, the pulse must be checked. For an infant, the brachial pulse is used. An infant's neck is short and chubby, which makes it difficult to feel the carotid pulse. The brachial pulse can be found on the inside of the upper arm midway between the armpit and elbow. Feeling for the brachial pulse in an infant requires the use of the index and middle fingers of one hand. Place your thumb on the outside of the infant's arm midway between the shoulder and elbow. Place the tips of your index and middle fingers on the inside of the infant's arm opposite your thumb. The thumb is used to help with hand placement only, not to feel for the victim's pulse. Light pressure is applied toward the underlying bone to feel for the pulse. While checking the brachial pulse, keep your other hand on the infant's forehead to maintain the head-tilt position.

Should a pulse exist but breathing is absent, continue rescue breathing. A rescue breath is given once every three seconds or 20 times a minute. After 20 breaths, you should activate the EMS.

Chest Compressions

An infant without a pulse requires both rescue breathing and external chest compressions. The proper chest compression point in an infant is the midsternum. To locate this area, imagine a line connecting the infant's nipples. Place three fingers (index, middle, and ring) with the index finger next to the imaginary nipple line on the infant's feet side. Lift the index finger off the chest.

Use the two remaining fingers to apply the chest compressions. Press the infant's midsternum (area between the nipples) one-half to one inch into the chest with the middle and ring finger. Either place your other hand under the infant's shoulder to provide support or keep it on the infant's forehead to keep the head tilted. If the infant is carried during CPR, the length of the body is on the rescuer's forearm with the head kept level with the trunk.

An infant's heart rate is faster than an adult's and so the rate of compressions must also be faster. The infant compression rate is 100 per minute. External chest compressions must always be combined with rescue breathing. The ratio of compressions to breaths is 5 to 1. Each series of five compressions is performed while the rescuer says aloud "One, two, three, four, five." After the fifth

compression, the rescuer opens the victim's airway and gives one breath.

After the first minute of CPR, and if a second rescuer is not available, activate the EMS. Every few minutes feel the pulse.

The procedures for performing rescue breathing and external chest compressions on an infant are as follows:

1. Determine responsiveness by tapping the victim; if the infant is lying facedown, turn him or her onto their back.

2. Make sure the victim's head is positioned with a moderate head-tilt/chin-lift to open the airway.

3. Check for breathing.

4. If breathing is absent, form an airtight seal over the victim's nose and mouth, and give two slow breaths using shallow puffs of air; watch to see if the victim's chest rises. Remove your mouth to allow the air to come out and move your head away as you take another breath. If the first breath did not go in, retilt the victim's head and try a second breath. If breaths do not go in, see the section on unconscious choking management on page 101.

5. Check for a pulse at the brachial pulse point. If the breaths went in and the victim has a pulse, continue giving rescue breathing. Because infants breathe faster than adults, breathe into an infant once every three seconds or 20 times a minute. Between breaths, remove your mouth from the victim's to allow air to flow out of the victim's lungs. As you remove your mouth, turn your head to the side to see if the victim's chest fell after each breath. For rescue breathing, breathe into the infant for the first second, count "one–one thousand" for the second, then take a breath yourself for the third second.

6. If a pulse is absent, begin chest compressions.

7. After one minute of CPR, activate the EMS if another rescuer has not.

Airway Obstruction—Infant

People, especially children and infants, inhale all kinds of objects. Foods such as hot dogs, candy, peanuts, and grapes are major offenders because of their shape and consistencies. Non-food choking deaths are caused by balloons, balls and marbles, toys, and coins. Balloons are the top cause of non-food choking deaths in children.

If you see a motionless infant . . .

1

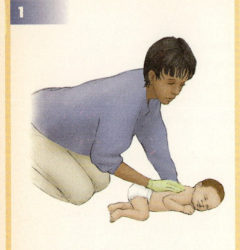

Check responsiveness
- If spine injury is suspected, move only if absolutely necessary.
- Tap infant's shoulder.

2

Send bystander, if available, to activate EMS. If you are alone, give rescue breathing or CPR for 1 minute before activating EMS.

3

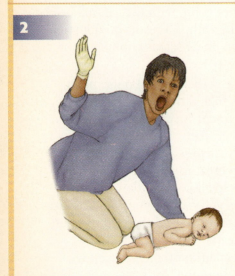

Roll infant onto back
Gently roll infant's head, body, and legs over at the same time (avoid twisting).

4

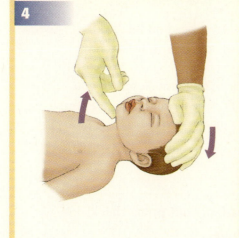

Open airway (use head-tilt/chin-lift method)

- Place your hand nearest infant's head on infant's forehead and apply backward pressure to tilt head back (known as the "sniffing" or neutral position).
- Place fingers of other hand under bony part of jaw near chin and lift. Avoid pressing on soft tissues under jaw.
- Tilt head backward without closing infant's mouth.
- Do not use your thumb to lift the chin.

If you suspect a spine injury

Do not move infant's head or neck. First try lifting chin without tilting head back. If breaths do not go in, slowly and gently bend the head back until breaths can go in.

5

Check for breathing (take 3–5 seconds)

- Place your ear over infant's mouth and nose while keeping airway open.
- Look at infant's chest to check for rise and fall; listen and feel for breathing.

6

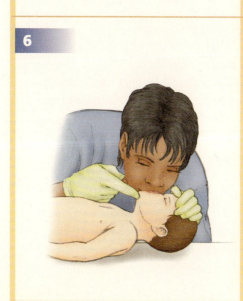

Give 2 slow breaths

- Keep head tilted back with head-tilt/chin-lift to keep airway open.
- With your mouth make a seal over infant's mouth and nose.
- Give 2 slow breaths, each lasting 1 to 1½ seconds (you should take a breath after each breath given).
- Watch chest rise to see if your breaths go in.
- Allow for chest deflation after each breath.

If first breath did not go in

Retilt the head and try another breath. If second breath is unsuccessful, suspect choking, also known as foreign body airway obstruction (refer to the section *Unconscious Infant with Foreign Body Airway Obstruction (Choking)*).

7

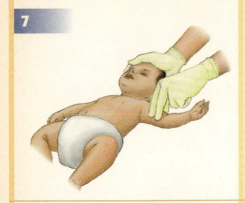

Check for pulse
- Maintain head tilt with hand nearest head on forehead.
- Feel for pulse on the inside of the upper arm between the elbow and armpit (the brachial).
- Press gently with 2 fingers on inside of arm closest to you.
- Place thumb of same hand on outside of infant's upper arm.

8

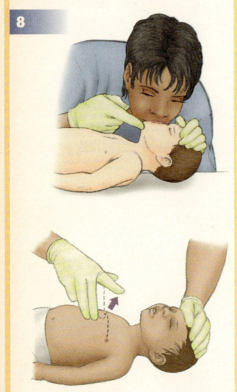

Perform rescue procedures based on your pulse check.

If there is a pulse but no breathing

Give rescue breaths every 3 seconds. Use the same techniques for rescue breathing given in Step 6 but give only one breath. If you are alone, activate the EMS after the first minute. Every minute (20 breaths), stop and check the pulse to make sure there is one. Continue until:

- Infant starts breathing on his or her own.

OR

- Trained help, such as emergency medical technicians (EMTs), arrives and relieves you.

OR

- You are completely exhausted.

If there is no pulse, give CPR

- Locate fingers' position.
  1. Maintain a head tilt.
  2. Imagine a line connecting the nipples.
  3. Place 3 fingers on sternum with index finger touching but below imaginary nipple line.
  4. Raise your index finger and use other 2 fingers for compression. If you feel the notch at the end of the sternum, move your fingers up a little.
- Give 5 compressions.
  1. Do 5 chest compressions at rate of 100 per minute. Count as you push down, "one, two, three, four, five."
  2. Press sternum ½ to 1 inch or about ⅓ to ½ of the depth of the chest.
  3. Keep fingers pointing across the infant's chest away from you. Keep fingers in contact with infant's chest.
  4. Maintain head tilt with hand nearest head on forehead.

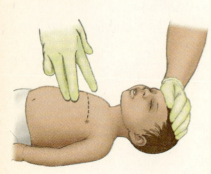

8

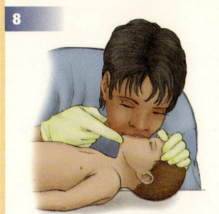

- Give 1 breath.
- Complete 20 cycles of 5 compressions and 1 breath (takes about 1 minute), then check the pulse. If you are alone, activate the EMS. If there is no pulse, restart CPR with chest compressions. Recheck the pulse every few minutes. If there is a pulse, give rescue breathing.
- Give CPR until:
  Infant revives.

OR

  Trained help, such as emergency medical technicians (EMTs), arrives and relieves you.

OR

  You are completely exhausted.

As discussed before, the airway may be partially or completely blocked. With a partial airway obstruction, an infant is able to make persistent coughing efforts that should not be hampered. If good air exchange becomes a poor exchange or poor air exchange occurs initially, the victim should be managed as having a complete airway obstruction. Poor air exchanges are indicated by ineffective coughing, high-pitched noises, breathing difficulty, and blueness of the lips and fingernail beds.

Unconscious Victim

Choking management of a completely obstructed airway in an unconscious infant consists of the combination of back blows and chest thrusts. Abdominal thrusts are not advisable for infants because of possible injury to the abdominal organs. Finger sweeps of the mouth in an unconscious infant should be done only if the object can be seen. Finger sweeps should not be done with any conscious victim.

Back Blows and Chest Thrusts

To perform back blows on an infant, straddle the victim facedown over your forearm. The infant's head should be lower than the trunk. Your hand should be around the jaw and neck of the infant giving support to the infant's head. For more support, rest your forearm under the infant on your thigh. Using the heel of the other hand, you are ready to give five rapid back blows between the infant's shoulder blades.

To give chest thrusts, turn the infant onto his or her back. After delivering the five back blows, immediately place your free hand on the back of the infant's head and neck while the other hand remains in place. Using both hands and forearms to sandwich the infant—one supporting the jaw, neck, and chest, and the other the back—turn the infant over. Once turned onto the back, the infant should be resting on your thigh. The infant's head should be lower than the trunk. With the infant positioned, give five chest thrusts in rapid succession. The thrusts are given to the sternum (between the nipples), using two fingers. The technique used to locate and perform chest thrusts is the same as that used to perform external chest compressions for CPR.

Finger Sweeps

As stated earlier, do not perform blind finger sweeps of an infant. However, if the foreign body is visible,

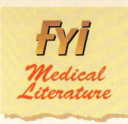

Balloons: Serious Choking Hazard for Children Ordinary balloons can be deadly if they are inhaled while inflated, partially inflated, or after bursting into fragments, according to a study of 449 children who died from choking on foreign objects. Balloons were responsible for more deaths than any other nonfood object. Balls and marbles were next on the hazard list. Balloons pose a greater threat than solid objects that are swallowed because balloons conform to the shape of the breathing passage and thus block it more completely.

Source: F. L. Rimell, et al., "Characteristics of Objects that Cause Choking in Children," *Journal of the American Medical Association.* 274:1763, December 13, 1995.

you should try to remove it, taking great care to avoid pushing it farther down into the airway.

The infant's mouth should be opened by means of the tongue-jaw lift. To perform the tongue-jaw lift, place your thumb in the victim's mouth over the tongue. Then grasp the victim's tongue and lower jaw between your thumb and fingers and lift them upward. If you can see a foreign body, sweep it out of the victim's mouth with your little finger.

Unconscious Choking Victim Management

To help an unconscious choking infant, you should:

- Determine responsiveness.
- Call out for help.
- Open the victim's airway—use the head-tilt/chin-lift method.
- Determine if the victim is breathing by looking at the chest and listening for air coming out of the mouth and nose.
- Give two slow breaths. If the first breath does not go in, retilt the infant's head and try a second breath. *The breaths not going in indicates choking.*
- Give five back blows with the infant facing downward and head below the trunk.
- Give chest thrusts with the infant facing upward and head below the trunk.
- Using one hand, open the victim's mouth with the tongue-jaw lift. If a foreign object is seen, use the little finger of the other hand to finger

sweep the mouth and remove any reachable foreign body.

- Reposition the victim in a head-tilt/chin-lift position and give one breath.
- If unsuccessful, repeat the following steps until the airway is clear or until the victim becomes conscious: five back blows, five chest thrusts, look for object and if seen use a finger sweep, one breath.

Conscious Victim

Help for a conscious infant also consists of the combined use of back blows and chest thrusts. These maneuvers are performed in the same manner as for an unconscious infant. They should be given when an infant has complete airway obstruction as evidenced by the inability to breathe, cough, or cry. No finger sweeps or rescue breaths should be attempted.

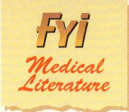

CPR Training and HIV

With concerns about the human immunodeficiency virus (HIV) and other infectious agents, many people are wondering whether disinfection procedures are adequate to prevent the transmission of diseases by way of manikins used for CPR training. A report suggests that even less-than-thorough disinfection with 70 percent isopropyl alcohol is enough to prevent the spread of the virus that causes AIDS. In fact, the study suggests that just wiping the manikin with a dry cloth may be sufficient.

Although there have been no cases to date of HIV transmitted by CPR manikins, the virus is found in saliva and can survive for a time on plastic material. And other diseases, such as herpes, have been contracted during CPR training. While the risk is minimal, it is important to ease fears about disease transmission if widespread CPR training nationwide is to be promoted.

The currently preferred method of disinfecting equipment is to use a bleach solution, with isopropyl alcohol available as an option. When isopropyl alcohol is used, it is supposed to be applied to the manikin for 60 seconds. To test the effectiveness of these agents, the researchers applied a concentrated dose of HIV-infected white blood cells—a much denser concentration than would be found in saliva—to the face mask of a CPR manikin. They then used alcohol to disinfect the manikin, but they disinfected for only 5 or 10 seconds. They also looked at the effects of simply wiping with a dry cloth. After each cleaning, the researchers checked the manikin to determine whether any infected white blood cells remained.

The study reported that even with sloppy cleaning, decontamination was effective. "Our data suggest that one should not refrain from CPR training out of fear of contracting HIV infection," the researchers concluded.

Source: I.B. Corless, A. Lisker, R.W. Buckheit, "Decontamination of an HIV-infected CPR Manikin," *American Journal of Public Health.* 82:1542–43 (1992).

If infant is conscious and cannot cough, cry, or breathe . . .

1

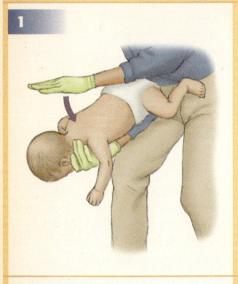

Give up to 5 back blows
- Hold infant's head and neck with 1 hand by firmly supporting infant's jaw between your thumb and fingers.
- Lay infant face down over your forearm with head lower than his or her chest. Brace your forearm and infant against your thigh.
- Give up to 5 distinct and separate back blows between shoulder blades with the heel of your hand.

2

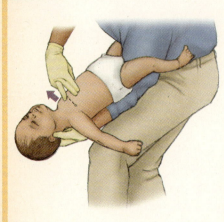

Give up to 5 chest thrusts
- Support the back of infant's head.
- Sandwich infant between your hands and arms, turn on back, with head lower than chest. If you are small, you may need to support infant on your lap.
- Imagine a line connecting infant's nipples.
- Place 3 fingers on sternum with your ring finger next to imaginary nipple line on the infant's feet side.
- Lift your ring finger off chest. If you feel the notch at the end of the sternum, move your fingers up a little.
- Give up to 5 separate and distinct thrusts with index and middle fingers on sternum in a manner similar to CPR chest compressions, but at a slower rate.
- Keep fingers in contact with chest between chest thrusts.

3

Repeat
- Give up to 5 back blows, then
- Give up to 5 chest thrusts until
Infant becomes unconscious.

OR
Object is expelled, and infant begins to breathe or cough forcefully.

Unconscious Infant with Foreign Body Airway Obstruction (Choking)

1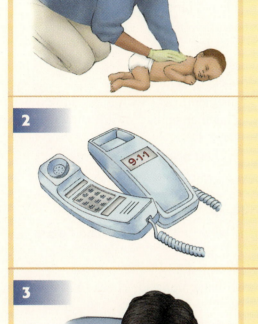

Check responsiveness
- If spine injury is suspected, move infant only if absolutely necessary.
- Tap infant's shoulder.

2

Send bystander, if available, to activate EMS. If you are alone, resuscitate for 1 minute before activating EMS.

3

Give 2 slow breaths
- Open the airway with head-tilt/chin-lift.
- Seal your mouth over infant's mouth and nose.
- Give 2 slow breaths (1 to 1½ seconds each).

If first breath did not go in, retilt the head and try 1 more slow breath.

4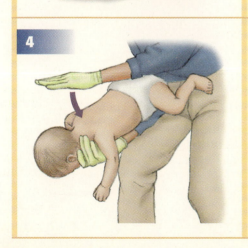

Give up to 5 back blows
- Hold infant's head and neck with 1 hand by firmly supporting infant's jaw between your thumb and fingers.
- Lay infant face down over your forearm with head lower than chest. Brace your forearm and infant against your thigh.
- Give up to 5 distinct and separate back blows between shoulder blades with the heel of your hand.

5

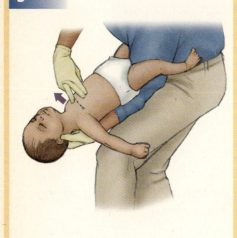

Give up to 5 chest thrusts

- Support the back of infant's head.
- Sandwich infant between your hands and arms, then turn infant on back, with head lower than chest. If you are small, you may need to support infant on your lap.
- Imagine a line connecting infant's nipples.
- Place 3 fingers on sternum with your ring finger next to imaginary nipple line on the infant's feet side.
- Lift your ring finger off chest. If you feel the notch at the end of the sternum, move your fingers up a little.
- Give up to 5 separate and distinct thrusts with index and middle fingers on sternum in a manner similar to CPR chest compressions but at a slower rate.
- Keep fingers in contact with chest between chest thrusts.

6

Check mouth for foreign object

- Grasp both tongue and jaw between your thumb and fingers and lift up.
- If object is visible, remove it with a finger sweep by sliding your little finger of the other hand alongside cheek to base of tongue using a hooking action.
- Do *not* try to remove an object you cannot see (a "blind finger sweep").
- Do not push object deeper.

7

Repeat

1. Give 1 slow breath.
2. Give up to 5 back blows.
3. Give up to 5 chest thrusts.
4. Check mouth for foreign object. If object is visible, use finger sweep.

Repeat until object is expelled or EMS arrives. If you are alone and after 1 minute the object has not been expelled, take infant with you and call the EMS.

Infant Basic Life Support Proficiency Checklist

S = self-check / P = partner check / I = instructor check

Infant Rescue Breathing

	S	P	I
1. Check responsiveness.	☐	☐	☐
2. Send a bystander, if available, to call EMS.	☐	☐	☐
3. Roll infant onto back.	☐	☐	☐
4. Airway open.	☐	☐	☐
5. Breathing check.	☐	☐	☐
6. 2 slow breaths.	☐	☐	☐
7. Check pulse at brachial.	☐	☐	☐
8. Rescue breathing (1 every 3 seconds).	☐	☐	☐
9. If alone, call EMS after 1 minute.	☐	☐	☐
10. Recheck pulse and breathing after first minute, then every few minutes.	☐	☐	☐

Infant CPR

	S	P	I
1. Check responsiveness.	☐	☐	☐
2. Send a bystander, if available, to call EMS.	☐	☐	☐
3. Roll infant onto back.	☐	☐	☐
4. Airway open.	☐	☐	☐
5. Breathing check.	☐	☐	☐
6. 2 slow breaths.	☐	☐	☐
7. Check pulse at brachial.	☐	☐	☐
8. Find fingers' position.	☐	☐	☐
9. 5 chest compressions.	☐	☐	☐
10. 1 slow breath.	☐	☐	☐
11. Continue CPR for 1 minute (19 more cycles, for total of 20).	☐	☐	☐
12. If alone, call EMS after 1 minute.	☐	☐	☐
13. Recheck pulse.	☐	☐	☐
14. Continue CPR (start with compressions).	☐	☐	☐
15. Recheck pulse after first minute, then every few minutes.	☐	☐	☐

Conscious Infant Choking Management

	S	P	I
1. Recognize choking.	☐	☐	☐
2. Up to 5 back blows (head and face down).	☐	☐	☐
3. Up to 5 chest thrusts (head down with face up).	☐	☐	☐
4. Repeat Steps 2 and 3.	☐	☐	☐

Unconscious Infant Choking Management

	S	P	I
1. Check responsiveness.	☐	☐	☐
2. Send a bystander, if available, to call EMS.	☐	☐	☐
3. Roll infant onto back.	☐	☐	☐
4. Airway open.	☐	☐	☐
5. Breathing check.	☐	☐	☐
6. Try 2 slow breaths. (If first breath unsuccessful, retilt head and try 1 more breath.)	☐	☐	☐
7. Up to 5 back blows (head and face down).	☐	☐	☐
8. Up to 5 chest thrusts (head down and face up).	☐	☐	☐
9. Check mouth for foreign object (finger sweep only if object is visible).	☐	☐	☐
10. Try 1 slow breath.	☐	☐	☐
11. Repeat sequence of 5 blows, 5 thrusts, mouth check, 1 breath.	☐	☐	☐

CPR Review

Action	Infant (0–1 year)	Child (1–8 years)	Adult (>8 years)
How to open airway?	Head-tilt/chin-lift	Head-tilt/chin-lift	Head-tilt/chin-lift
How to check breathing?	Look at chest and listen and feel for air (3–5 seconds).	Look at chest and listen and feel for air (3–5 seconds).	Look at chest and listen and feel for air (3–5 seconds).
What kinds of breaths?	Slow, make chest rise and fall	Slow, make chest rise and fall	Slow, make chest rise and fall
Where to check pulse?	Brachial artery (5–10 seconds)	Carotid artery (5–10 seconds)	Carotid artery (5–10 seconds)
Hand position for chest compressions?	1 finger's width below imaginary line between nipples	1 finger's width above tip of sternum	1 finger's width above tip of sternum
Compress with?	2 fingers	Heel of 1 hand	Heels of 2 hands, one hand on top of the other
Compression depth?	½–1 inch	1–1½ inches	1½–2 inches
Compression rate?	100 per minute	100 per minute	80–100 per minute
Compression:breath ratio?	5:1	5:1	15:2
How to count for compression rate?	1,2,3,4,5, breathe	1, 2, 3, 4, 5, breathe	1 and, 2 and, 3 and, 4 and, 5 and, 6 and, . . . 15 and, breathe, breathe
How often to reassess?	After the first minute, then every few minutes	After the first minute, then every few minutes	After the first minute, then every few minutes
After reassessment, resume CPR with?	Compressions	Compressions	Compressions
How often to give only breaths during rescue breathing?	Every 3 seconds	Every 3 seconds	Every 5 seconds

STUDY QUESTIONS 5

Name _HRTAL BHAYANI_ Course _____ Date _____

Activities

Activity 1

Choose the best answer.

_a_ 1. Are chest compressions likely to work if the victim is on a soft surface?
  a. Yes, a soft surface is okay.
  b. No, the surface should be hard.

_B_ 2. When you tip the head with the chin lift, where do you place your fingertips?
  a. Under the soft part of the throat near the chin
  b. Under the bony part of the jaw near the chin

_C_ 3. Which is the safer way to open the airway of a person who may have a spine injury?
  a. Push the jaw forward from the corners.
  b. Stabilize head and lift the chin.
  c. Use either method.

_A_ 4. How should you check for stopped breathing?
  a. Look at the chest; listen and feel for air coming out of the mouth.
  b. Look at the pupils of the eyes.
  c. Check the pulse.

_____ 5. When you give breaths to an adult, the breaths should be:
  a. Slow
  b. Fast

_A_ 6. Before deciding whether to give CPR, check the victim's pulse for:
  a. 1–3 seconds
  b. 3–5 seconds
  c. 5–10 seconds
  d. 10–20 seconds

_B_ 7. To find where to push on the chest for chest compressions, you should measure up:
  a. Two hand-widths from the navel
  b. One finger-width from the middle finger on the sternum's tip

_B_ 8. Give chest compressions:
  a. With a quick jerk
  b. Smoothly and regularly

_B_ 9. Push on a victim's chest:
  a. At an angle
  b. Straight down

_B_ 10. Compress an adult's chest at least:
  a. ½ to 1 inch
  b. 1½ to 2 inches

_B_ 11. In one-rescuer CPR, give chest compressions to an adult at the rate, per minute, of:
  a. 100–120
  b. 80–100
  c. 60–80
  d. 40–60

_A_ 12. What is the pattern of compressions and breaths in one-rescuer CPR for an adult victim?
  a. 15 compressions, 2 breaths
  b. 15 compressions, 1 breath
  c. 5 compressions, 2 breaths
  d. 5 compressions, 1 breath

Activity 2

Choose the best answer.

_B_ 1. An adult victim is coughing forcefully. Should you give back blows and thrusts?
  a. Yes
  b. No

_A_ 2. A person is coughing weakly and making wheezing noises. You should:
  a. Give abdominal thrusts.
  b. Let the person alone and watch closely.

_B_ 3. A victim who seems to be choking _can_ speak. Should you give abdominal thrusts?
  a. Yes
  b. No

_A_ 4. A conscious person is coughing force-fully, trying to dislodge an object. Then the person stops coughing and cannot speak. You should:
    a. Give abdominal thrusts.
    b. Let the person alone and watch closely.

_C_ 5. When you give abdominal thrusts to a conscious victim, what part of your fist do you place against the victim?
    a. The palm side
    b. The little finger side
    c. The thumb side

_A_ 6. Give abdominal thrusts quickly:
    a. Inward and upward
    b. Straight back

_B_ 7. Where do you place your fist to give abdominal thrusts?
    a. Over the breastbone
    b. Slightly above the navel
    c. Below the navel

_A_ 8. To give abdominal thrusts to a victim who is lying down, place the heel of one hand:
    a. Slightly above the navel
    b. On the edge of the breastbone
    c. Below the navel

_B_ 9. For a victim who is obese or in advanced pregnancy, it is better to give:
    a. Abdominal thrusts
    b. Chest thrusts

Activity 3
Choose the best answer.

_A_ 1. How should you check for stopped breathing?
    a. Look at the chest; listen and feel for air coming out of the mouth.
    b. Look at the pupils of the eyes.
    c. Check the pulse.

_B_ 2. If your amount of breath is enough:
    a. The stomach will form a pouch.
    b. The chest will rise.
    c. Your air backs up against incoming air.

_A_ 3. Check a baby's pulse at the:
    a. Middle of the upper arm
    b. Wrist
    c. Neck

_A_ 4. To give a baby chest compressions use:
    a. 2 or 3 fingers
    b. The heel of one hand

_A_ 5. Push on the chest of a child or baby one finger-width:
    a. Above nipple line
    b. Below nipple line
    c. Above xiphoid process

_B_ 6. How far should you compress a baby's chest?
    a. 1½ to 2 inches
    b. ½ to 1 inch

_A_ 7. Give a baby chest compressions at the rate per minute of:
    a. 100
    b. 80
    c. 60

_D_ 8. Give babies and children:
    a. 15 compressions, 2 breaths
    b. 5 compressions, 2 breaths
    c. 15 compressions, 1 breath
    d. 5 compressions, 1 breath

_A_ 9. When giving chest compressions to a child, use:
    a. 2 or 3 fingers or heel of one hand
    b. The heel of one hand and the other hand on top

Activity 4
Choose the best answer.

_D_ 1. You believe a baby has an object caught in its airway; it cannot cough or cry. What do you do first?
    a. Let it alone and watch closely.
    b. Give abdominal thrusts.
    c. Give chest thrusts.
    d. Give back blows.

2. Use your finger to remove an object from an unconscious baby or child's mouth:
   a. Whenever back blows and chest thrusts fail
   b. Only if you see the object

Case Situations

Case 1

You find a 50-year-old male lying in an office building hallway, suffering from cardiac arrest.

1. Describe how to locate the proper hand positioning for giving CPR.

2. Describe:

_2_ a. How many hands should you compress an adult's chest with?

_1½-2"_ b. Compression depth in inches

_15_ c. Compressions per minute

_15:2_ d. Compression to ventilation ratio

3. List four common CPR compression mistakes:

a. Miscounting of the compressions

b. the victims heart compressed to hard

c. the victims heart compressed to soft

d. the Rescuers may have incorrect hand placement

Case 2

At a family picnic you find an uncle unconscious. You open his airway and unsuccessfully attempt to give one rescue breath.

1. What do you do now?

a. Reach out for the head lilt & chin lift again & try giving another rescue breath.

b. Ask standbyers to go call for EMS

2. If that fails, what should you do?

If that fails try giving him abdominal thrusts.

3. If that fails, what should you try next?

keep trying – give him some more abdominal thrust.

4. Then what, if you are still unsuccessful?

keep trying until EMS takes over or until you get exhausted.

Case 3

A six-year-old, whose face is cyanotic, appears to be choking and violently gasping for air.

1. What is the immediate emergency care to alleviate the problem? What should be done?

Ask the child if he or she could speak. If not one should start giving an abdominal thrusts

2. Describe the proper procedure for the immediate emergency care necessary in this situation.

_____
_____
_____
_____
_____
_____

Case 4

A frantic mother calls to report that her infant suddenly has stopped breathing. Within seconds, you cross the street to her house and find the mother giving rescue breathing. A check of the infant's pulse reveals no pulse.

1. What is the immediate emergency care in this situation?

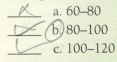 Ask the mother to go call EMS. check the ABC's Start giving CPR to the Crd.

2. For an infant, how many cardiac compressions per minute should you complete?
   - ✗ a. 60–80
   - ✗ (b.) 80–100
   - ✓ c. 100–120

3. For a small infant, how many inches down should you compress the chest wall?
   - ✗ a. ¼
   - ✗ b. ¼ to ½
   - ✓ c. ½ to 1
   - ✗ d. 1 to 1½

4. When taking an infant's pulse, the best location to use is the:
   - ✗ a. carotid artery
   - ✗ b. left nipple
   - ✓ c. brachial artery
   - ✗ d. femoral artery

Case 5

While eating at a local fast-food restaurant, you see a young male kneeling against a table bench, grasping his throat with one hand. You find that he is cyanotic about the lips. He is unable to speak. The victim's friends tell you that he is allergic to aspirin.

1. This victim is most likely experiencing:
   - a. an acute asthma attack
   - B b. an airway obstruction
   - c. an allergic reaction
   - d. a respiratory infection

2. Immediate care of this victim would include:
   - a. giving two rescue breaths
   - b. hitting him repeatedly between the shoulder blades
   - c. trying to dislodge the food with your finger
   - D d. if he is sitting or standing, applying upward, inward abdominal thrusts with your hands

NOTES

CHAPTER

6

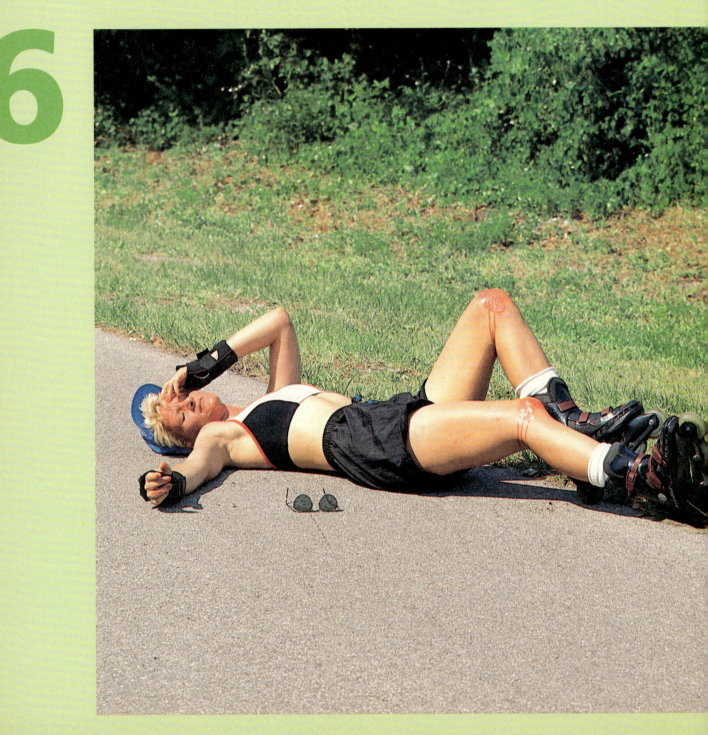

BLEEDING AND SHOCK

Bleeding

The average-size adult has about five to six quarts (10–12 pints) of blood and can safely give up a pint during a blood donation. However, rapid blood loss of one quart or more can lead to shock and death. A child who loses one pint of blood is in extreme danger.

External Bleeding

External bleeding occurs when blood can be seen coming from an open wound. The term **hemorrhage** refers to a large amount of bleeding in a short time.

Types of External Bleeding

External bleeding can be classified into three types according to its source. In **arterial bleeding,** blood spurts (up to several feet) from the wound. Arterial bleeding is the most serious type of bleeding because blood is lost at a fast rate, leading to a large blood loss. Arterial bleeding also is less likely to clot because blood can clot only when it is flowing slowly or not at all. However, unless a very large artery has been cut, it is unlikely that a person will bleed to death before the flow can be controlled. Nevertheless, arterial bleeding is dangerous, and some external means of control must be used to stop it.

In **venous bleeding,** blood from a vein flows steadily or gushes. Venous bleeding is easier to control than arterial bleeding. Most veins collapse when cut. Bleeding from deep veins, however, can be as copious and as hard to control as arterial bleeding.

In **capillary bleeding,** blood oozes from capillaries. The most common type of bleeding, capillary bleeding usually is not serious and is controlled easily. Quite often, this type of bleeding will clot off by itself.

Each type of blood vessel—artery, vein, capillary—contains blood of a different shade of red. An inexperienced person may have difficulty detecting the difference. Bleeding can be controlled by the same methods no matter what its source, so being able to identify the type of bleeding by its color is unnecessary.

The body naturally responds to bleeding by the following actions:

- *Blood vessel spasm.* Arteries contain small amounts of muscle tissue in their walls. If a blood vessel is completely severed, it draws back into the tissue, constricts its diameter, and slows the bleeding dramatically. If an artery is only partially cut across its diameter, however, constriction is incomplete. The vessel may not contract, and the loss of blood may not slow as dramatically.

- *Clotting.* Special elements (platelets) in blood form a clot. Clotting serves as a protective covering for a wound until the tissues underneath can repair themselves. In a healthy individual, initial clot formation normally takes about 10 minutes. Clotting time lengthens in persons who have lost a great deal of blood over a prolonged period of time, are taking aspirin or anticoagulants, are anemic, are hemophiliacs, or have severe liver disease.

What to Do

Regardless of the type of bleeding or the type of wound, first aid is the same. First, and most important, you must control the bleeding:

1. Protect yourself against disease by wearing latex gloves. If latex gloves are not available, use sev-

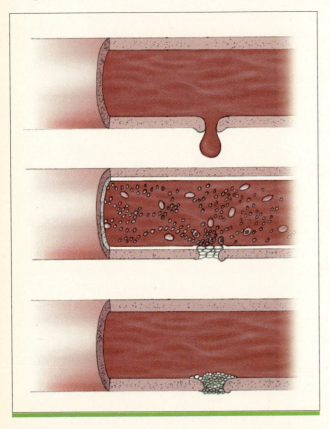

Clotting begins as soon as a break in a blood vessel wall occurs (top). Platelets (the oval disks in the middle drawing) stick to the vessel wall and release adenosine diphosphate (ADP) (the smaller, round objects), which recruits more platelets. Finally, the temporary platelet plug is replaced by a tough fibrin clot (bottom).

CAUTION: DO NOT

- touch a wound with your bare hands. If you must use your bare hands, do so only as a last resort. After the bleeding has stopped and the wound has been cared for, vigorously wash your hands with soap and water.
- use direct pressure on an eye injury, a wound with an embedded object, or a skull fracture.
- contact blood with your bare hands. Protect yourself with latex gloves, extra gauze pads, or clean cloths, or have the victim apply the direct pressure.
- remove a blood-soaked dressing. Apply another dressing on top and keep pressing.

eral layers of gauze pads, plastic wrap, a plastic bag, or waterproof material. You can even have the victim apply pressure with his or her own hand.

2. Expose the wound by removing or cutting the clothing to see where the blood is coming from.

3. Place a sterile gauze pad or a clean cloth (e.g., handkerchief, washcloth, or towel) over the entire wound and apply direct pressure with your fingers or the palm of your hand. The gauze or cloth allows you to apply even pressure. Direct pressure stops most bleeding. Applying direct pressure to the wound helps the body's natural clotting mechanisms to work. Be sure the pressure remains constant, is not too light, and is applied to the bleeding source. If you apply direct pressure and the bleeding doesn't stop, continue to apply pressure. Do not remove blood-soaked dressings; simply apply new dressings over the old ones.

    If, after a few minutes, the bleeding remains uncontrolled, continue to the next step.

4. If bleeding does not stop in 10 minutes, the pressure may be too light or in the wrong location. Press harder over a wider area for another 10 minutes. If the bleeding is from an arm or leg, while still applying pressure, elevate the injured area above heart level to reduce blood flow. Elevation allows gravity to make it difficult for the body to pump blood to the affected extremity. Elevation alone, however, will not stop bleeding and must be used in combination with direct pressure over the wound.

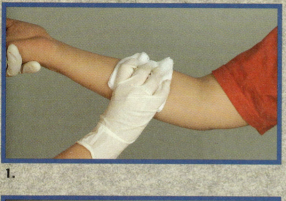

1.

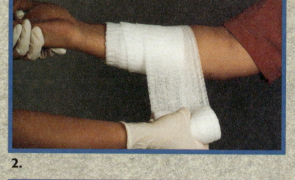

2.

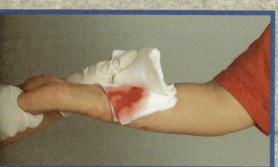

3.

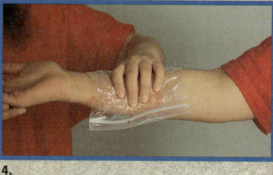

4.

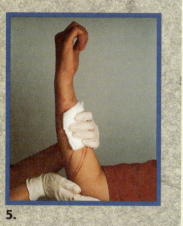

5.

1. Direct pressure stops most bleeding. Wearing disposable gloves, place sterile gauze pad or clean cloth over wound. If bleeding does not stop in 10 minutes, press harder over a wider area.
2. A pressure bandage can free you to attend to other injuries or victims.
3. Do not remove a blood-soaked dressing. Add more on top.
4. If disposable gloves are not available, use another barrier or extra gauze pads or cloths.
5. If bleeding persists, use elevation to help reduce blood flow. Combine with direct pressure over the wound.
6. If bleeding still continues, apply pressure at a pressure point to slow blood flow. Locations are: **(a)** brachial or **(b)** femoral. Use with direct pressure over the wound.

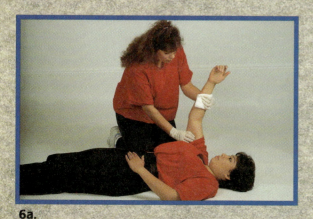

6a.

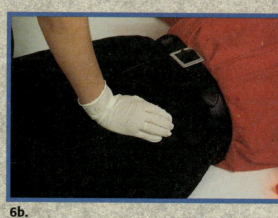

6b.

5. If the bleeding continues, apply pressure at a pressure point to slow the flow of blood, in combination with direct pressure over the wound. A pressure point is where an artery is near the skin's surface and where it passes close to a bone, against which it can be compressed. Two pressure points on both sides of the body are the most accessible: the brachial point in the upper inside arm and the femoral point in the groin. Using pressure points requires skill, and unless the exact location of the pulse point is used, the pressure-point technique is useless. Many first aiders cannot locate the pressure-point location. Most bleeding, however, is stopped by direct pressure.

6. After the bleeding stops or to free you to attend to other injuries or victims, use a pressure bandage to hold the dressing on the wound. Wrap a roller gauze bandage tightly over the dressing and above and below the wound site.

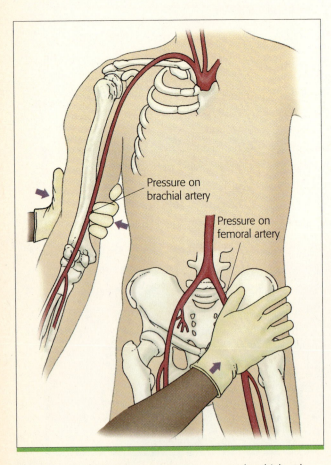

Proper hand positions for applying pressure on brachial and femoral arteries

CAUTION: DO NOT

- apply a pressure bandage so tight that it cuts off circulation. Check the radial pulse if the bandage is on an arm; for a leg, check the pulse between the inside ankle bone knob and the Achilles tendon (posterior tibal).
- use a tourniquet. They are rarely needed and can damage nerves and blood vessels. Use of a tourniquet may cause the loss of an arm or leg. If you do use one, apply wide, flat materials—never rope or wire—and do not loosen it. Remember: Use of a tourniquet usually means the extremity will have to be amputated.

7. When direct pressure cannot be applied (e.g., in the case of a protruding bone, skull fracture, or embedded object) use a doughnut-shaped (ring) pad to control bleeding. To make a ring pad, wrap one end of a narrow bandage (roller or cravat) several times around your four fingers to form a loop. Pass the other end of the bandage through the loop and wrap it around and around until the entire bandage is used and a ring has been made.

Some people panic when they see even the smallest amount of blood. The sight of more than a couple of tablespoonfuls of blood generally is enough to scare victims and bystanders. Take time to reassure the victim that everything possible is being done. Don't belittle the victim's concerns.

Internal Bleeding

Internal bleeding occurs when the skin is unbroken and blood is not visible. It can be difficult to detect and can be life threatening. Internal bleeding comes from injuries that do not break the skin or from nontraumatic disorders such as ulcers.

What to Look For

The signs of internal bleeding may take days to appear:

- bruises or contusions of the skin
- painful, tender, rigid, bruised abdomen
- fractured ribs or bruises on chest
- vomiting or coughing up blood
- stools that are black or contain bright red blood

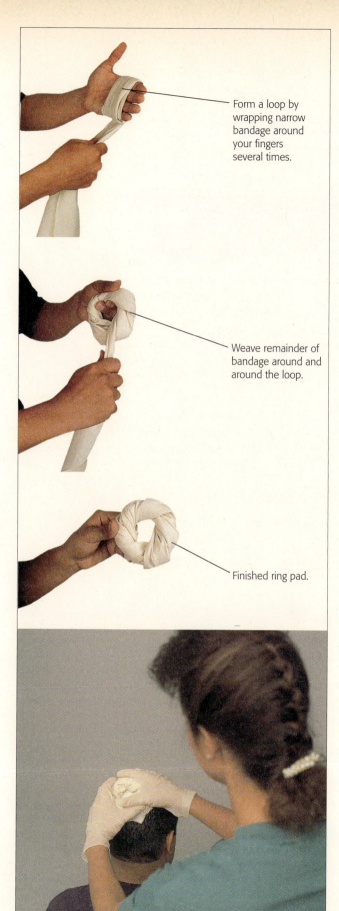

Form a loop by wrapping narrow bandage around your fingers several times.

Weave remainder of bandage around and around the loop.

Finished ring pad.

Control bleeding with a ring pad.

What to Do

For severe internal bleeding, follow these steps:

1. Monitor the ABCs.
2. Expect vomiting. If vomiting occurs, keep the victim lying on his or her left side for drainage, to prevent inhalation of vomitus, and to prevent expulsion of vomit from the stomach.
3. Treat for shock by raising the victim's legs 8–12 inches and cover the victim with a coat or blanket to keep warm. See page 118 for when to use other body positions.
4. Seek immediate medical attention.

CAUTION: DO NOT

- give a victim anything to eat or drink. It could cause nausea and vomiting, which could result in aspiration. It could cause complications if surgery is needed.

Bruises are a form of internal bleeding but are not life threatening. To treat bruises:

1. Apply an ice pack for 20 minutes. Protect the victim's skin from frostbite by placing a wet cloth between the ice and the skin. The wet cloth transfers cold better than a dry one, which insulates.
2. If the bruise is on an arm or leg, raise the limb if it is not broken.
3. If an arm or a leg is involved, apply an elastic bandage with a pad between the bandage and the bruised skin.

Shock (Hypoperfusion)

Shock refers to circulatory system failure, which happens when oxygenated blood is not provided in sufficient amounts for every body part. Because every injury affects the circulatory system to some degree, first aiders should automatically treat injured victims for shock. Shock is one of the most common causes of death in an injured victim.

The damage caused by shock depends on which body part is deprived of oxygen and for how long. For example, without oxygen, the brain will be irreparably damaged in 4 to 6 minutes, the abdominal organs in 45 to 90 minutes, and the skin and muscle cells in 3 to 6 hours.

BLEEDING

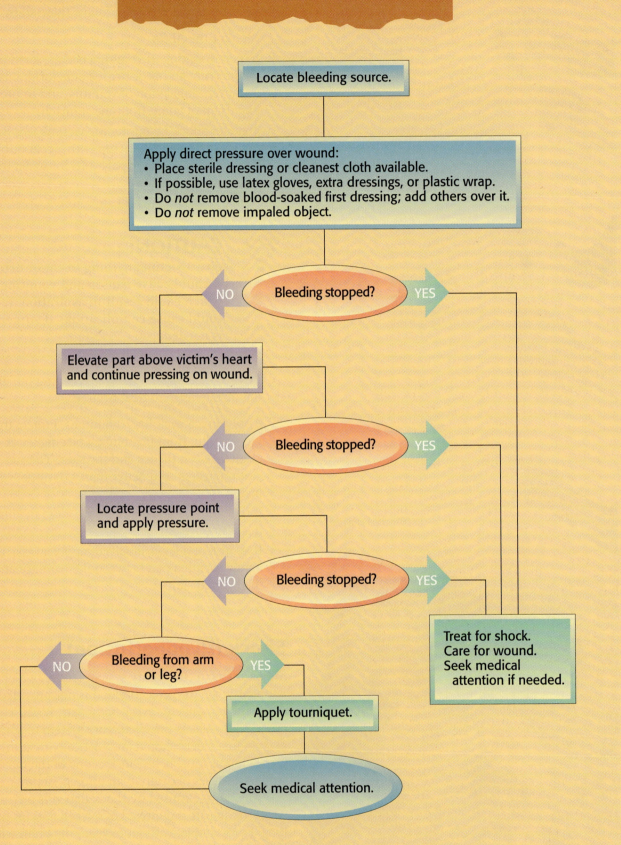

Locate bleeding source.

Apply direct pressure over wound:
- Place sterile dressing or cleanest cloth available.
- If possible, use latex gloves, extra dressings, or plastic wrap.
- Do *not* remove blood-soaked first dressing; add others over it.
- Do *not* remove impaled object.

Bleeding stopped? — NO / YES

Elevate part above victim's heart and continue pressing on wound.

Bleeding stopped? — NO / YES

Locate pressure point and apply pressure.

Bleeding stopped? — NO / YES

Bleeding from arm or leg? — NO / YES

Apply tourniquet.

Treat for shock.
Care for wound.
Seek medical attention if needed.

Seek medical attention.

To understand shock, think of the circulatory system as having three components: a working pump (the heart), a network of pipes (the blood vessels), and an adequate amount of fluid (the blood) pumped through the pipes. Damage to any of those components can deprive tissues of blood and produce the condition known as shock.

Shock can be classified as one of three types according to which component has failed.

- *Pump failure.* **Cardiogenic shock** results from a failure of the heart to pump sufficient blood. For example, a major heart attack can cause damage to the heart muscle so the heart cannot squeeze and therefore cannot push blood through the blood vessels.

- *Fluid loss.* **Hypovolemic shock** happens with the loss of a significant amount of fluid from the system. If the lost fluid is blood, this type of shock is best known as **hemorrhagic shock.** People experiencing dehydration due to vomiting, diarrhea, diabetes, insufficient fluid intake, or misuse of diuretics can lose large amounts of fluid. Profuse sweating can also result in a sizable amount of fluid loss.

- *Pipe failure.* When the nervous system is damaged (e.g., the spinal cord is damaged or the victim has taken an overdose of certain drugs), **neurogenic shock** may result. In neurogenic shock, the blood vessels (pipes) enlarge and the blood supply is insufficient to fill them.

Septic shock develops in some victims with bacterial infection when damaged blood vessels

Table 6-1: Signs of Shock	
Signs (in order of appearance)	**Reason**
1. Altered mental status: • anxiety • restlessness • combativeness	Brain not receiving enough oxygen.
2. Skin: • pale • cold • clammy	Body attempts to correct problem by diverting blood from nonvital to vital organs (i.e., from skin to heart and brain).
3. Nausea and vomiting	Blood diverted from digestive system, which causes nausea and occasional vomiting.

4. Changes in vital signs	As body tries to pump more blood:
	• pulse rapid—
	  60 to 100 = normal;
	  >120 = serious.
	• respirations rapid—
	  12 to 20 = normal;
	  >24 = serious.

5. Other signs: • thirst • dilated pupils • sometimes cyanosis (blue color), especially of lips and nail beds	

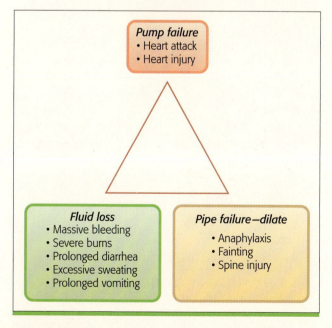

Causes of shock

lose their ability to contract. First aiders seldom see cases of septic shock because victims usually are already hospitalized for a serious illness, injury, or operation.

Shock resulting from blood or fluid loss is the most common type.

What to Look For

- altered mental status: anxiety and restlessness
- pale, cold, and clammy skin, lips, and nail beds
- nausea and vomiting
- breathing and pulse rapid
- unresponsiveness when shock is severe

What to Do

Even if an injured victim does not have signs or symptoms of shock, first aiders should treat for shock. You can prevent shock from getting worse; you cannot reverse it.

1. Treat life-threatening injuries and other severe injuries.
2. Lay the victim on his or her back.

> ⚠ **CAUTION: DO NOT**
> - raise the legs of victims with head injuries or strokes. Slightly raise the victim's head if no spine injury is suspected.
> - place victims with breathing difficulties, chest injuries, penetrating eye injuries, or heart attack on their backs. Place them in a half-sitting position to help breathing.
> - place victims rated as V, P, or U (see page 53) or vomiting victims on their backs. Use the recovery position (see page 72). If a spine injury is suspected, do *not* move the victim.
> - place an advanced (third trimester) pregnant woman on her back—instead, place her on her left side to avoid pressing the vena cava.

3. Raise the victim's legs 8–12 inches. Raising the legs allows the blood to drain from the legs back to the heart.

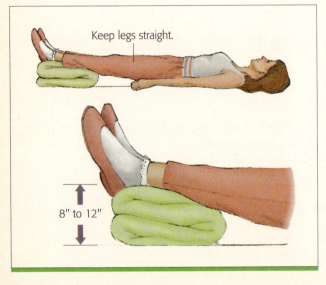

Keep legs straight.

8" to 12"

Elevate the legs to circulate blood to the vital organs.

"If the face is red,
Raise the head.
If the face is pale,
Raise the tail."

Old first aid axiom

> ⚠ **CAUTION: DO NOT**
> - raise the legs more than 12 inches since that would affect the victim's breathing by having the abdominal organs push up against the diaphragm.
> - lift the foot of a bed or stretcher—breathing will be affected, and the blood flow from the brain may be retarded and lead to brain swelling.
> - raise the legs of a victim with head injuries, stroke, chest injuries, breathing difficulty, unconsciousness. Place the victim in the proper position, as described above.

4. Prevent body heat loss by putting blankets and coats under and over the victim.

Emergency Blankets

At rest, 75 percent of a body's heat production is lost by radiation and convection from the body surface. Such heat loss can be detrimental to an injured victim. An inexpensive—but controversial—"emergency" blanket now has scientific backing. These aluminized covers or blankets reduce body heat loss by protecting the body surface from exposure to cool temperatures and air currents and by blocking the escape of radiant body heat to the atmosphere.

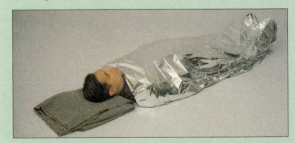

Sources: R. S. Erickson et al., "Effect of Aluminized Covers on Body Temperature," *Heart and Lung* 20(3):255–264 (May 1991); K. B. Hindsholm et al., "Reflective Blankets Used for Reduction of Heat Loss," *British Journal of Anaesthesia* 68:531–533 (1992).

HYPOVOLEMIC SHOCK

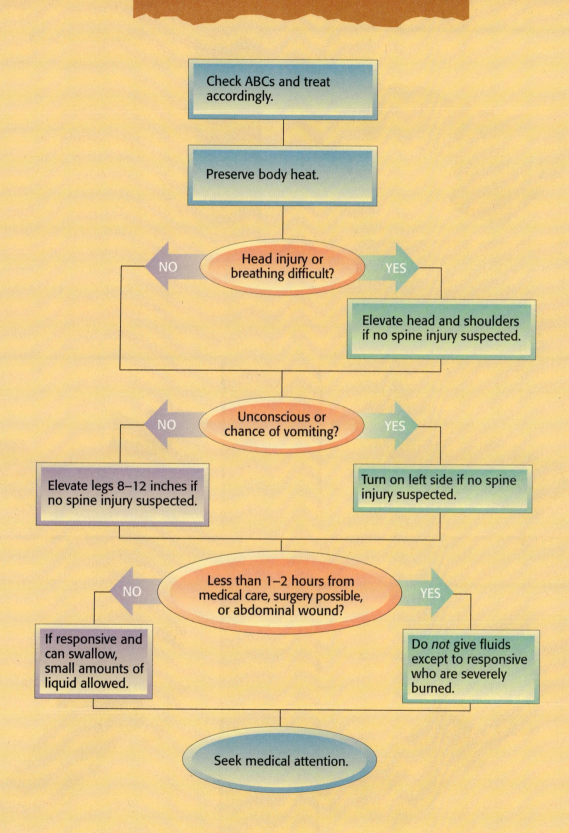

Check ABCs and treat accordingly.

Preserve body heat.

Head injury or breathing difficult?

NO / YES

Elevate head and shoulders if no spine injury suspected.

Unconscious or chance of vomiting?

NO / YES

Elevate legs 8–12 inches if no spine injury suspected.

Turn on left side if no spine injury suspected.

Less than 1–2 hours from medical care, surgery possible, or abdominal wound?

NO / YES

If responsive and can swallow, small amounts of liquid allowed.

Do *not* give fluids except to responsive who are severely burned.

Seek medical attention.

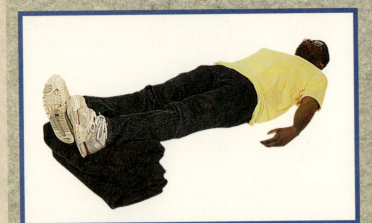

1.

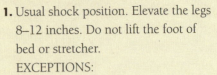

1. Usual shock position. Elevate the legs 8–12 inches. Do not lift the foot of bed or stretcher.
EXCEPTIONS:
2. Elevate the head for injuries or stroke.
3. Lay an unconscious, unresponsive, or vomiting victim on his or her left side.
4. Use a half-sitting position for those with breathing difficulties, chest injuries, or a heart attack.
5. Keep victim flat if a neck or spine injury is suspected or victim has leg fractures.

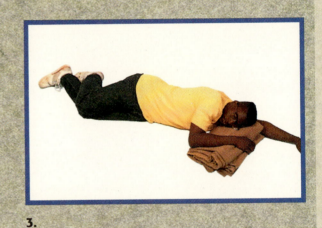

2.

3.

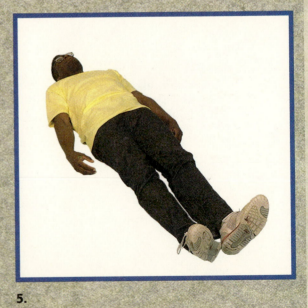

4.

5.

Anaphylaxis

Allergies are usually thought of as causing rashes, itching, or some other short-term discomfort that disappears when the offending agent is removed from contact with the allergic person. However, a more powerful reaction to substances ordinarily eaten or injected can occur within minutes or even seconds. This reaction, called **anaphylaxis,** can cause death if it is not treated immediately.

Anaphylaxis is a massive allergic reaction by the body's immune system. Normally, the immune system's function is to recognize and eliminate foreign materials such as bacteria and viral particles. In the case of anaphylaxis, however, the immune system forms an antibody to a foreign protein when it is first exposed to that foreign material. When the individual is again exposed to the foreign protein (an antigen), the preformed antibody immediately attempts to neutralize the exposure by binding with the antigen. When the antibody and the antigen combine, they form an antigen-antibody complex. That triggers certain cells in body tissues and in the bloodstream to release a series of chemicals. Those released chemicals are the cause of the severe cardiac, respiratory, skin, and gastrointestinal signs and symptoms that occur in anaphylaxis.

Common Causes of Anaphylaxis

Like less severe allergic reactions, anaphylaxis is an abnormal response to an antigen that doesn't bother most people but causes symptoms in those who have a hypersensitivity to it. Well-known antigens that can cause anaphylaxis include:

- medications (penicillin and related drugs, aspirin, sulfa drugs)
- food and food additives (shellfish, nuts, eggs, monosodium glutamate, nitrates, nitrites)
- insect stings (honeybee, yellow jacket, wasp, hornet, fire ant)
- plant pollen
- radiographic dyes

Since the mid-1900s, penicillin has been by far the most common cause of anaphylaxis. Most allergic reactions to penicillin are local skin reactions (e.g., hives or a rash) or systemic reactions (wheezing, swelling, redness).

Insect stings are another major cause of anaphylactic death. Hymenoptera (honeybees, bumble-

Hero CITATION

Roger Lindsay saved David Triplett from drowning, Isleta, New Mexico, May 7, 1990. Triplett, 37, attempted to swim across Sunrise Lake but began to struggle midway. He yelled for help. Fishing nearby from the bank, Lindsay, 30, was alerted to Triplett's plight. Although he had not swum for several years, following an accident which resulted in a leg being amputated below the knee, Lindsay, wearing a prosthesis, dived into the lake and swam about 150 feet to Triplett, who had by then submerged. Lindsay pulled Triplett to the surface of the water and began to swim back to the bank, towing him. He tired en route, his prosthetic leg pulling him down, and began to struggle. When he reached the bank, others pulled Triplett out of the water. He was revived and taken to the hospital for treatment.

bees, wasps, hornets, yellow jackets, and fire ants) are the offending insects. Although millions of people in the United States are allergic to insect venom, and hundreds of thousands of them have allergic reactions to stings each year, the number of deaths reported from those reactions is estimated at only 50 to 100 per year.

The best way to prevent anaphylaxis is to avoid the instigator (e.g., bees, aspirin, certain foods).

What to Look For

Anaphylaxis typically comes on within minutes of exposure to the offending substance, peaks in 15 to 30 minutes, and is over within hours.

The first symptom is usually a sensation of warmth followed by intense itching, especially on the soles of the feet and the palms of the hands. The skin flushes, hives may appear, and the face may swell. Breathing becomes difficult, and the victim may feel faint and anxious. Convulsions, shock, unconsciousness, even death may follow. Other signs and symptoms of anaphylaxis include:

- sneezing, coughing, wheezing
- shortness of breath
- tightness and swelling in the throat
- tightness in the chest
- increased pulse rate
- swelling of the mucous membranes (tongue, mouth, nose)
- blueness around lips and mouth
- dizziness
- nausea and vomiting

⚠ CAUTION: DO NOT

- mistake anaphylaxis for other reactions such as hyperventilation, anxiety attacks, alcohol intoxication, or low blood sugar.

About 60 to 80 percent of anaphylactic deaths are caused by the victims' inability to breathe because swollen airway passages obstruct airflow to the lungs. The second most common cause of anaphylactic deaths—about 24 percent by one estimate—is shock, caused by insufficient blood circulating through the body's dilated blood vessels.

What to Do

Since the main causes of death resulting from anaphylaxis are the collapse of the circulatory system and respiratory compromise, first aiders must focus on the care of those two body systems. Rapid identification of breathing difficulty and shock will allow the appropriate first aid to be started.

Rescue breathing or CPR may be needed. If a bee sting is involved, remove the stinger by scraping, not squeezing. An ice pack to the sting area may decrease the absorption of more antigen.

Epinephrine

The drug epinephrine can reverse many of the life-threatening processes of anaphylaxis on the circulatory and respiratory systems (vessel dilation and bronchospasm). Epinephrine produces bronchodilation, increases cardiac output, and constricts blood vessels. Injectable epinephrine for use by a first aider is available only through a victim's

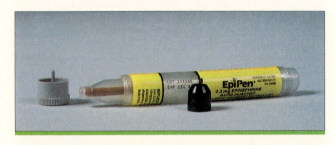

Doctor-prescribed preloaded epinephrine autoinjector

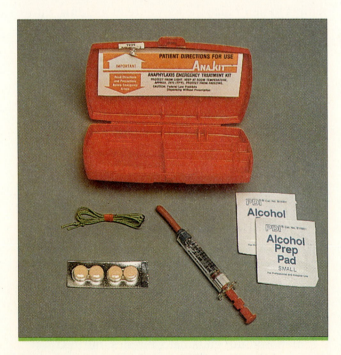

Doctor-prescribed preloaded epinephrine with 2 shots

physician-prescribed emergency epinephrine kit. Two such kits are available: AnaKit® and EpiPen®. The AnaKit's advantage is that two separate injections in prefilled syringes are available. The EpiPen's advantage is that it has a prefilled syringe with the needle hidden from view.

The recommended injection site when using an EpiPen is the front outside part of the thigh. Do not inject into the buttock or into a vein. To use an EpiPen, remove the device's safety cap and place the autoinjector's tip against the thigh, at a right angle to the leg. Push the autoinjector firmly until it activates, then hold it in place for about 10 seconds. That allows time for the medication to be injected. Remove the injector and massage the site for several seconds. Some relief of symptoms may appear as soon as one or two minutes after administration.

Should you believe that you or a family member is susceptible to anaphylaxis, consult your physician about the need to have an epinephrine kit. Should you face a situation that has all the signals of a severe allergic reaction and the victim's breathing is being affected, ask the victim or anyone else around if the victim has a physician-prescribed epinephrine kit. While most emergency situations are not life threatening, anaphylaxis is—so be prepared.

Parents, relatives, neighbors, family friends, and school personnel must be taught how to recognize and handle an attack. In addition to injectable epinephrine, the allergic victim should wear a medical-alert tag or necklace at all times. If food is the culprit, food labels and restaurant menus must be scrutinized for potential allergens. If flying insects (e.g., bees) are the culprit, sensitive individuals must avoid them and not wear perfume, cologne, or bright colors, which attract the insects.

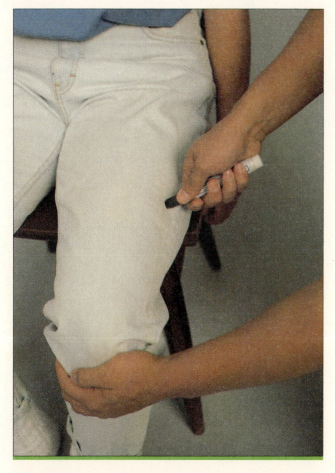

Push the autoinjector against the thigh and hold in place until medication is injected (10 seconds).

ANAPHYLAXIS
(known as severe allergic reaction and anaphylactic Shock)

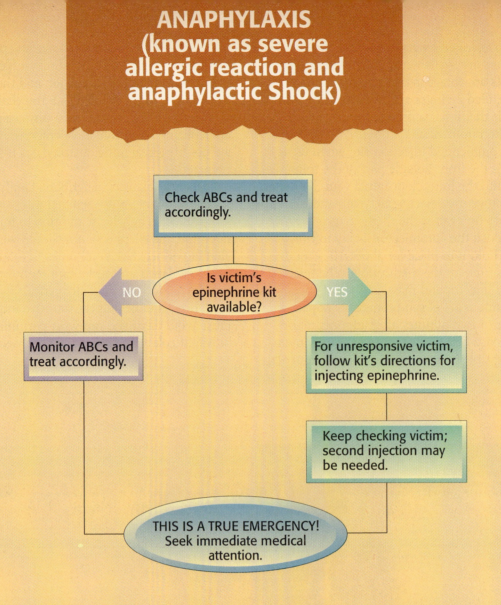

Check ABCs and treat accordingly.

Is victim's epinephrine kit available?

NO

YES

Monitor ABCs and treat accordingly.

For unresponsive victim, follow kit's directions for injecting epinephrine.

Keep checking victim; second injection may be needed.

THIS IS A TRUE EMERGENCY! Seek immediate medical attention.

CHAPTER

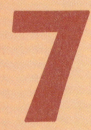

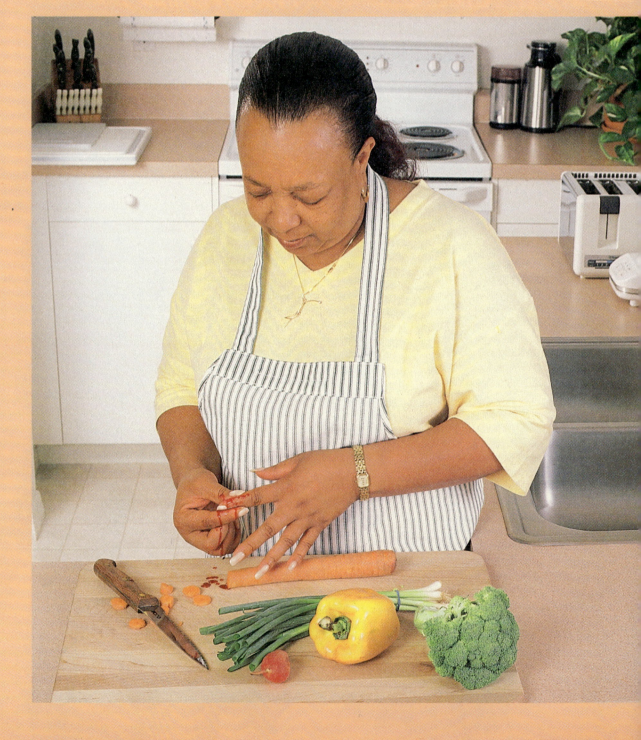

WOUNDS

Open Wounds

An open wound is a break in the skin's surface in which there is external bleeding. Victims of open wounds are susceptible to blood loss and infection.

There are several types of open wounds. With an **abrasion,** the top layer of skin is removed, with little or no blood loss. Abrasions tend to be painful, because the nerve endings often are abraded along with the skin. Ground-in debris may be present. This type of wound can be serious if it covers a large area or if foreign matter becomes embedded in it. An abrasion is also known as a "scrape," "road rash," and "rug burn."

A **laceration** is cut skin with jagged, irregular edges. This type of wound is usually caused by a forceful tearing away of skin tissue.

Incisions tend to be smooth edged, resembling a surgical cut or a paper cut. The amount of bleeding depends on the depth, the location, and the size of the wound.

Punctures are usually deep, narrow wounds in the skin and underlying organs. An example is a stab wound from a nail or a knife. The entrance is usually small, and the risk of infection is high. The object causing the injury may remain impaled in the wound.

With an **avulsion,** a flap of skin is torn loose and is either hanging from the body or completely removed. This type of wound can bleed heavily. If the flap is still attached and folded back, lay it flat and realign it into its normal position. Avulsions most often involve ears, fingers, and hands.

An **amputation** involves the cutting or tearing off of a body part, such as a finger, toe, hand, foot, arm, or leg.

What to Do

1. Protect yourself against disease by wearing latex gloves. If latex gloves are not available, use several layers of gauze pads, plastic wrap or bags, or waterproof material. You can even have the victim apply pressure with his or her own hand. Your bare hand should be used *only* as a last resort.

2. Expose the wound by removing or cutting the clothing to see where the blood is coming from.

3. Control bleeding by using direct pressure and, if needed, the other methods described in Chapter 6.

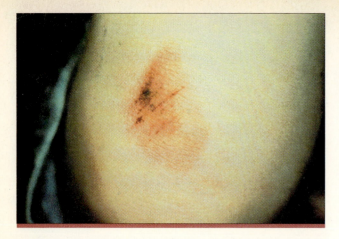

Abrasion

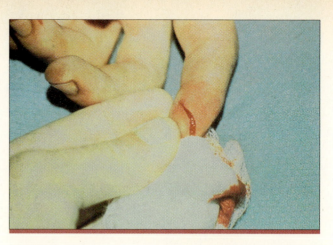

Laceration

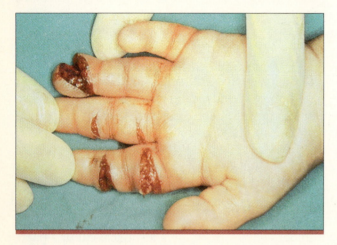

Incision

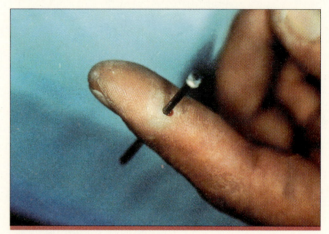

Puncture

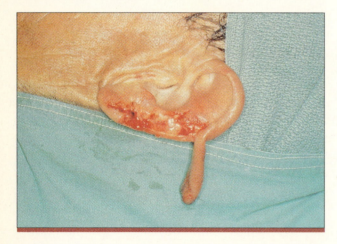

Avulsion

Cleaning a Wound

A victim's wound should be cleaned to help prevent infection. Wound cleaning may restart bleeding, but it should be done anyway. For severe bleeding, leave the pressure bandage in place until you are certain that bleeding has stopped.

1. Scrub your hands vigorously with soap and water. Then, if they are available, put on latex gloves.
2. Clean the wound.
   For a shallow wound (e.g., laceration, incision):
   • Wash inside it with soap and water.
   • Irrigate the wound with water (use water that is clean enough to drink). Run water directly into the wound and allow it to run out. Irrigation with water needs pressure (minimum 5 to 8 psi) for adequate tissue cleansing. Water from a faucet provides the pressure and the amount needed. Pouring the water or using a bulb syringe is not forceful enough.

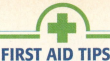

FIRST AID TIPS

Wound Care: What the Medical Literature Says
- Soaking wounds is not effective.
- Scrubbing wounds is debatable.
- Irrigating wounds need a minimum of 5–8 psi of pressure for tissue cleansing.
- Not closing a wound (e.g., with butterfly bandages, Steri-strips), especially a dirty wound, reduces the risk of infection.
- Applying antiseptic solutions (e.g., Merthiolate, Mercurochrome, iodine, isopropyl alcohol, hydrogen peroxide) can injure wounded tissues.
- Applying antibiotic ointment (e.g., Neosporin, Polysporin) reduces the risk of infection.

Source: J. M. Howell et al., "Outpatient Wound Preparation and Care: A National Survey," *Annals of Emergency Medicine* 21: 976–981 (1992).

For a wound with a high risk for infection (e.g., an animal bite, a very dirty or ragged wound, a puncture), seek medical attention for wound cleaning. If you are in a remote setting (greater than one hour from medical attention), clean the wound as best you can. If desired and it is available, apply Betadine 10-percent prep solution (not the surgical scrub solution) that has been diluted to 1 percent. Undiluted Betadine will damage tissue and affect wound healing.

3. With sterile tweezers, remove small objects not flushed out by irrigation. A dirty abrasion or other wound that is not cleaned will leave a "tattoo" on the victim's skin.

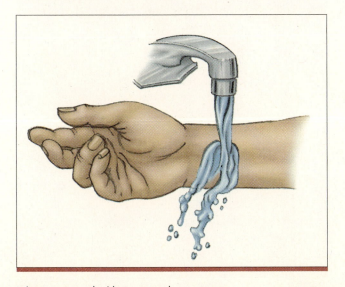

Irrigate a wound with water under pressure.

CAUTION: DO NOT
- clean large, extremely dirty, or life-threatening wounds. Let hospital emergency department personnel do the cleaning.
- scrub a wound. Scrubbing a wound is debatable, and it can bruise the tissue.

---

4. Cover the wound with a sterile and, if possible, nonstick dressing. Keep the dressing clean and dry. To keep the dressing in place on an arm or leg, use a self-adhering roller bandage or tape; on other parts of the body, tape the four sides of the dressing onto the skin. For a shallow wound, an antibiotic ointment can be applied.
5. Change the dressing daily, more often if it gets wet or dirty.

CAUTION: DO NOT
- irrigate a wound with full-strength iodine preparations (e.g., Betadine 10%) or isopropyl alcohol (70%). They kill body cells as well as bacteria and are painful. Also, some people are allergic to iodine.
- use hydrogen peroxide. It does not kill bacteria, and it adversely affects capillary blood flow and wound healing.
- use antibiotic ointment on wounds that require sutures or on puncture wounds (the ointment may prevent drainage). Use an antibiotic ointment only on abrasions and shallow wounds.
- soak a wound to clean it. No evidence supports the effectiveness of soaking.
- close the wound with tape (e.g., butterfly tape, Steri-strips). Infection is more likely when bacteria are trapped in the wound. If an unsightly scar later develops, it can be fixed later by a plastic surgeon. An extremity (e.g., hand, foot) wound can be sutured within 6 to 8 hours of the injury. Suturing of a head or trunk wound can wait up to 24 hours after the injury. Some wounds can be sutured 3 to 5 days after the injury.
- breathe on a wound or the dressing.

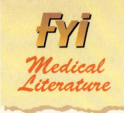

Wound Irrigation Prevents Wound Infection

Emergency physicians treat an estimated 10 million traumatic wounds annually in the United States. Different methods of wound management have been developed to help minimize wound infection. Use of systemic and topical antibiotics remains controversial. Numerous studies show the benefits of high-pressure irrigation of wounds. One study used 531 patients with traumatic wounds to compare three of the more commonly used wound irrigants in preventing wound infections: normal saline, 1-percent Betadine, and Shur-Clens. The researchers concluded that no difference in infection rates between the three irrigants existed and that the mechanical action of high-pressure irrigation, not the solution used, is the most important method of preventing wound infection.

Source: D. J. Dire, "A Comparison of Wound Irrigation Solutions Used in the Emergency Department," *Annals of Emergency Medicine* 19(6):704–708 (June 1990).

Covering a Wound

For a small wound that does not require sutures, cover it with a thin layer of antibiotic ointment (e.g., Neosporin or Polysporin). Such ointments can kill a great many bacteria and rarely cause allergic reactions. They are available without prescription.

Cover the wound with a sterile dressing, a non-stick type. Do not close the wound with tape (butterflies or Steri-strips). Bacteria may remain, leading to a greater chance of infection than if the wound were left open and covered by a sterile dressing. Closing a wound should be left to a physician.

Dressings and bandages are two different kinds of first aid supplies. A **dressing** is applied over a wound to control bleeding and prevent contamination. A **bandage** holds the dressing in place. Dressings should be sterile or as clean as possible; bandages need not be.

If a wound bleeds after a dressing has been applied and the dressing becomes stuck, leave it on as long as the wound is healing. Pulling the scab loose to change the dressing retards healing and increases the chance of infection. If a dressing must be re-moved, soak it in warm water to help soften the scab and make removal easier.

If a dressing becomes wet, change it. A wet dressing is an excellent breeding ground for bacteria. Dirty dressings should be changed for a better appearance.

When to Seek Medical Attention

High-risk wounds should receive medical attention. Examples of high-risk wounds include those with embedded foreign material (such as gravel), animal and human bites, puncture wounds, and ragged wounds. Sutures, if needed, are best placed within six to eight hours after the injury. Anyone who has not had a tetanus vaccination within 10 years, 5 years in the case of a dirty wound, should seek medical attention within 72 hours to update his or her tetanus inoculation status.

Wound Infection

Any wound, large or small, can become infected. Once an infection begins, damage can be extensive, so prevention is the best way to avoid the problem. A wound should be cleaned using the procedures described above.

It is important to know how to recognize and treat an infected wound. Most infected wounds swell and become reddened. They may give a sensation of warmth and develop a throbbing pain and

OTC Treatment for Wounds (Days to Heal)

Polysporin™—8.2 days
Neosporin™—9.2 days
Johnson & Johnson First Aid Cream™—9.8 days
Mercurochrome—13.1 days
No treatment—13.3 days
Bactine™ spray—14.2 days
Merthiolate—14.2 days
Hydrogen peroxide (3%)—14.3 days
Campho-Phenique—15.4 days
Tincture of iodine—15.7 days

Source: J. J. Leyden, "Comparison of Topical Antibiotic Ointments, a Wound Protectant, and Antiseptics for the Treatment of Human Blister Wounds Contaminated with *Staphylococcus aureus,*" *Journal of Family Practice* 24(6):601–604 (1987).

a pus discharge. The victim may develop a fever and swelling of the lymph nodes. One or more red streaks may appear, leading from the wound toward the heart. This is a serious sign that the infection is spreading and could cause death. If chills and fever develop, the infection has reached the circulatory system (known as blood poisoning).

Factors that increase the likelihood for wound infection include:

- dirty and foreign material left in the wound
- ragged or crushed tissue
- injury to an underlying bone, joint, or tendon
- bite wounds (human or animal)
- hand and foot wounds
- puncture wounds or other wounds that cannot drain

In the early stages of an infection, a physician may allow a wound to be treated at home. Such home treatment would include:

- keeping the area clean
- soaking the wound in warm water or applying warm, wet packs
- elevating the infected part
- applying antibiotic ointment
- changing dressings daily
- seeking medical help if the infection persists or becomes worse

Tetanus

Tetanus is also called "lockjaw" because of its best-known symptom, tightening of the jaw muscles. Tetanus is caused by a toxin produced by a bacterium. The bacterium, which is found throughout the world, forms a spore that can survive in a variety of environments for years. The World Health Organization reports that tetanus causes at least 50,000—perhaps even up to one million—deaths each year.

Millions of adults in the United States have let their tetanus immunizations lapse; a smaller number have never been vaccinated. In addition, antibody levels in immunized children decline over time; one-fifth of youngsters ages 10 to 16 do not have protective levels. Only 50 cases a year of tetanus are reported. Tetanus is not communicable from one person to another.

The bacterium by itself does not cause tetanus. But when it enters a wound that contains little oxygen (e.g., a puncture wound), the bacterium can produce a **toxin,** which is a powerful poison. The toxin travels through the nervous system to the brain and the spinal cord. It then causes contractions of certain muscle groups (particularly in the jaw). There is no known antidote to the toxin once it enters the nervous system.

It is not just stepping on a rusty nail that can bring on the disease. Tetanus bacteria are commonly found in soil, street dust, organic garden fertilizers, and pet feces, and even minor cuts can introduce them into the bloodstream.

A vaccination can completely prevent tetanus. Everyone needs an initial series of vaccinations to prepare the immune system to defend against the toxin. Then a booster shot once every 5 to 10 years is sufficient to jog the immune system's memory.

The guidelines for tetanus immunization boosters are as follows:

- Anyone with a wound who has never been immunized against tetanus should be given a tetanus vaccine and booster immediately.
- A victim who was once immunized but has not received a tetanus booster within the last 10 years should receive a booster.
- A victim with a dirty wound who has not had a booster for over 5 years should receive a booster.
- Tetanus immunization shots must be given within 72 hours of the injury to be effective.

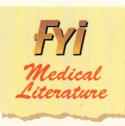

Tetanus Prevalence

Despite the wide availability of immunization against tetanus in the United States, many people are inadequately protected against that uncommon but often lethal disease. Protection was found in only 70 percent of people studied, with levels of immunity varying widely.

About 50 cases of tetanus occur in the United States each year, principally among the elderly and those who never received a primary series of vaccinations. Adults should have booster shots for tetanus every 10 years.

Source: P. J. Gergen et al., "A Population-Based Serologic Survey of Immunity to Tetanus in the United States," *New England Journal of Medicine* 332:761 (March 1995).

Amputations

Eighty to 90 percent of amputated extremities can be successfully replanted (reattached after complete amputation) so that blood flow is restored to a severely damaged but still attached extremity.

Types of Amputations

Amputations usually involve fingers, hands, and arms rather than legs. Amputations are classified according to the type of injury:

- A **guillotine amputation** is a clean-cut, complete detachment. Examples would include a finger cut off with an ax or an arm severed with a saw.
- A **crushing amputation** occurs when an extremity separates by being crushed or mashed off. An example would be a hand being caught in a roller machine.
- **Degloving** is when the skin is peeled off, much as you would take off a glove.

A crushing amputation, the most common type, has a poor chance of reattachment. A guillotine type has a much better chance because it is clean cut. Microsurgical techniques allow amputated parts to be effectively reattached 80–90 percent of the time so they function normally or nearly so.

A complete amputation may not involve heavy blood loss. That is because blood vessels tend to go into spasm, recede into the injured body parts, and shrink in diameter, resulting in a surprisingly small blood loss. More blood is seen in a partial amputation.

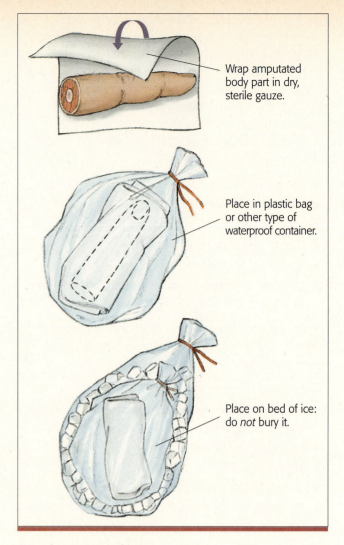

Wrap amputated body part in dry, sterile gauze.

Place in plastic bag or other type of waterproof container.

Place on bed of ice: do *not* bury it.

Care of an amputated part

What to Do

1. Control the bleeding with direct pressure and elevate the extremity. Apply a dry dressing or bulky cloths. Be sure to protect yourself against disease. Tourniquets are rarely needed and if used will destroy tissue, blood vessels, and nerves necessary for replantation.
2. Treat the victim for shock.
3. Recover the amputated part and, whenever possible, take it with the victim. However, in multicasualty cases, in reduced lighting conditions, or when untrained people transport the victim, someone may be requested to locate and take the severed body part to the hospital after the victim's departure.

4. To care for the amputated body part:
   - If possible, rinse it with clean water to remove any debris; do not scrub. The amputated portion does not need to be cleaned.
   - Wrap the amputated part with a dry sterile gauze or other clean cloth.
   - Put the wrapped amputated part in a plastic bag or other waterproof container (e.g., a cup or glass).
   - Place the bag or container with the wrapped part on a bed of ice.
5. Seek medical attention immediately.

Amputated body parts without cooling for more than 6 hours have little chance of survival; 18 hours is probably the maximum time allowable for a part that has been cooled properly. Muscles without blood lose viability within 4 to 6 hours. Fingers with tendons and ligaments can tolerate a longer amputated time period than limbs.

AMPUTATION

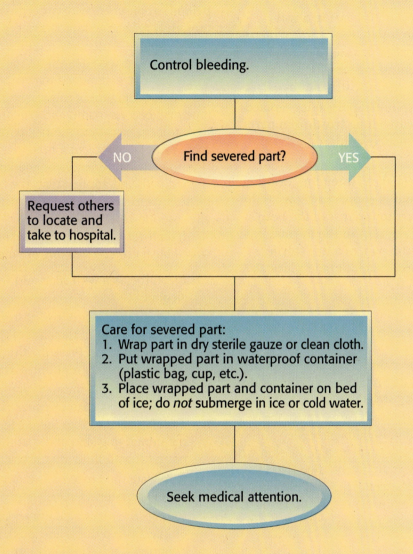

Control bleeding.

Find severed part?

NO

YES

Request others to locate and take to hospital.

Care for severed part:
1. Wrap part in dry sterile gauze or clean cloth.
2. Put wrapped part in waterproof container (plastic bag, cup, etc.).
3. Place wrapped part and container on bed of ice; do *not* submerge in ice or cold water.

Seek medical attention.

Blisters

A blister is a collection of fluid in a "bubble" under the outer layer of skin. (This section applies only to friction blisters and does not apply to blisters from burns, frostbite, drug reactions, insect or snake bites, or contact with a poisonous plant.)

Repeated rubbing of a small area of the skin will produce a blister. Blisters are so common that many people assume they are a fact of life. But blisters are avoidable, and life for many people could be more comfortable if they knew how to treat and prevent blisters.

Rubbing—as between a sock and a foot—causes stress on the skin's surface because the supporting tissue remains stationary. The stress separates the skin into two layers, and the resulting space fills with fluid. The fluid may collect either under or within the skin's outer layer, the epidermis. Because of differences in skin, blister formation varies considerably from person to person.

What to Do

When caring for a friction blister, try to (1) avoid the risk of infection, (2) minimize the victim's pain and discomfort, (3) limit the blister's development, and (4) help a fast recovery.

The best care for a particular blister is determined mainly by its size and location.

If an area on the skin becomes a "hot spot" (painful, red area), tightly apply a piece of silver aluminum duct tape, or cover it with a doughnut-shaped moleskin secured by tape.

If a blister on a foot is closed and not very painful, a conservative approach is to tape the blister tightly with duct tape or waterproof adhesive tape. The tape must remain on the blister for several days; otherwise, tearing of the blister's roof when the tape is removed may expose unprotected skin. One limitation of this approach is that the tape may become damp and contaminated and have to be replaced, at the risk of tearing the blister roof. You could also cut a hole in a piece of moleskin to fit around the blister, making a doughnut-shaped pad, and apply it over the blister. Small blisters, especially on weight-bearing areas, generally respond better if left alone.

If a blister on the foot is open, or a very painful closed blister affects walking or running:

1. Clean the area with soap and water or rubbing alcohol.
2. Drain all fluid out of the blister by making several small holes at the base of the blister with a sterilized needle. Press the fluid out. Do not remove the blister's roof unless it is torn.
3. Apply antibiotic ointment and cover it tightly with a nonstick pad or gauze pad. The pressure dressing ensures that the blister's roof sticks to the underlying skin and that the blister does not refill with fluid after it has been drained.
4. Duplicate the procedures described for treating a closed blister.
5. Change the dressing daily and check for signs of infection (redness and pus). Seek medical attention if infection develops.

With few exceptions, the blister's roof, which is the best and most comfortable "dressing," should be removed only when an infection is present. Once a blister has been opened, the area should be washed with soap to prevent further infection. For 10 to 14 days, or until new skin forms, a protective bandage or other cover should be used. A popular temporary cover is a synthetic porous membrane known as Spenco Second Skin™. Available over the counter, it is designed to absorb pressure and reduce friction against the blister site.

Even with no evidence of infection, you should consider removing the blister's roof when a partially torn blister roof may tear skin adjacent to the blister site, resulting in an even larger open wound. In

BLISTERS

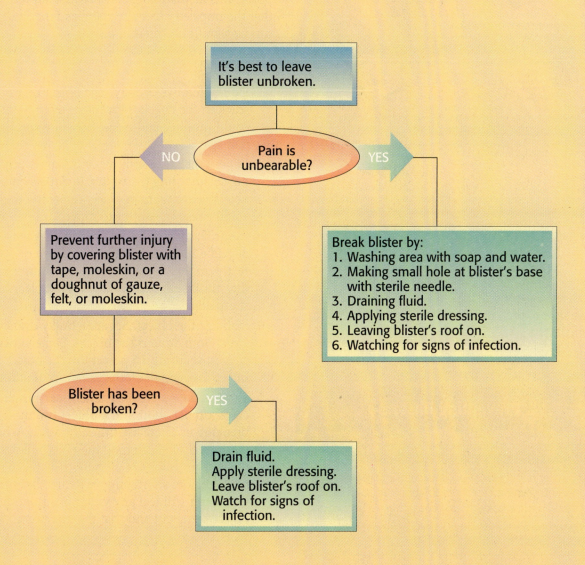

It's best to leave blister unbroken.

Pain is unbearable?

NO

YES

Prevent further injury by covering blister with tape, moleskin, or a doughnut of gauze, felt, or moleskin.

Break blister by:
1. Washing area with soap and water.
2. Making small hole at blister's base with sterile needle.
3. Draining fluid.
4. Applying sterile dressing.
5. Leaving blister's roof on.
6. Watching for signs of infection.

Blister has been broken?

YES

Drain fluid.
Apply sterile dressing.
Leave blister's roof on.
Watch for signs of infection.

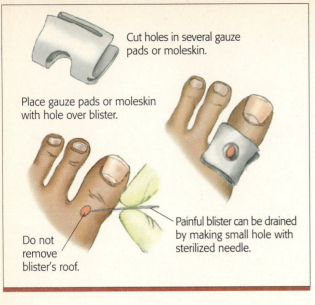

Cut holes in several gauze pads or moleskin.

Place gauze pads or moleskin with hole over blister.

Do not remove blister's roof.

Painful blister can be drained by making small hole with sterilized needle.

Blister care

such cases, use sterilized scissors to remove the loose skin of the blister's roof up to the edge of the normal tissue.

Preventing Blisters

Keeping the skin lubricated and protected will reduce the likelihood of a blister forming. Applying duct or adhesive tape to problem areas, such as around a big toe, can help reduce blister formation by allowing the sock to rub against the tape instead of directly against the skin.

Wearing proper clothing also can prevent blisters. For example, acrylic socks are considered superior to cotton socks in avoiding foot blisters because they are made in layers that are designed to absorb friction. Socks with CoolMax™ construction are highly recommended. Avoid tube socks made of any material because their less precise fit tends to cause more friction than regular, fitted socks. Wear gloves to protect the skin on your hands.

Anything that can be done to keep the skin dry can also reduce blister formation. Moist skin is more susceptible to blisters than either very dry or very wet skin. One method is to wear socks that wick moisture from the skin. Interestingly, the application of antiperspirants to the feet has been shown to reduce the formation of serious blisters.

Impaled Objects

Impaled objects come in all shapes and sizes, from pencils and screwdrivers to knives, glass, fence posts, and cactus spines. Proper first aid requires that the impaled object be stabilized, because there can be significant internal damage.

What to Do

1. Do not remove or move the object unless it is stuck in the cheek. Movement of any kind could produce additional bleeding and tissue damage.
2. Expose the area. Remove or cut away any clothing surrounding the injury. If clothes cover the object, leave them in place; removing them could cause the object to move.
3. Control any bleeding with direct pressure. Straddle the object with gauze. Do not press directly on the object or along the wound next to the cutting edge, especially if the object has sharp edges.
4. Stabilize the object. Secure a bulky dressing or clean cloth around the object. Some experts suggest securing 75 percent of the object with bulky dressing or cloths to reduce motion.
5. Shorten the object only if necessary. In most cases, do not shorten the object by cutting or breaking it. There are times, however, when cutting off or shortening the object allows for easier transportation. Be sure to stabilize the object before shortening it. Remember that the victim will feel any vibrations from the object being cut and that the injury could be worsened.

Impaled Object in the Cheek

The only time it is safe to remove an impaled object outside a medical setting is when the object is in the victim's cheek.

What to Do

1. Examine the injury inside the mouth. If the object extends through the cheek and you are more than one hour from medical help, consider removing it.
2. Remove the object. Place two fingers next to the object, straddling it. Gently pull it in the direction from which it entered. If it cannot be removed easily, leave it in place and secure it with bulky dressings.

3. Control bleeding. After you have removed the object, place dressings over the wound inside the mouth, between the cheek and the teeth. The dressings will help control bleeding and will not interfere with the victim's airway. Also place a dressing on the outside wound.

Impaled Object in the Eye

If an object is impaled in the eye, it is vital that pressure not be put on the eye. The eyeball consists of two chambers, each filled with fluid. *Do not exert any pressure against the eyeball;* fluid can be forced out of it, worsening the injury.

What to Do

1. Stabilize the object. For a long protruding object, stabilize it with bulky dressings or clean cloths. For short objects, surround the eye without touching the object with a doughnut-shaped (ring) pad covered with a roller bandage. You can place a protective paper cup over the affected eye to prevent accidental bumping of the object.
2. Cover the unaffected eye. Most experts suggest that the unaffected eye also be covered to prevent sympathetic eye movement (i.e., the injured eye moving if the unaffected one does, thereby aggravating the injury). Remember that the victim is unable to see when both eyes are covered and may be anxious. Make sure you explain to the victim everything you are doing.
3. Seek medical attention immediately.

Slivers

Small slivers of wood or metal can be painful and irritating. They also can cause infection. Because of their size and common location in the fingers, removal usually can be done easily with tweezers. Sometimes, it is necessary to tease one end of the object with a sterile needle to place it in a better position for removal with tweezers. After you have removed the sliver, clean the site with soap and water and apply an adhesive strip (Band-Aid™).

Cactus Spines

Cacti are a part of the desert ecology. They also are used as ornamental plants. Infection from cactus-spine punctures is rare. Removing cactus spines is tedious because they usually are acquired in bunches, are difficult to see, and are designed by

nature to resist removal. Usually spines can easily, yet tediously, be removed with tweezers.

Another method for removing a large number of cactus spines is to coat the area with a thin layer of white woodworking glue or rubber cement and allow it to dry for at least 30 minutes. Slowly roll up the dried glue from the margins. If the glue is applied in strips rather than puddles, the rolling procedure goes more smoothly. A single layer of gauze gently pressed onto the still damp glue helps its removal after it has dried. Using tweezers and glue will remove most of the spines.

Using adhesive tape, duct tape, or Scotch tape, while quick and easy, removes only 30 percent of the spines, even after multiple attempts. Do not use Super Glue (or other similar product) to remove cactus spines. Not only does it fail to roll up when applied to the skin, it welds the spines to the skin. There is also the risk that the skin will permanently bond to anything it touches.

Fishhooks

Tape an embedded fishhook in place and do *not* try to remove it if injury to a nearby body part (e.g., eye) or an underlying structure (e.g., blood vessel or nerve) is possible or if the victim is uncooperative.

If only the point and not the barb of a fishhook has penetrated the skin, remove the fishhook by backing it out. Then treat the wound like a puncture wound. Seek medical advice for a possible tetanus shot.

If the hook's barb has entered the skin, follow these procedures:

1. If medical care is near, transport the victim and have a physician remove the hook.
2. If you are in a remote area, far from medical care, remove the hook by either the pliers method or the fishline method.

Pliers Method ("Push and Cut")

Use extreme care with the pliers method of fishhook removal because it can produce further severe injury if the hook is pushed into blood vessels, nerves, or tendons. Use pliers with tempered jaws that can cut through a hook. The proper kind of pliers is usually unavailable, or sometimes the barb is buried too deep to be pushed through. Test the pliers by first cutting a similar fishhook.

1. Use cold or hard pressure around the hook to provide temporary numbness.

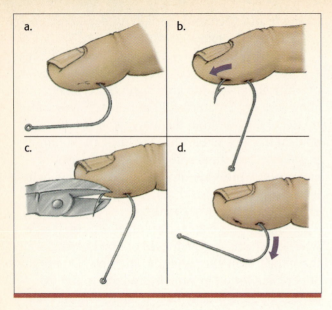

Fishhook removal: Pliers method

2. Push the embedded hook further in, in a shallow curve, until the point and the barb come out through the skin.
3. Cut the barb off, then back the hook out the way it came in.
4. After removing the hook, treat the wound and seek medical attention for a possible tetanus shot.

Fishline Method ("Push and Pull")

1. Loop a piece of fishline over the bend or curve of the embedded hook.
2. Stabilize the victim's hooked body area.
3. Use cold or hard pressure around the hook to provide temporary numbness.
4. With one hand, press down on the hook's shank and eye while the other hand sharply jerks the fishline that is over the hook's bend or curve. The jerk movement should be parallel to the skin's surface. The hook will neatly come out of the same hole it entered, causing little pain.

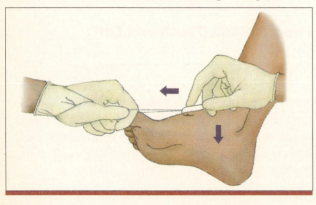

Fishhook removal: Fishline method

5. After removing the hook, treat the wound and seek medical attention for a possible tetanus shot.

Closed Wounds

A closed wound happens when a blunt object strikes the body. The skin is not broken, but tissue and blood vessels beneath the skin's surface are crushed, causing bleeding within a confined area. There are three types of closed wounds:

- **Bruises and contusions** occur when blood collects under the skin in the injured area. The victim will experience pain and swelling (immediately or within 24–48 hours). As blood accumulates, a black-and-blue mark may appear.
- A **hematoma** is a clot of blood under the skin. There may be a lump or bluish discoloration.
- **Crush injuries** are caused by extreme forces, which can injure vital organs and bones without breaking open the skin. Crush injuries may indicate an underlying problem such as a fracture. Signs and symptoms include discoloration, swelling, pain, and loss of use.

What to Do

1. Control bleeding by applying an ice pack for no more than 20 minutes.
2. Apply an elastic bandage with a gauze pad between the bandage and the skin.
3. Check for a possible fracture.
4. Elevate an injured extremity above the victim's heart level to decrease pain and swelling.

Wounds That Require Medical Attention

At some point, you probably will have to decide about obtaining medical assistance for a wounded victim. As a guideline, seek medical attention for the following conditions:

- arterial bleeding
- uncontrolled bleeding
- a deep incision, laceration, or avulsion that
  • goes into the muscle or bone
  • is located on a body part that bends (e.g., elbow or knee)

- tends to gape widely
- is located on the thumb or palm of the hand (nerves may be affected)
- a large or deep puncture wound
- a large embedded object or a deeply embedded object of any size
- foreign matter left in the wound
- human or animal bite
- possibility of a noticeable scar (sutured cuts usually heal with less scarring than unsutured ones)
- a wide, gaping wound
- an eyelid cut (to prevent later drooping)
- a slit lip (easily scarred)
- internal bleeding
- any wound you are not certain how to treat
- victim's immunization against tetanus not up to date

Sutures (Stitches)

If sutures are needed, they should be made by a physician within six to eight hours of the injury. Suturing wounds allows faster healing, reduces infection, and lessens scarring.

Some wounds do not usually require sutures:

- wounds in which the skin's cut edges tend to fall together
- cuts less than one inch long that are not deep

Rather than close a gaping wound with butterfly bandages or Steri-strips, cover the wound with sterile gauze. Closing the wound might trap bacteria inside, resulting in an infection. In most cases, a physician can be reached in time for sutures to be made; if not, a wound without sutures will still heal but with scars. Scar tissue can be attended to later by a plastic surgeon.

Gunshot Wounds

Guns are abundant in the United States. It is estimated that about one-half of all American homes have a firearm.

A bullet causes injury in the following ways, depending on its velocity, or speed:

- *Laceration and crushing.* When the bullet penetrates, the tissue is crushed and forced apart. That is the main effect of low-velocity bullets. The crushing and laceration caused by the passage of the bullet usually is not serious unless vital organs or major blood vessels are injured. The bullet damages only those tissues with which it comes into direct contact, and the wound is comparable to that caused by weapons such as knives.
- *Shock waves and temporary cavitation.* When a bullet penetrates, a shock wave exerts outward pressure from the bullet's path. That pushes tissues away. A temporary cavity is created, which can be as much as 30 times the diameter of the bullet. As the cavity is formed, a negative pressure develops inside, creating a vacuum. The vacuum then draws debris in with it. Temporary cavitation occurs only with high-velocity bullets and is the main reason for their immensely destructive effect. The cavitation lasts only a millisecond but can damage muscles, nerves, blood vessels, and bone.

In a *penetrating* wound, there is a bullet entry point but no exit. In a *perforating* wound, there are both entry and exit points. The exit wound of a high-velocity bullet is larger than the entrance wound; the exit wound from a low-velocity bullet is about the same size as the entry wound. In a bullet wound at very close range, the entrance wound may be larger than the exit wound because the gases from the gun's muzzle contribute to the surface tissue damage.

Bullets sometimes hit hard tissue (i.e., bone) and may bounce around in the body cavities and cause a great deal of damage to tissue and organs. Moreover, bone chips can be forced to other body areas and cause damage. A split or misshapen bullet does greater damage than a smooth bullet going in a straight line because it tumbles, exerting its force over a greater diameter.

What to Do

Regardless of the type of wound, initial care is roughly the same as for any other wound.

1. Check the ABCDs.
2. Expose the wound(s). Look for entrance and exit wounds.
3. Control bleeding with direct pressure.
4. Apply dry, sterile dressing(s) to the wound(s) and bandage securely in place.
5. Treat for shock.
6. Keep the victim calm and quiet.
7. Seek immediate medical care.

CAUTION: DO NOT

- try to remove material from a gunshot wound. The hospital emergency department personnel will clean the wound.

Legal Aspects

Because gunshot wounds will involve contact with law enforcement agencies and possibly testifying in court, carefully observe the scene and the victim. Keep an accurate record of your observations. Preserve possible evidence, such as cartridge casings or shells, for the police. Do not touch or move anything unless absolutely necessary to treat the victim. All gunshot wounds must be reported to the police regardless of whether they are intentional (suicide, assault, murder, self-defense) or accidental.

DRESSINGS AND BANDAGES

Dressings

A dressing covers an open wound—it touches the wound. Whenever possible, a dressing should be:

- sterile. If a sterile dressing is not available, use a clean cloth (e.g., handkerchief, washcloth, towel)
- larger than the wound
- thick, soft, and compressible so pressure is evenly distributed over the wound
- lint free

A dressing's purposes are to:

- control bleeding
- prevent infection and contamination
- absorb blood and wound drainage
- protect the wound from further injury

CAUTION: DO NOT

- use fluffy cotton or cotton balls as a dressing. Cotton fibers can get in the wound and be difficult to remove.
- remove a blood-soaked dressing until the bleeding stops. Cover it with a new dressing.
- pull off a dressing stuck to a wound. If it needs to be removed, soak it off in warm water.

Types of Dressings

Use commercial dressings whenever possible. Dressings used in most first aid situations are commercially prepared, but dressings may need to be improvised.

- *Gauze pads* are used for small wounds. They come in separately wrapped packages of various sizes (e.g., 2 inch by 2 inch; 4 inch by 4 inch) and are sterile, unless the package is broken. Some gauze pads have a special coat-

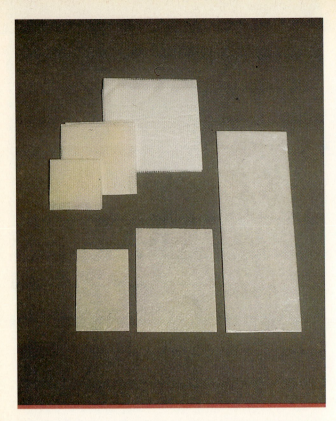

Gauze pads

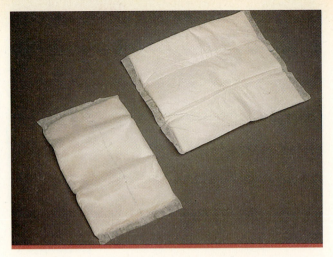

Trauma dressings

ble (e.g., handkerchief, towel). Either use the cleanest cloth available or, in some conditions and if time allows, sterilize a cloth by boiling it and allowing it to dry, by ironing it for several minutes, or by soaking it in rubbing alcohol and allowing it to dry.

ing to keep them from sticking to the wound and are especially helpful for burns or wounds secreting fluids.

- *Adhesive strips* (e.g., Band-Aids™) are used for small cuts and abrasions and are a combination of both a sterile dressing and a bandage.
- *Trauma dressings* are made of large, thick, absorbent, sterile materials. Individually wrapped sanitary napkins can serve because of their bulk and absorbency, but they usually are not sterile.
- When commercial sterile dressings are not available, an *improvised dressing* should be as clean, absorbent, soft, and free of lint as possi-

Applying a Sterile Dressing
What to Do

1. If possible, wash your hands.
2. Use a dressing large enough to extend beyond the wound's edges. Hold the dressing by a corner. Place the dressing directly over the wound. Do not slide it on.
3. Cover the dressing with one of the types of bandages described on pages 151–152.

▼ **CAUTION: DO NOT**
- **touch any part of the wound or any part of the dressing that will be in contact with the wound.**
- **cough, breathe, or talk over the wound or dressing.**

Bandages

A bandage can be used to:

- hold a dressing in place over an open wound
- apply direct pressure over a dressing to control bleeding
- prevent or reduce swelling
- provide support and stability for an extremity or joint

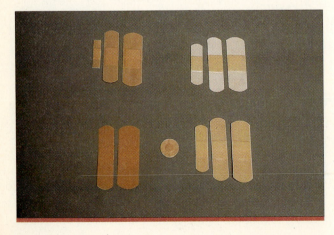

Adhesive strips

A bandage should be clean but need not be sterile.

CAUTION: DO NOT

- apply a bandage directly over a wound. Put a sterile dressing on first.
- bandage so tightly as to restrict blood circulation. Always check the extremity's pulse. If you cannot feel the pulse, loosen the bandage.
- bandage so loosely that the dressing will slip. This is the most common bandaging error. Bandages tend to stretch after a short time.
- leave loose ends. They might get caught.
- cover fingers or toes unless they are injured. They need to be observed for color change should circulation be impaired.
- use elastic bandages over a wound. First aiders have a tendency to apply them too tightly.
- apply a circular bandage around a victim's neck—strangulation may occur.
- start a roller bandage above the wound. Instead, start below the wound and work upward.

Signs that a bandage is too tight:

- blue tinge of the fingernails or toenails
- blue or pale skin color
- tingling or loss of sensation
- coldness of the extremity
- inability to move the fingers or toes

Bandages should be applied firmly enough to keep dressings and splints in place but not so tight as to cause injury to the part or to impede blood circulation.

A square knot is preferred because it is neat, attractive, holds well, and can be easily untied. However, the type of knot is not important. If the knot or the bandage is likely to cause the victim discomfort, a pad should be placed between the knot or bandage and the body.

Types of Bandages

There are four basic types of bandages:

- *Roller bandages* come in various widths, lengths, and types of material. For best results, use different widths for different body areas:
  - 1-inch width for fingers
  - 2-inch width for wrists, hands, feet
  - 3-inch width for ankles, elbows, arms
  - 4-inch width for knees, legs

  Self-adhering, conforming bandages come as rolls of slightly elastic, gauzelike material in various widths. Their self-adherent quality makes them easy to use.

  Gauze rollers are cotton, rigid, and nonelastic. They come in various widths (1, 2, and 3 inches) and usually are 10 yards long.

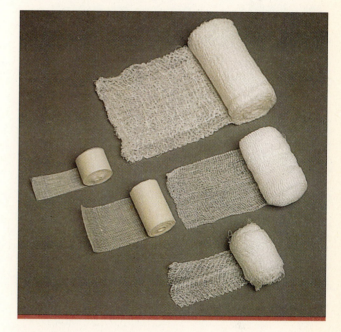

Self-adhering conforming bandages of various sizes

  Elastic roller bandages are used for compression on sprains, strains, and contusions and comes in various widths. Elastic bandages are not usually applied over dressings covering a wound.

  When commercial roller bandages are unavailable, you can make *improvised bandages* from belts, neckties, or strips of cloth torn from a sheet or other similar material.

- *Triangular bandages* are available commercially or can be made from a 36- to 40-inch square of preshrunk cotton muslin material that is cut diagonally from corner to corner to produce two triangular pieces of cloth. The longest side is called the *base*; the corner directly across from the base is the *point*; the other two corners are called *ends*. A triangular bandage may be applied two ways:

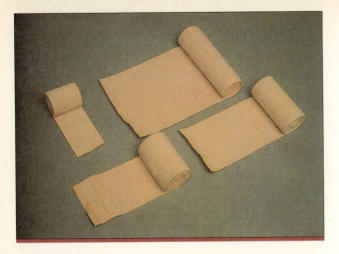

Elastic bandages of various sizes

- Fully opened (not folded). Best used for an arm sling. When used to hold dressings in place, fully opened triangular bandages do not apply sufficient pressure on the wound.
- As a cravat (folded triangular). The point is folded to the center of the base and folded in half again from the top to the base to form a cravat. It is used to hold splints in place, to apply pressure evenly over a dressing, or as a swathe (binder) around the victim's body to stabilize an injured arm in an arm sling.
- *Adhesive tape* comes in rolls and in a variety of widths. It is often used to secure roller bandages and small dressings in place. For those allergic to adhesive tape, use paper tape or special dermatologic tape.

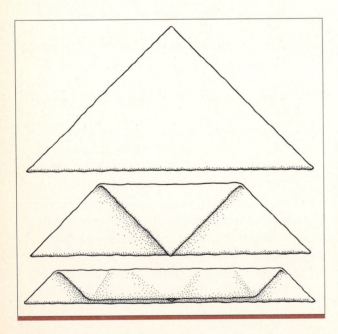

Triangular bandage folded into a cravat

FIRST AID TIPS

Removing Adhesive Tape

When you first apply the tape, fold over one end (sticky sides together) to make a tab. Then when it comes time to remove the tape, you can grasp the starter tab. No need to pick at the tape (and the victim's skin) to get the strip started.

To remove adhesive tape from the skin, gently lift the tape with one hand and with the other gently push the skin down and away from the tape.

Save time and frustration by leaving a tab on the end of the roll of tape for quick access the next time you need it.

Adhesive Bandage

To make an adhesive bandage snug on a chin, knee, or elbow, first cut the adhesive parts of the bandage lengthwise, but do not cut into the pad. Place the pad horizontally over the cut or wound. Then bring the bottom strips of the adhesive up and smooth them on the skin. Bring the top parts of the adhesive strips down and smooth them on the skin. Result: an adhesive bandage that contours to the wound.

CAUTION: DO NOT

- apply adhesive tape over or to clothing or other material because it can slip. Adhesive tape should be applied directly to the skin.

- *Adhesive strips* are used for small cuts and abrasions and are a combination of a dressing and a bandage.

  To apply an adhesive strip:

  1. Remove the wrapping and hold the dressing, pad-side down, by the protective strips.

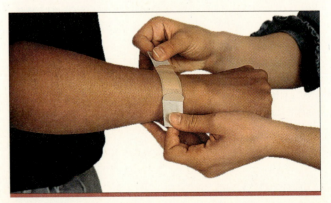

Applying an adhesive strip

2. Peel back, but do not remove, the protective strips. Without touching the dressing pad, place it directly onto the wound.
3. Carefully pull away the protective strips. Press the ends and edges down.

Applying a Roller Bandage

With a little ingenuity, you can apply a roller bandage to almost any body part. Self-adhering, conforming roller bandages eliminate the need for many of the complicated bandaging techniques required with standard gauze roller, cravat, and triangular bandages.

Circular Method: Forehead, Ear, Eyes (3- or 4-inch roller)

The roller bandage encircles the part with several layers of bandage on top of the previous ones. For an injured eye, cover both eyes to prevent the injured eye from moving.

What to Do

1. Place end of bandage over dressing covering the wound (or eyes) and wrap the bandage around the head.
2. When wrapping a roller bandage around the head, keep the bandage near the eyebrows (except for the eyes when they are covered) and low on the back of the head to prevent the bandage from slipping.

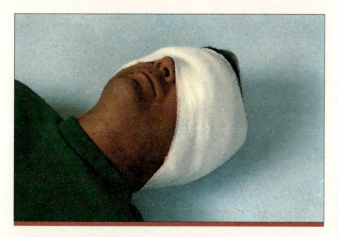

Bandaging both eyes stops eye movement.

Spiral Method: Arm or Leg (3-inch roller for arm; 4-inch roller for leg)

What to Do

1. Start at the narrow part of an arm or leg and wrap upward toward the wider part to make the bandage more secure. Start below and at the edge of the dressing.
2. Make two straight anchoring turns with the bandage.

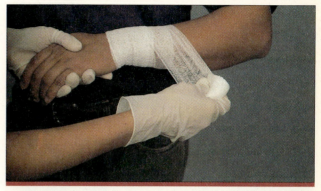

3. Make a series of spiral turns, working up the arm or leg. Each turn should overlap the preceding one by about three-fourths of the previous turn's width. If more support is needed or if the wrapping applies uneven pressure, wrap the part with criss-cross (figure-8) turns.

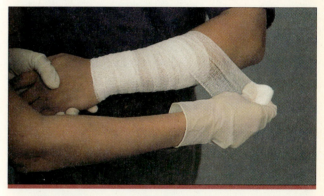

4. Finish with two straight turns and secure the bandage.

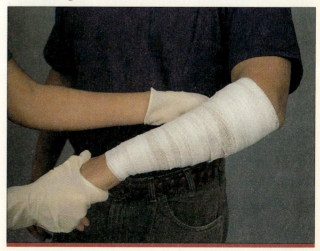

Figure-8 Method

Use this method of applying a roller bandage to hold dressings or to provide compression at or near a joint (e.g., ankle). The figure-8 method involves continuous spiral loops of bandage, one up and one down, crossing each other to form an "8."

Elbow or Knee   (3-inch roller for elbow; 4-inch roller for knee)

What to Do

1. Bend the elbow or knee slightly and make two straight anchoring turns with the bandage over the elbow point or kneecap.

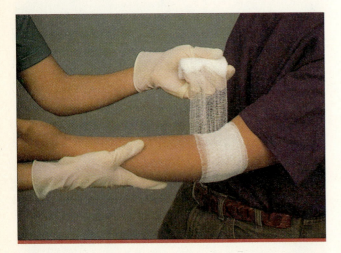

2. Bring the bandage above the joint to the upper arm or leg, and make one turn, covering half to three-fourths of the bandage from the first turn.

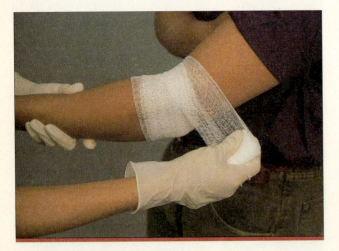

3. Bring the bandage just under the joint and make one turn around the lower arm or leg, covering half to three-fourths of the first straight turn.

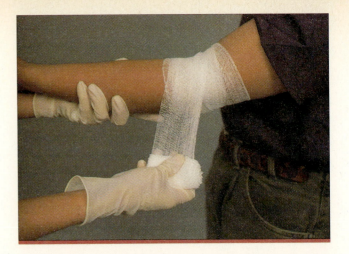

4. Continue alternating the turns in a figure-8 maneuver by covering only half to three-fourths of the previous layer each time.
5. Finish by making two straight turns and secure the end.

Hand (2- or 3-inch roller)

What to Do

Method 1

1. Make two straight anchoring turns with the bandage around the palm of the hand.

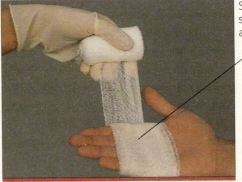

Start with 2 straight turns around palm.

2. Carry the bandage diagonally across the back of the hand and then around the wrist and back across the palm.

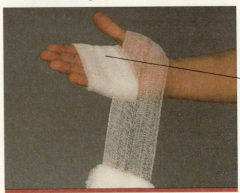

Diagonal turn across back of hand, around wrist, and back across palm.

3. Complete several figure-8 turns, overlapping each by about three-fourths of the previous bandage width.

Make several figure-8 turns, overlapping ¾ of previous layer.

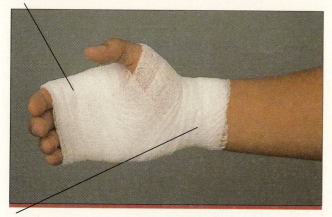

Make 2 straight turns at wrist and secure the end.

4. Make two straight turns around the wrist, and secure the bandage.

Method 2

1. Make two straight anchoring turns with the bandage around the wrist.

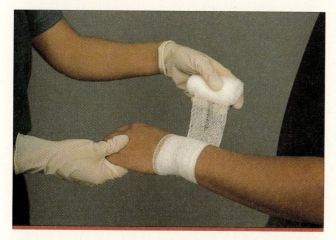

2. Proceed diagonally across the dressing (could be on palm or back of hand).

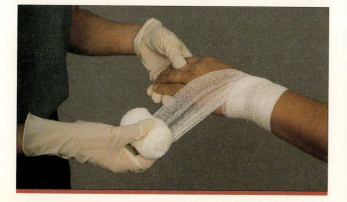

3. Circle around the lower ends of the fingers and up diagonally back across the dressing to the wrist to complete the figure-8.

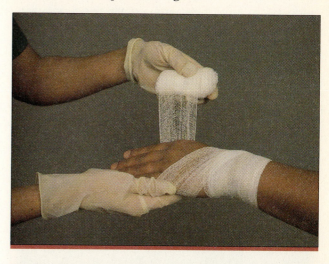

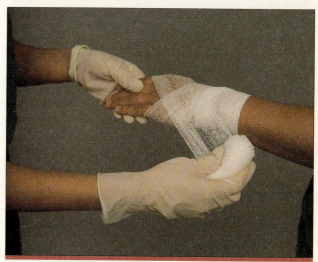

4. Repeat the figure-8 process, overlapping each by about three-fourths of the previous bandage width, until the area is sufficiently covered. Work up toward the wrist, leaving the thumb free.

5. Finish with two straight turns around the wrist and secure the bandage.

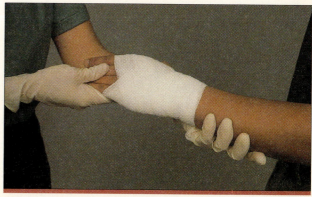

Ankle or Foot (2- or 3-inch roller) This wrapping is to hold a dressing or apply compression for treating a sprained ankle, not for supporting the ankle and foot during sports activity, which involves additional maneuvers.

What to Do

1. Make two straight anchoring turns with the bandage around the foot's instep.

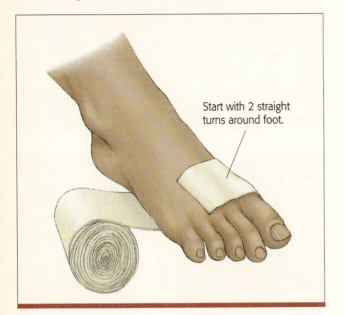

Start with 2 straight turns around foot.

2. Make several figure-8 turns by taking the bandage diagonally across the front of the foot, around the ankle, and again diagonally across the foot and under the arch.

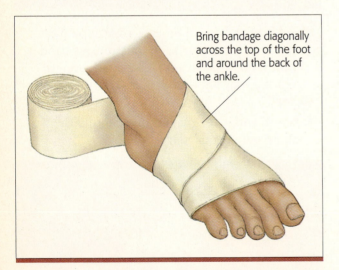

Bring bandage diagonally across the top of the foot and around the back of the ankle.

3. Make several of these figure-8 turns, each turn overlapping the previous one by about three-fourths the width of the bandage. The bandage advances up the leg.

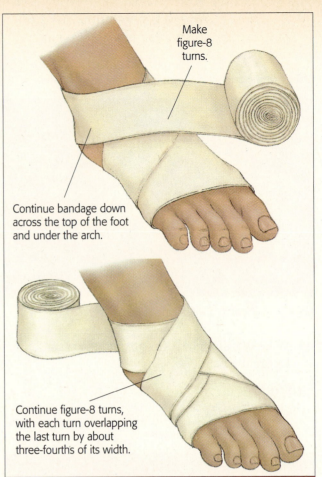

Make figure-8 turns.

Continue bandage down across the top of the foot and under the arch.

Continue figure-8 turns, with each turn overlapping the last turn by about three-fourths of its width.

4. Finish with two straight turns around the leg and secure the bandage.

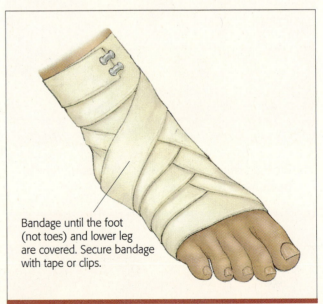

Bandage until the foot (not toes) and lower leg are covered. Secure bandage with tape or clips.

To securely fasten a roller bandage:

- Apply adhesive tape.
- Use safety pin(s).
- Use special clips provided with elastic bandage.

- Tie by either of these two methods:
  - *Loop method.* Reverse the direction of the bandage by looping it around a thumb or finger and continue back to the opposite side of the body part. Encircle the part with the looped end and the free end; tie them together.
  - *Split-tail method.* Split the end of the bandage lengthwise for about 12 inches, then tie a knot to prevent further splitting. Pass the ends in opposite directions around the body part and tie.

Applying a Triangular Bandage

A triangular bandage can be used as a sling. Slings support and protect the upper extremities. A sling is not a bandage but is used as a support for an injury to the shoulder or arm.

An arm sling can be used to support the upper arm, forearm, and hand when there are injuries to the upper extremity.

Arm Sling

What to Do

1. Support the injured arm slightly away from the chest, with the wrist and hand slightly higher than the elbow.
2. Place an open triangular bandage between the forearm and chest with its point toward the elbow and stretching well beyond it.

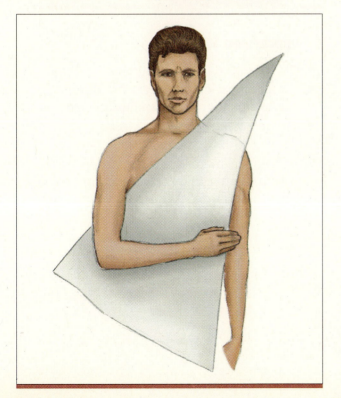

3. Pull the upper end over the shoulder on the uninjured side and around the neck to rest on the collarbone on the injured side.
4. Bring the lower end of the bandage over the hand and forearm and tie to the other end at the hollow above the collarbone.

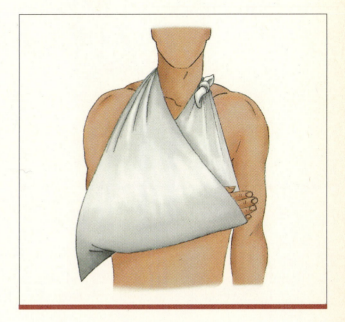

5. Bring the point around to the front of the elbow, and secure it to the sling with a safety pin or twist it into a "pigtail," which can be tied into a knot or tucked away. Placing a swathe (binder) around the arm and body further stabilizes the arm.

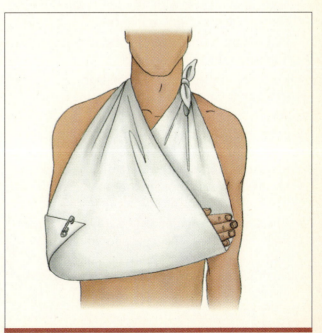

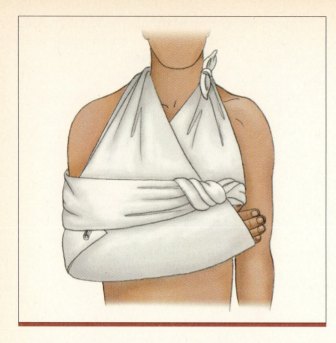

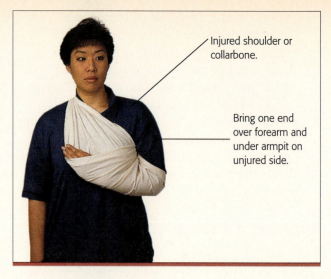

Injured shoulder or collarbone.

Bring one end over forearm and under armpit on unjured side.

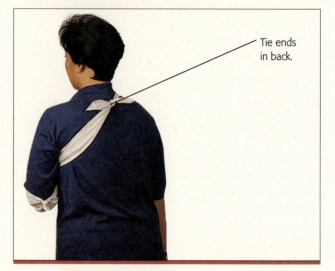

Tie ends in back.

6. Check for signs of circulation loss (e.g., pulse, fingernail color). The hand should be in a thumbs-up position within the sling and slightly above the level of the elbow (about 4 inches).

Collarbone/Shoulder Sling

What to Do

1. Support the injured arm slightly away from chest with the wrist and hand slightly higher than the elbow.
2. Place an open triangular bandage between the forearm and chest with its point toward the elbow and stretching well beyond it.
3. Pull the upper end over the shoulder on the uninjured side.
4. Bring the lower end of the bandage over the forearm and under the armpit on the injured side.
5. Continue bringing the lower end of the bandage around the victim's back where it is tied to the upper end of the triangular bandage. Placing a swathe (binder) around the arm and body further stabilizes the arm.
6. Check for signs of circulation loss (e.g., pulse, fingernail color). The hand should be in a thumbs-up position within the sling and slightly above the level of the elbow (about 4 inches).

Improvised Slings

- Place the hand inside a buttoned jacket.
- Use a belt, necktie, or other clothing item looped around the neck and the injured arm.
- Pin the sleeve of the shirt or jacket to the clothing in the desired position.
- Turn up the lower edge of the victim's jacket or shirt over the injured arm and pin it to the upper part of the jacket or shirt.

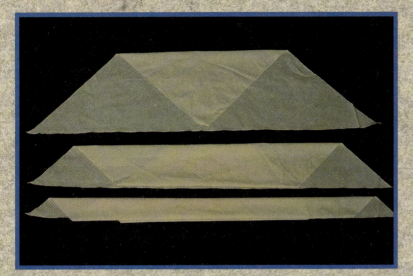

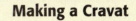

Making a Cravat

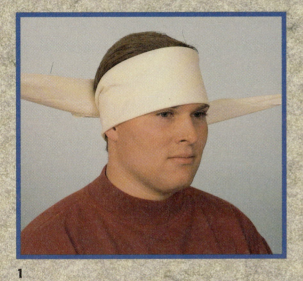

1

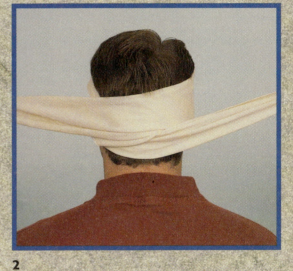

2

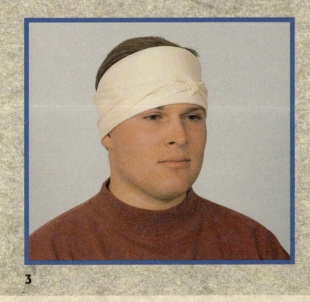

3

Cravat Bandage for Head, Ears, or Eyes

1. Place middle of bandage over the dressing covering the wound.
2. Cross the two ends snugly over each other.
3. Bring the ends back around to where the dressing is and tie the ends in a knot.

Cravat Bandage for Arm or Leg

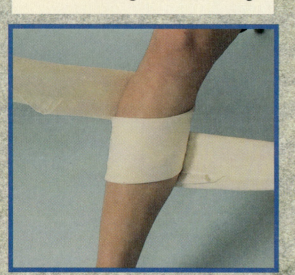

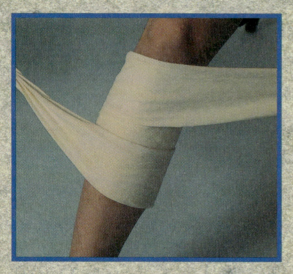

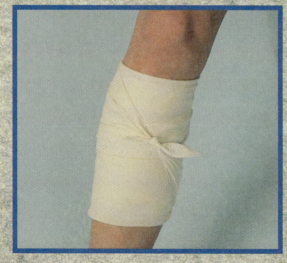

Cravat Bandage for Elbow or Knee

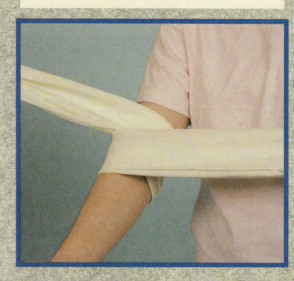

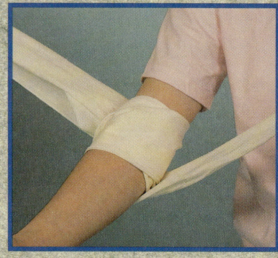

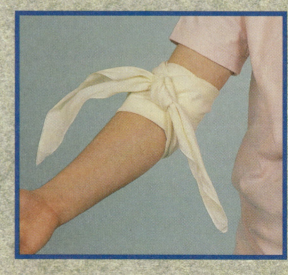

SKILL SCAN: Bandaging—Roller (Self-adhering), Figure-8

Roller Bandage for Hand: Method 1

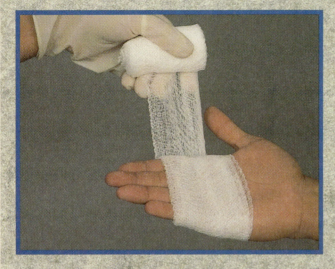

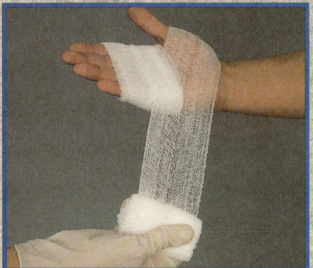

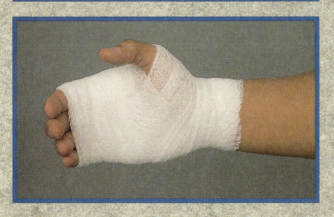

Roller Bandage for Hand: Method 2

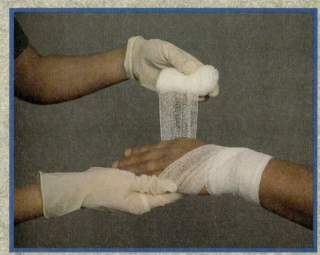

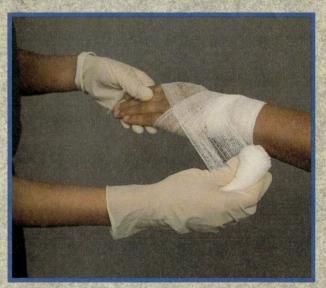

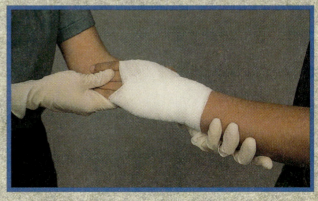

Roller Bandage for Elbow or Knee

Roller Bandage for Ankle

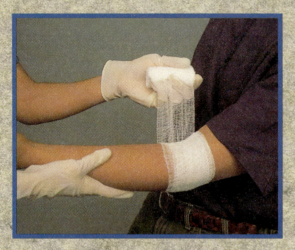

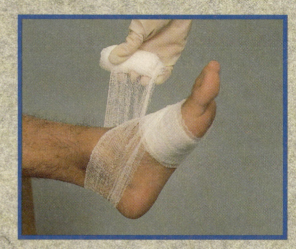

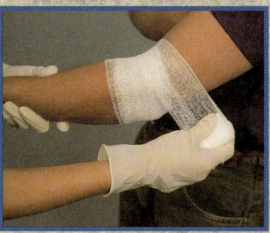

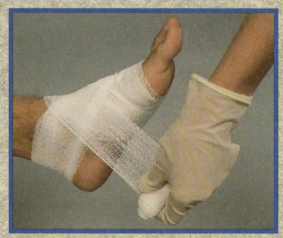

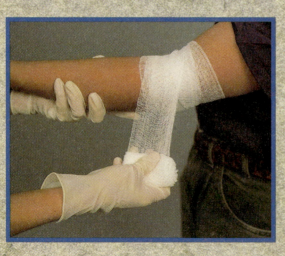

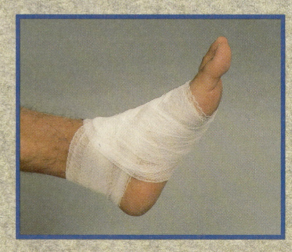

NOTES

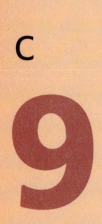

C H A P T E R

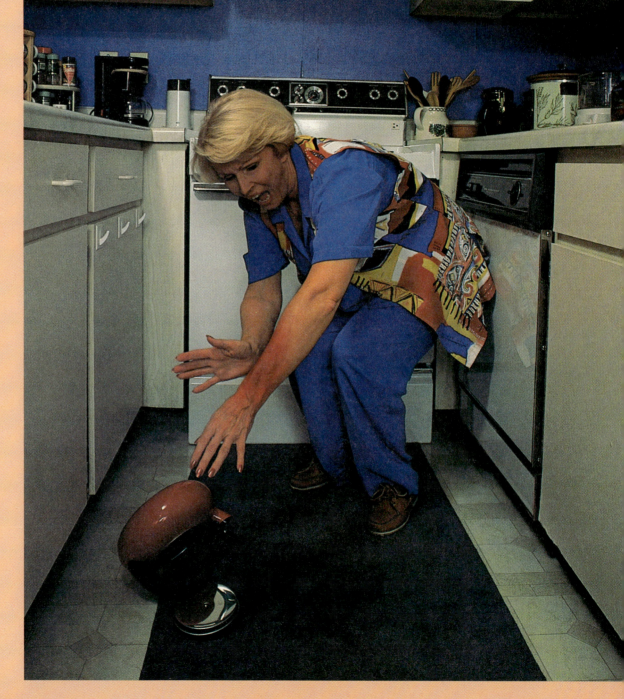

BURNS

Severe burns can be an overwhelming experience. An estimated 2 million burn injuries occur each year in the United States, resulting in 75,000 hospitalizations and more than 4,000 deaths. Burns occur in every age group, across all socioeconomic levels, at home and in the workplace, and in urban, suburban, and rural settings.

It has been estimated that about 70 percent of all burn injuries occur in the home, with house fires responsible for the majority of fire deaths. Most burn victims are injured as a result of their own actions.

The highest-risk age groups for burn injuries are children younger than 5 years and adults over 55. Both groups may have a limited ability to recognize and escape from a fire or burn incident. Their relatively thinner skin predisposes them to more serious injuries. Death and complications increase dramatically for burn victims older than 55 due to the likelihood of preexisting health problems and their immune systems' decreased ability to fight infection.

Skin death and injury occur as the applied heat exceeds the body's ability to handle it. That point starts at about 113°F. The amount and depth of skin damage depend on the heat's intensity, the duration of contact, and the skin thickness.

Burn injuries can be classified as thermal (heat), chemical, or electrical.

- *Thermal burns*. Not all thermal burns are caused by flames. Contact with hot objects, flammable vapor that ignites and causes a flash or an explosion, and steam or hot liquid are other common causes of burns. Just three seconds of exposure to water at 140°F can cause a full-thickness (third-degree) burn in an adult. At 156°F the same burn occurs in one second.

- *Chemical burns*. A wide range of chemical agents is capable of causing tissue damage and death on contact with the skin. As with thermal burns, the amount of tissue damage depends on the duration of contact, the skin thickness in the area of exposure, and the strength of the chemical agent. Chemicals will continue to cause tissue destruction until the chemical agent is removed. Three types of chemicals—acids, alkalis, and organic compounds—are responsible for most chemical burns. Alkalis produce deeper, more extensive burns than acids.

- *Electrical burns*. The injury severity from exposure to electrical current depends on the type of current (direct or alternating), the voltage, the area of the body exposed, and the duration of contact.

Electricity can induce ventricular fibrillation (a type of cardiac arrest), cause respiratory arrest, or "freeze" the victim to the electrical contact point with powerful muscle spasms that increase the length of exposure. Victims of low-voltage electrical injuries may have no skin burns at all yet suffer cardiac or respiratory arrest.

Historically, burns have been described as *first-degree, second-degree,* and *third-degree* injuries. The terms *superficial, partial thickness,* and *full thickness* are often used by burn-care professionals because they are more descriptive of the tissue damage.

- **First-degree (superficial) burns** affect the skin's outer layer (epidermis). Characteristics include redness, mild swelling, tenderness, and pain. Healing occurs without scarring, usually within a week. The outer edges of deeper burns often are first-degree burns.

- **Second-degree (partial-thickness) burns** extend through the entire outer layer and into the inner skin layer. Blisters, swelling, weeping of fluids, and severe pain characterize these burns, which occur because the capillary blood vessels in the dermis are damaged and give up fluid into surrounding tissues. Intact blisters provide a sterile waterproof covering. Once a blister breaks, a weeping wound results and infection risk increases.

- **Third-degree (full-thickness) burns** are severe burns that penetrate all the skin layers, into the underlying fat and muscle. The skin looks leathery, waxy, or pearly gray and sometimes charred. There is a dry appearance, because capillary blood vessels have been destroyed and no more fluid is brought to the area. The skin does not blanch after being pressed because the area is dead. The victim feels no pain from a third-degree burn because the nerve endings have been damaged or destroyed. Any pain that is felt is from surrounding burns of lesser degrees. A third-degree burn requires medical care, which involves removal of the dead tissue and a skin graft to heal properly.

Respiratory-tract damage caused by heat associated with a burn remains the leading cause of death after a victim is hospitalized. Respiratory damage may result, for example, from breathing heat or the products of combustion; from being burned by a flame while in a closed space; or from being in an

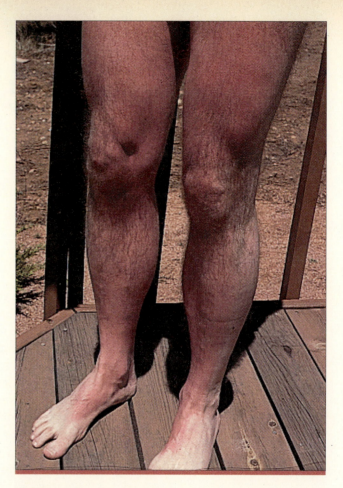
First-degree burn

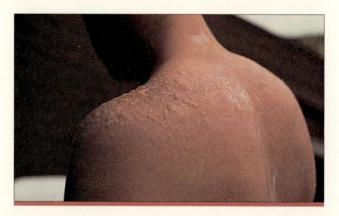
Second-degree burn blisters

explosion. In those instances, even if there is no burn injury, there may be respiratory damage. It is rare that the upper respiratory tract or the lungs are actually burned. That is because they are constructed to cool or warm air to prepare it for inhalation. The superheated air from a flame or from a hot steam explosion will be absorbed by the upper respiratory tract (the area from the nose through to

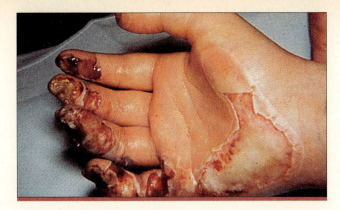
Second- and third-degree burns

the trachea), resulting in inflammation. Swelling results in 2 to 24 hours, restricting or even completely shutting off the airway so that air cannot reach the lungs. *All respiratory injuries must receive medical care.*

Burns can aggravate existing medical conditions such as diabetes, heart disease, and lung disease, as well as other medical problems. Concurrent injuries such as fractures, internal injuries, and open wounds increase the severity of a burn.

Thermal Burns

What to Do

1. Stop the burning! Burns can continue to injure tissue for a surprisingly long time. If clothing has ignited, have the victim roll on the ground using the "stop, drop, and roll" method. Smother the flames with a blanket or douse the victim with water. Stop a person whose clothes are on fire from running; running only serves to fan the flames. Nor should the victim remain standing, because a standing victim is more apt to inhale flames. Once the fire is dead, remove all smoldering clothing; the burning may continue if the clothing is left on. Remove hot or burned clothing immediately. If possible, remove jewelry, since heat may be held near the skin and cause more damage.

2. Check the ABCs.

3. Determine the depth of the burn. It is difficult to tell a burn's depth because the destruction varies within the same burn. Even experienced physicians will not know the depth for several days after the burn. However, making an assessment of burn depth will help you decide whether to seek medical care for the victim.

> **CAUTION: DO NOT**
> - remove clothing stuck to the skin. Cut around the areas where clothing sticks to the skin.
> - pull on stuck clothing—pulling will further damage the skin.
> - forget to remove jewelry as soon as possible—swelling could make jewelry difficult to remove later.

4. Determine the extent of the burn. Skin will not ignite unless heated to thousands of degrees. However, if clothing ignites or skin is kept in contact with a heat source, such as scalding water, large areas of the skin will be injured. Determining the extent of a burn means estimating how much body surface area the burn covers. A rough guide known as the **rule of nines** assigns a percentage value to each part of an adult's body. The entire head is 9 percent, one complete arm is 9 percent, the front torso is 18 percent, the complete back is 18 percent, and each leg is 18 percent. The rule of nines must be modified to take into account the different proportions of a small child. In small children and infants, the head accounts for 18 percent and each leg is 14 percent.

For small or scattered burns, use the **rule of the palm.** The victim's hand, excluding the fin-

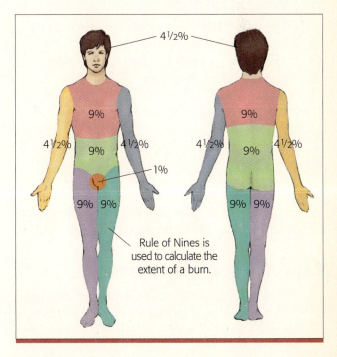

Rule of Nines

gers and the thumb, represents about 1 percent of his or her total body surface. For a very large burn, estimate the *unburned* area in number of hands and subtract from 100 percent.

5. Determine what parts of the body are burned. Burns on the face, hands, feet, and genitals are more severe than on other body parts. A circumferential burn (one that goes around a finger, toe, arm, leg, neck, or chest) is considered more severe than a noncircumferential one because of the possible constriction and tourniquet effect on circulation and, in some cases, breathing. All these burns require medical care.

6. Determine if other injuries or preexisting medical problems exist or if the victim is elderly (over 55) or very young (under 5). A medical problem or belonging to one of those age groups increases a burn's severity.

7. Determine the burn's severity. This forms the basis for how to treat the burned victim. After you have evaluated the burn according to Steps 3 through 6, use the American Burn Association (ABA) guidelines to determine the burn's severity. Most burns are minor, occur at home, and can be managed outside a medical setting. Seek medical attention for all moderate and severe burns, as classified by the ABA, or if any of the following conditions applies:

   - The victim is under 5 or over 55 years of age.
   - The victim has difficulty breathing.
   - Other injuries exist.
   - An electrical injury exists.
   - The face, hands, feet, or genitals are burned.
   - Child abuse is suspected.
   - The surface area of a second-degree burn is greater than 15 percent of the body surface area.
   - The burn is third degree.

Burn Care

Burn care aims to reduce pain, protect against infection, and prevent evaporation. All burn wounds are sterile for the first 24–48 hours after injury.

Care of First-Degree Burns

1. Relieve pain by immersing the burned area in cold water or by applying a wet, cold cloth. Apply cold until the part is pain free both in and out of the water (usually in 10 minutes, but it may take up to 45 minutes). Cold also stops the

Table 9-1: Burn Severity

Minor Burns

First-degree burn covering < 50% BSA*

Second-degree burn covering <15% BSA in adults

Second-degree burn covering <10% BSA in children/ elderly persons

Third-degree burn covering <2% BSA

Moderate Burns

First-degree burn covering >50% BSA

Second-degree burn covering 15%–30% BSA in adults

Second-degree burn covering 10%–20% BSA in children/elderly persons

Third-degree burn covering <10% BSA

Critical Burns

Second-degree burn covering >30% BSA in adults

Second-degree burn covering >20% BSA in children/ elderly persons

Third-degree burn covering >10% BSA

Burns of hands, face, eyes, feet, or genitalia; also most inhalation injuries, electrical injuries, and burns accompanied by major trauma or significant preexisting conditions

*BSA = body surface area

Source: Adapted with permission from the American Burn Association categorization.

CAUTION: DO NOT

- apply cold to more than 20 percent of an adult's body surface (10 percent for children)—widespread cooling can cause hypothermia. Burn victims lose large amounts of heat and water.
- leave wet packs on wounds for long periods.
- use an ice pack unless it is the only source of cold. If you must use one, apply it for only 10–15 minutes, since frostbite and hypothermia can develop.
- apply salve, ointment, grease, butter, cream, spray, home remedy, or any other coating on a burn until it has been cooled. Such coatings are unsterile and can lead to infection. They also can seal in heat, causing further damage.

Table 9-2: First Aid for Burns

Type of Burn	Do ...	Don't ...
First-degree Burn (redness, mild swelling, and pain)	... apply cold water and/or dry sterile dressing.	... apply butter, oleomargarine, etc.
Second-degree Burn (deeper injury; blisters develop)	... immerse in cold water, blot dry with sterile cloth for protection. ... apply bacitracin. ... treat for shock. ... obtain medical attention if severe.	... break blisters. ... remove shreds of tissue. ... use antiseptic preparation, ointment spray, or home remedy on severe burn. ... remove charred clothing that is stuck to burn. ... apply ice. ... use home medication.
Third-degree Burn (deeper destruction; skin layers destroyed)	... cover burn with sterile cloth to protect it. ... treat victim for shock. ... watch for breathing difficulty. ... obtain medical attention quickly.	
Chemical Burn	... remove chemical by flushing with large quantities of water for at least 20 minutes or longer. ... remove surrounding clothing.	

Source: Adapted from U.S. Coast Guard.

burn's progression into deeper tissue. If cold water is unavailable, use any cold liquid you drink to reduce the burned skin's temperature.

2. Relieve pain and inflammation with aspirin or ibuprofen. Acetaminophen relieves pain but not inflammation.

3. Apply an aloe vera gel or an inexpensive moisturizer to keep the skin moistened and to avoid itching and peeling. Aloe vera has antimicrobial properties and is an effective analgesic.

⚠ CAUTION: DO NOT

- use a dressing. Most first-degree burns do not need a dressing.
- use anesthetic sprays because they may sensitize the skin to "-caine" anesthetics.

Care of Second-Degree Burns

1. Relieve pain by immersing the burned area in cold water or by applying a wet, cold cloth. Apply cold until the part is pain free both in

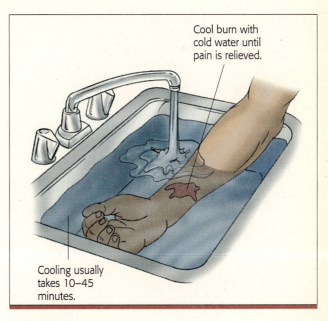

Cool burn with cold water until pain is relieved.

Cooling usually takes 10–45 minutes.

Immerse the burn in cold water.

and out of the water (usually in 10 minutes, but it may take up to 45 minutes). Cold also stops the burn's progression into deeper tissue. If cold water is unavailable, use any cold liquid you drink to reduce the burned skin's temperature.

Burn Care **169**

HEAT BURNS

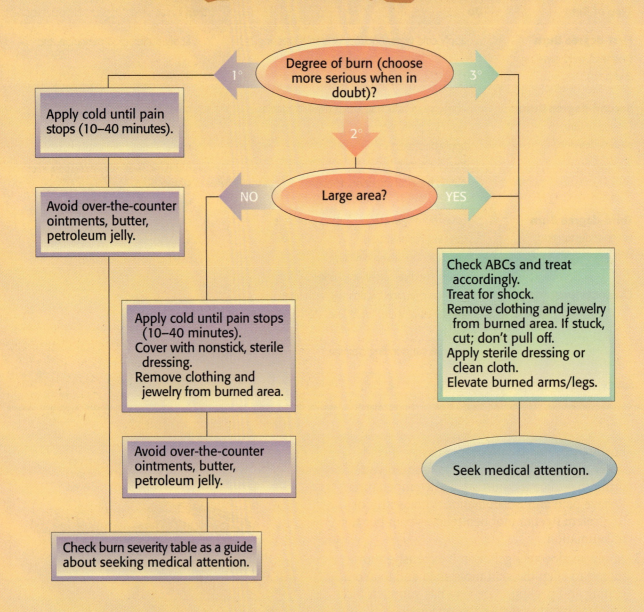

Degree of burn (choose more serious when in doubt)?

1°

Apply cold until pain stops (10–40 minutes).

Avoid over-the-counter ointments, butter, petroleum jelly.

2°

Large area?

NO

Apply cold until pain stops (10–40 minutes).
Cover with nonstick, sterile dressing.
Remove clothing and jewelry from burned area.

Avoid over-the-counter ointments, butter, petroleum jelly.

Check burn severity table as a guide about seeking medical attention.

3°

YES

Check ABCs and treat accordingly.
Treat for shock.
Remove clothing and jewelry from burned area. If stuck, cut; don't pull off.
Apply sterile dressing or clean cloth.
Elevate burned arms/legs.

Seek medical attention.

CAUTION: DO NOT

- cool more than 20 percent of an adult's body surface area (10 percent for a child) except to extinguish flames.

2. Relieve pain and inflammation with aspirin or ibuprofen. Acetaminophen relieves pain but not inflammation. Keep a burned extremity elevated to reduce gravity-induced swelling.

3. Apply a thin layer of ointment such as bacitracin. Topical antibiotic therapy like bacitracin does not sterilize a wound, but it does decrease the number of bacteria to a level that can be controlled by the body's defense mechanisms and prevents the entrance of bacteria. Physicians may prescribe Silvadene™, which is the agent of choice for burn wounds. However, bacitracin works as well, does not require a physician's prescription, and is much less expensive.

CAUTION: DO NOT

- break any blisters. Intact blisters serve as excellent burn dressings. Cover a ruptured blister with bacitracin ointment and a dry, sterile dressing.
- apply salve, ointment, grease, butter, cream, spray, home remedy, or any other coating on a burn until it has cooled. Such coatings are unsterile and may lead to infection. They can also seal in heat, causing further damage. For moderate and severe burns, a physician will have to scrape off the coating, which will cause the victim unnecessary additional pain.
- place a moist dressing over a burn since it will dry out quickly. A wet dressing over a large area can induce hypothermia. A cold wet pack can be used to cool a burn initially, but it should not serve as a dressing.
- use plastic as a dressing (its only advantage is that it will not stick to the burn), since it will trap moisture and provide a good place for bacteria to grow.

4. Cover the burn with a dry, nonsticking, sterile dressing or a clean cloth. Covering the burn reduces the amount of pain by keeping air from the exposed nerve endings. The main purpose of a dressing over a burn is to keep the burn clean, prevent evaporative loss, and reduce the pain.

Care of Third-Degree Burns

It usually is not necessary to apply cold to third-degree burns since pain is absent. Any pain felt with a third-degree burn comes from accompanying first- and second-degree burns, for which cold applications can be helpful.

1. Cover the burn with a dry, nonsticking, sterile dressing or a clean cloth.

CAUTION: DO NOT

- apply salve, ointment, grease, butter, cream, spray, home remedy, or any other coating on a burn. Such coatings are unsterile and may lead to infection. They can also seal in the heat, causing further damage. For moderate and severe burns, a physician will have to scrape off the coating, which will cause the victim unnecessary additional pain.

2. Treat the victim for shock by elevating the legs and keeping the victim warm with a clean sheet or blanket.

Scald Burns

Scald burns are the result of contact with hot liquids. Scald burns can be divided into two types: immersion burns and spill burns. An **immersion burn** results when an area of the body is fully im-

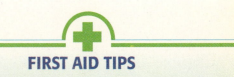

FIRST AID TIPS

Burned Tongue
A few grains of sugar sprinkled on the tongue can relieve the misery of a tongue burned by hot food or drink. Repeat as often as needed. Sucking on ice chips or a Popsicle can cool the burn.

mersed in a hot liquid. It generally has definite demarcations between healthy and injured tissue. This type of burn tends to be deep and is often full thickness. The cause of this type of injury is generally abuse and is seen most often in children.

A **spill burn** occurs when a liquid spills, drops, or is thrown on a person. The pattern of this type of burn generally is irregular and may be scattered across large body areas. A spill burn usually is not as deep as an immersion burn.

Neglect and nonsupervison of children in the kitchen and the bathtub are frequent causes of spill burns in children. Scalds in adults are more often in the elderly population, who generally have decreased sensation. For that reason, many elderly victims are scalded in their bath.

Later Burn Care

For after-burn care, follow a physician's recommendations, if there are any (many burns are never seen by a doctor). The following suggestions may apply:

- Wash hands thoroughly before changing any dressing.
- Leave unbroken blisters intact.
- Change dressings once or twice a day unless a physician instructs otherwise.
- To change a dressing:
  1. Remove old dressing. If a dressing sticks, soak it off with cool, clean water.
  2. Cleanse area gently with mild soap and water.
  3. Pat area dry with clean cloth.
  4. Apply a thin layer of antibiotic (bacitracin) ointment to the burn.
  5. Apply nonsticking sterile dressing.
- Watch for signs of infection. Call a physician if any of these appear:
  - increased redness, pain, tenderness, swelling, or red streaks near burn
  - pus
  - elevated temperature (fever)
- Keep the area and dressing as clean and dry as possible.
- Elevate the burned area, if possible, for the first 24 hours.
- Give pain medication, if necessary.

Sunburn

Sunburn is the skin's response to the trauma of ultraviolet radiation (UVR) that results mainly from exposure to ultraviolet B (UVB) radiation or, rarely, to UVA (ultraviolet A) radiation. Sunburn may be the most common burn suffered by humans, and probably all persons have had one at some time or another. True sunburn reaction begins two to eight hours after UVR exposure. The amount of ultraviolet light the skin has received is difficult to gauge accurately. Not until after exposure (4–12 hours later) does the redness, tenderness, and discomfort of sunburned skin confirm the overexposure. Painful blistering and swelling peak about 24 hours later.

Sunburn results in first- or second-degree burns. A third-degree burn can occur from a sunburn, but it is rare. The redness of a sunburn is caused by the dilation of the small blood vessels. Blister formation comes from plasma leakage.

Human skin displays marked differences in its response to UVR exposure. Some individuals always burn and never tan, while others rarely experience a painful sunburn. The variability is largely attributed to the degree of pigmentation (melanin) that the skin contains. Darker-hued individuals generally are more resistant to the sun's rays than are those with light complexions, but all human beings eventually will burn if exposed to enough UVB. Other variables that contribute to individual sensitivity include the area of the body exposed, the underlying condition of the skin, the degree of tanning, and the role of various photosensitizing medicines.

Various skin types respond differently to ultraviolet light:

- Type I skin always burns easily and never tans. An example is Irish people, who often have blue eyes, red hair, and freckles.
- Type II skin burns easily, tans slightly.
- Type III skin sometimes burns, always tans gradually and moderately.
- Type IV skin minimally burns, always tans well. Examples include Hispanics, Asians.
- Type V skin rarely burns, tans deeply. Examples include Middle Easterners, Indians (heavily pigmented).
- Type VI skin does not burn, is deeply pigmented (although it can burn or peel with significant exposure). An example is blacks.

Sunburn Prevention

The best protection against the damaging effects of UVR is to limit exposure to sunlight. That is done most easily with protective clothing, such as hats, long-sleeved shirts, and long pants. Wet, white cotton will transmit UVR light, so persons can be sunburned while wearing those clothes. People should avoid prolonged exposure during times of the day when radiation is most intense (usually between 10 A.M. and 2 P.M.) and apply effective sunscreens.

Sunscreens are readily available and offer the best protection against sunburn, development of skin cancers, and other long-term skin injury. The proper use of sunscreens will protect an individual from the harmful effects of the sun. Sunscreens must be applied correctly. That generally means applying the sunscreen at least 20 minutes before you go out, so it will "bond" to your skin, and reapplying it every few hours. Use waterproof sunscreen if you sweat a lot or if you are going to be in and out of the water. It is important to note that sunscreens do not promote tanning; they do, however, allow the user to tan gradually without serious burning.

To help consumers select an effective sunscreen, the system of rating products by the "skin protection factor" (SPF) has been developed. The higher the SPF number, the greater the protection against sunburn. However, a sunscreen that has an SPF of 30 is not twice as good as one with an SPF of 15. An SPF of 15 blocks out 95 percent of the most harmful rays; a sunscreen with an SPF of 30 gives you only another 3 percent of protection. But since most people usually use only half the amount of sunscreen that is effective, using a 15 SPF probably gets them a 7.5 SPF. If they use a sunscreen with a 30 SPF, they are probably getting the protection of 15.

Many "suntan lotions" have no sunscreen effect and serve only to keep the skin moist. Products such as baby oil and cocoa butter offer little protection against serious sunburn and may actually enhance burning.

Cool compresses for up to 45 minutes are quite soothing to sunburned skin. Frequent cool showers or soaking in a tub may provide remarkable relief. Some experts advise against the use of topical anal-gesics, sprays, or lotions, especially those containing benzocaine. Benzocaine may sensitize the skin, resulting in contact dermatitis that compounds the original problem. Topical anesthetic sprays or lotions may provide temporary relief, but they are expensive and generally ineffective. Over-the-counter analgesics, such as aspirin and especially ibuprofen, should suffice in most cases because they reduce pain and inflammation. Drinking lots of water is also suggested.

First- and second-degree sunburns can be quite painful. When a large area of skin is involved, the individual may feel ill with chills and fever. For first-degree sunburns and after the pain has subsided, the use of aloe vera or other body lotion (e.g., Noxzema™) can keep the skin moist. Do *not* use butter or petroleum jelly.

For aftercare of a second-degree sunburn, apply bacitracin (available as an over-the-counter medication) ointment in a thin layer. It is inexpensive, antimicrobial, widely available, easily applied, and adheres even to exposed areas such as the face.

If blisters break, thoroughly wash the area twice daily with soap and water and then cover with bacitracin and sterile gauze to prevent infection. If the burn becomes infected, contact a doctor. If the eyes are affected, contact a doctor.

Windburn resembles a first-degree sunburn. A greasy sunscreen can be used to prevent and treat it.

CAUTION: DO NOT

use topical over-the-counter burn ointments or sprays or anesthetic sprays because

- **Some products may cause allergic reactions.**
- **Most do not contain enough benzocaine or lidocaine to depress pain.**
- **The duration of any possible relief is relatively short (30–40 minutes). More than three or four applications per day of products containing local anesthetics is discouraged because toxicity can occur if the agents are used too frequently.**
- **They seal in the heat.**
- **They are expensive.**

Chemical Burns

A chemical burn is the result of a caustic or corrosive substance touching the skin. Since chemicals continue to "burn" as long as they are in contact with the skin, they should be removed from the victim as rapidly as possible.

First aid is the same for all chemical burns, except a few specific ones for which a chemical neutralizer has to be used. Alkalies (e.g., drain cleaners) cause more serious burns than acids (e.g., battery acid) because they penetrate deeper and remain active longer. Organic compounds (e.g., petroleum products) are another type of chemical in addition to acids and alkalies capable of burning.

What to Do

1. Immediately remove the chemical by flushing with water. If available, use a hose or a shower. Brush dry powder chemicals from the skin *before* flushing, unless large amounts of water are immediately available. Water may activate a dry chemical and cause more damage to the skin. Take precautions to protect yourself from exposure to the chemical.
2. Remove the victim's contaminated clothing while flushing with water. Clothing can hold chemicals, allowing them to continue to burn as long as they are in contact with the skin.

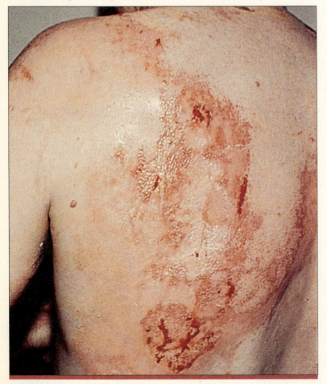

Chemical burn from sulfuric acid

 CAUTION: DO NOT

- waste time! A chemical burn is an emergency!
- apply water under high pressure—it will drive the chemical deeper into the tissue.
- try to neutralize a chemical even if you know which chemical is involved—heat may be produced, resulting in more damage. Some product labels for neutralizing may be wrong. Save the container or the label for the chemical's name.

3. Flush for 20 minutes or longer. Let the victim wash with a mild soap before a final rinse. Dilution with large amounts of water decreases the chemical concentration and washes it away.
4. Cover the burned area with a dry, sterile dressing or, for large areas, a clean pillowcase.
5. If the chemical is in an eye, flood it for at least 20 minutes, using low pressure.
6. Seek medical attention immediately for all chemical burns.

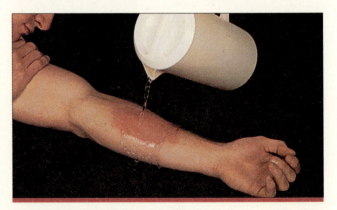

Flooding a chemical burn

Electrocution

Even a mild electrical shock can cause serious internal injuries. A current of 1,000 volts or more is considered high voltage, but even the 110 volts found in ordinary household current can be deadly.

There are three types of electrical injuries: thermal (flame), arc (flash), and true electrical injury (contact). A *thermal burn* (flame) results when clothing or objects in direct contact with the skin are ignited by an electrical current. These injuries

CHEMICAL BURNS

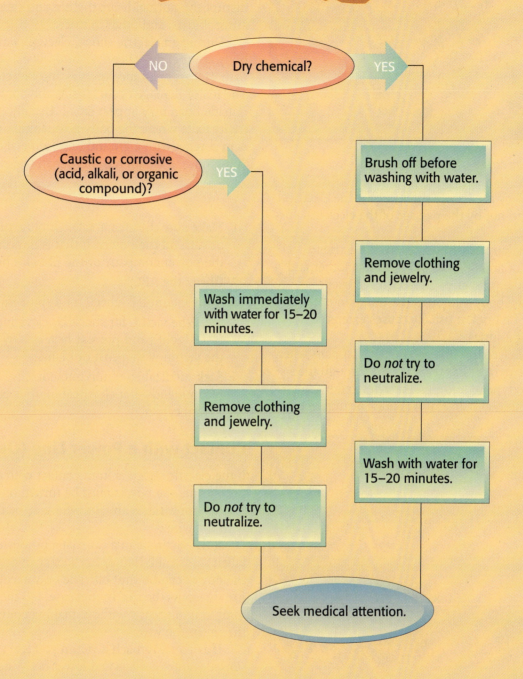

Dry chemical?

NO → (to Caustic or corrosive question)

YES → Brush off before washing with water.

Caustic or corrosive (acid, alkali, or organic compound)?

YES →

Wash immediately with water for 15–20 minutes.

Remove clothing and jewelry.

Do *not* try to neutralize.

Brush off before washing with water.

Remove clothing and jewelry.

Do *not* try to neutralize.

Wash with water for 15–20 minutes.

Seek medical attention.

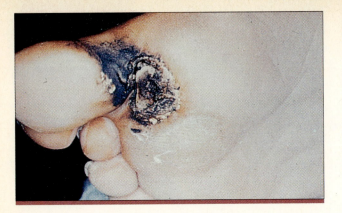

Electrical burn on toe

are caused by the flames produced by the electrical current and not by the passage of the electrical current or arc.

An *arc burn* (flash) occurs from electricity jumping, or arcing, from one spot to another and not from the passage of an electrical current through the body. Although the duration of the flash may be brief, it usually causes extensive superficial injuries.

A *true electrical injury* (contact) happens when an electric current has truly passed through the body. This type of injury is characterized by an entrance wound and an exit wound. The important

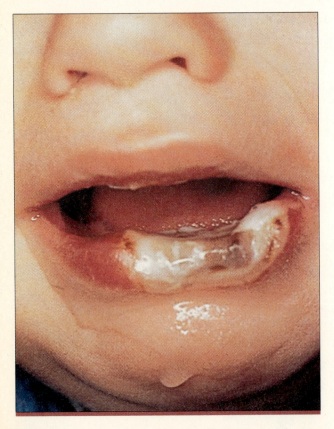

Electrical burn caused by chewing through electrical cord

factor with this type of injury is that the surface injury may be just the tip of the iceberg. High-voltage electrical currents passing through the body may disrupt the normal heart rhythm and cause cardiac arrest, burns, and other injuries.

During an electric shock, electricity enters the body at the point of contact and travels along the path of least resistance (nerves and blood vessels). The major damage occurs inside the body—the outside burn may appear small. Usually, the electricity exits where the body is touching a surface or is in contact with a ground (e.g., a metal object). Sometimes, a victim has more than one exit site.

What to Do

1. Make sure the area is safe. Unplug, disconnect, or turn off the power. If that is impossible, call the power company or the EMS for help.
2. Check the ABCs.
3. If the victim fell, check for a spine injury.
4. Treat the victim for shock by elevating the legs 8–12 inches and prevent heat loss by covering the victim with a coat or blanket.
5. Seek medical attention immediately. The ABA recommends that electrical injuries be treated in a burn center.

Contact with a Power Line (Outdoors)

If the electric shock is from contact with a downed power line, the power *must* be turned off before a rescuer approaches anyone who may be in contact with the wire.

If the victim is in a car that a power line has fallen across, tell him or her to stay in the car until the power can be shut off. The only exception is if fire threatens the car. In that case, tell the victim to jump out of the car without making contact with the car or the wire.

If as you approach a victim you feel a tingling sensation in your legs and lower body, stop. The sensation signals that you are on energized ground and that an electrical current is entering through one foot, passing through your lower body, and leaving through the other foot. Raise one foot off the ground, turn around, and hop to a safe place.

If you can safely reach the victim, do not attempt to move any wires, even with wooden poles, tools with wood handles, or tree branches. Do not use objects with a high moisture content and certainly not metal objects. The recommendation for not using wood-handled rakes, brooms, or shovels

ELECTROCUTION

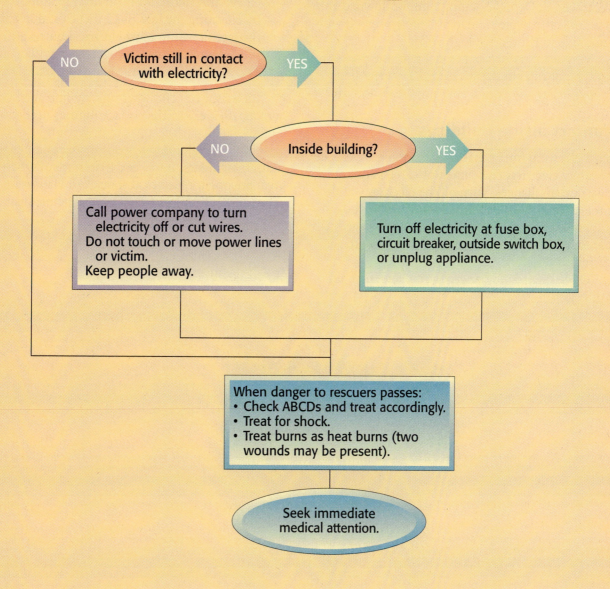

Victim still in contact with electricity?

NO / YES

Inside building?

NO / YES

Call power company to turn electricity off or cut wires.
Do not touch or move power lines or victim.
Keep people away.

Turn off electricity at fuse box, circuit breaker, outside switch box, or unplug appliance.

When danger to rescuers passes:
• Check ABCDs and treat accordingly.
• Treat for shock.
• Treat burns as heat burns (two wounds may be present).

Seek immediate medical attention.

is that if the voltage is high enough (you seldom will know how much voltage is involved) those objects can conduct electricity and the rescuer will be electrocuted. Do not attempt to move downed wires at all unless you are trained and are equipped with tools able to handle the high voltage.

Wait until trained personnel with the proper equipment can cut the wires or disconnect them. Prevent bystanders from entering the danger area.

Contact inside Buildings

Most electrical burns that occur indoors are caused by faulty electrical equipment or careless use of electrical appliances. Turn off the electricity at the circuit breaker, fuse box, or outside switch box or unplug the appliance if the plug is undamaged. Do not touch the appliance or the victim until the current is off.

Once there is no danger to rescuers, first aid can begin.

What to Do

1. Check the ABCs and treat accordingly.
2. Check the victim for burns and treat for shock by elevating the legs 8–12 inches and keeping the victim warm. Most electrical burns are third-degree burns, so cover them with a sterile dressing and elevate the affected part.

Electrical current flows quickly into the body's tissues, then exits. The surface injuries of the skin involve small surface areas (entrance and exit points); the major damage occurs deep under the skin. First aiders must keep that in mind when they treat anyone for electrical shock. All victims of electrical shock should receive immediate medical attention.

HEAD AND SPINE INJURIES

Head Injuries

Scalp Wounds

Scalp wounds bleed profusely because of the scalp's rich blood supply and the scalp's blood vessels do not constrict. A profusely bleeding scalp wound does not mean the blood supply to the brain is affected. The brain obtains its blood supply from arteries in the neck, not the scalp. Look into the wound for exposed skull bone or brain tissue and indentation of the skull. Suspect a spine injury to the neck.

What to Do

1. Control bleeding by gently applying direct pressure with a dry sterile dressing. If the dressing becomes blood-filled, do not remove it. Add another dressing on top of the first one.
2. If you suspect a skull fracture, apply pressure around the edges of the wound and over a broad area rather than on the center of the wound. A doughnut (ring) pad serves well in such an application.
3. Keep the head and shoulders slightly elevated to help control bleeding.

 CAUTION: DO NOT

- remove an embedded object; instead stabilize it in place with bulky dressings. If a skull fracture is suspected, do not clean a scalp wound or irrigate it since the fluid can carry debris and bacteria into the brain.

Skull Fracture

A skull fracture is a break or a crack in the cranium (bony case surrounding the brain). Skull fractures may be open or closed (i.e., with or without an accompanying scalp wound).

What to Look For

It is extremely difficult to determine a skull fracture except by x-ray unless the skull deformity is severe and obvious. Signs of a skull fracture include the following:

- Pain at the point of injury.
- Deformity of the skull.
- Bleeding from the ears or nose.
- Leakage of clear, pink, watery fluid—cerebrospinal fluid (CSF)—from an ear or the nose. To determine if CSF is leaking, have the suspected fluid drip onto a handkerchief, pillowcase, or other cloth. CSF will form a pink ring resembling a target around a slightly blood-tinged center; this is called the "halo sign" or "ring sign."
- Discoloration around the eyes ("raccoon eyes") appearing several hours after the injury.
- Discoloration behind an ear (known as "Battle's sign"), appearing several hours after the injury.
- Unequal pupils.
- Profuse scalp bleeding if skin is broken. A scalp wound may expose the skull or brain tissue.
- Penetrating wound (e.g., from a bullet) or impaled object.

What to Do

1. Monitor the ABCs.
2. Cover wounds with a sterile dressing.
3. Stabilize the victim's neck against movement.
4. Slightly elevate the victim's head and shoulders to help control bleeding.
5. Apply pressure around the edges of the wound, not directly on it.

CAUTION: DO NOT

- stop the flow of blood or CSF from an ear or nose. Blocking the flow could increase pressure within the skull.
- remove an impaled object from the head. Stabilize it in place with bulky dressings.
- clean an open skull fracture—infection into the brain could result.

Brain Injuries

Statistics from the insurance industry indicate that at least eight million head injuries are reported in the United States each year. It is not injury specifically to the head that causes most short- and long-term problems but injuries to the brain itself. Most head injuries come from motor vehicle accidents and falls. Many of these injuries are minor—shallow lacerations or localized bruising and swelling. However, 50,000 people die each year in the United States from head trauma, and twice that many suffer brain injuries that leave them with permanent damage.

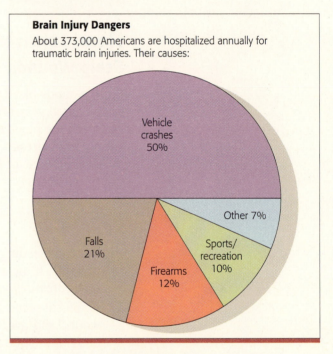

Brain Injury Dangers
About 373,000 Americans are hospitalized annually for traumatic brain injuries. Their causes:

- Vehicle crashes 50%
- Other 7%
- Sports/recreation 10%
- Firearms 12%
- Falls 21%

Source: Brain Injury Association

The brain is a delicate organ. When the head is struck with sufficient force, the brain is bounced around inside the skull. Brain injuries can be serious and difficult first aid emergencies to handle. The victim is often confused or unresponsive, making assessment difficult. Many brain injuries are life threatening. If a victim with a brain injury is mishandled, permanent damage or death can occur.

The brain, like other body tissue, will swell when injured. Unlike other tissue, the brain is confined in a rigid compartment, the skull, where little additional space exists to accommodate any swelling. Therefore, swelling of brain tissue or accumulation of blood inside the skull compresses the brain and increases the pressure inside the skull. That intracranial pressure causes changes that interfere with brain functioning. Furthermore, because the skull is hard, both the brain and the blood vessels on the brain's surface may be damaged if they strike the skull's inner surface, which can occur when the head is struck directly or is rapidly accelerated or decelerated. The phenomenon of a person "seeing stars" when struck on the back of the head results from the occipital lobe of the brain (the part that controls vision) banging against the back of the skull.

The nerve cells of the brain and the spinal cord, unlike most other cells in the body, are unable to regenerate. When those cells die, they are lost forever and are unable to regrow or be replaced by transplantation.

Injuries to the brain can be caused by a penetrating foreign object, by bony fragments from a skull fracture, or by the brain crashing into the skull after a person's head has hit a stationary object (such as the ground)—a *deceleration injury*—or been hit by something like a baseball bat or a teammate's knee—an *acceleration injury*.

Sometimes there will be two points of injury, one at the point of impact and one where the brain rebounds off the skull on the opposite side.

There are three types of commonly occurring brain injuries:

- A **concussion** is temporary loss of brain function, usually without permanent damage. No bleeding in the brain occurs, and there may not be any external cut or swelling. Concussion can cause a person to be "knocked out" (unconscious) or to have memory loss (amnesia). A concussion can be dangerous even if the person is not knocked out because it affects the brain. The longer the victim is unconscious or the longer the memory loss lasts, the more serious the concussion. Concussions usually are not serious, but occasionally they can result in permanent damage to the brain and even cause death.

- A **contusion** is a bruising of brain tissue.

- A **hematoma** is a localized collection of blood as a result of a broken blood vessel. A hematoma is the most serious type of brain injury.

Brain injuries produce varying degrees of local or generalized edema (swelling). As swelling increases or a hematoma expands, intracranial pressure increases. As pressure rises, the blood supply is shut off by compression of swollen vessels, and brain tissue is deprived of oxygen. The brain stem

Table 10-1: Evaluating and Managing a Concussion

Severity	Symptoms	Guidelines
Grade 1 (mild)	Confusion without amnesia (loss of memory); no loss of consciousness	Remove from activity. Examine immediately and every 5 minutes for dizziness, ringing sound in the ears, and loss of memory. Can return to activity if amnesia does not appear and no other symptoms appear for at least 20 minutes.
Grade 2 (moderate)	Confusion with amnesia (loss of memory); no loss of consciousness	Remove from activity and do not allow to return. Physician should examine frequently. Physician should reexamine the next day. Return to activity after one full week without symptoms.
Grade 3 (severe)	Loss of consciousness; (does not respond at the A, V, P levels)	Transport to nearest hospital by ambulance (with spine stabilized). Physician performs thorough neurologic evaluation. May be admitted to hospital. If findings are normal, physician will instruct family or friend about overnight observation. Return to activity only after two full weeks without symptoms.

Note: Prolonged unconsciousness, persistent altered mental status, worsening postconcussion symptoms, or abnormalities found during neurologic examination require urgent neurosurgical attention or transfer to a hospital emergency department.

Source: Adapted from Guidelines for the Management of Concussion in Sports, Colorado Medical Society, Sports Medicine Committee.

can be squashed by the pressure, affecting heart and lung function.

A young child has a relatively large head, supported by a weak neck and positioned on a small trunk. A child's brain tissues are thinner, softer, and more flexible than an adult's. The tissues' flexibility diffuses the impact of an injury, but because they are fragile, they damage easily. Thus, children are especially vulnerable to brain injuries. Small children, overbalanced by their large heads, tend to run leaning forward and thus often run into things or fall over. Immature motor development can make toddlers clumsy, liable to stumble over their own feet. Infants, left unattended, can tumble from beds, highchairs, and changing tables.

What to Look For

Assessment is directed at determining whether injured brain tissue is swelling because of intracranial pressure. The following signs and symptoms, which may go unnoticed for the first 6–18 hours after injury, are indicative of increased intracranial pressure:

- Level of responsiveness V, P, or U on the AVPU scale (see page 190). Loss of responsiveness may be short or may persist for hours or days. The victim may alternate between periods of responsiveness and unresponsiveness or be responsive but disoriented, confused, and incoherent.
- Memory loss.
- Vomiting and nausea.
- Headache.
- Vision disturbance. Victim sees "double," or eyes fail to move together.
- Unequal pupils.

- Weakness, loss of balance, or paralysis.
- Seizures.
- Blood or CSF leaking from ears or nose.
- Combativeness. The victim strikes out randomly and with surprising strength at the nearest person.

For a responsive victim, ask what day it is, where he or she is, and personal questions such as birthday and home address. If the victim cannot answer those questions, there may be a significant problem. Another useful test is to give a list of five or six numbers and ask the victim to repeat them in the same order. Lists of objects can also be used as short-term memory tests. Failing these short-term memory tests indicates a concussion.

What to Do

1. Seek immediate medical attention for all brain-injury victims.
2. Suspect a spine injury in an unresponsive victim until proved otherwise. Stabilize the victim's head and neck as you found them by one of the following methods:
   - Grasp the victim's clavicle and trapezius muscle (shoulder) and cradle the head between the inside of your forearms. Hold the victim's head and neck still until the EMS responds.
   - Grasp the victim's head over the ears and hold the head and neck still until the EMS responds.
   - If a long wait for the EMS to respond is anticipated or if you are tired from holding the victim's head in place, kneel with the victim's head between your knees or place objects on each side of the victim's head to prevent it from rolling from side to side.
3. Monitor the ABCs.
4. Control scalp bleeding by covering wounds with sterile dressings as a barrier against infection. If you suspect a skull fracture, apply pressure around the wound edges, not directly on the wound. Do not try to clean a scalp wound of a suspected skull fracture. Stabilize impaled objects in place. Do not try to stop blood or CSF draining from the ears or nose. Blocking either flow could increase pressure within the skull.
5. Brain-injury victims tend to vomit. Rolling the victim onto his or her side while stabilizing the neck against movement will help drain vomit while keeping the airway open.

HEAD INJURIES

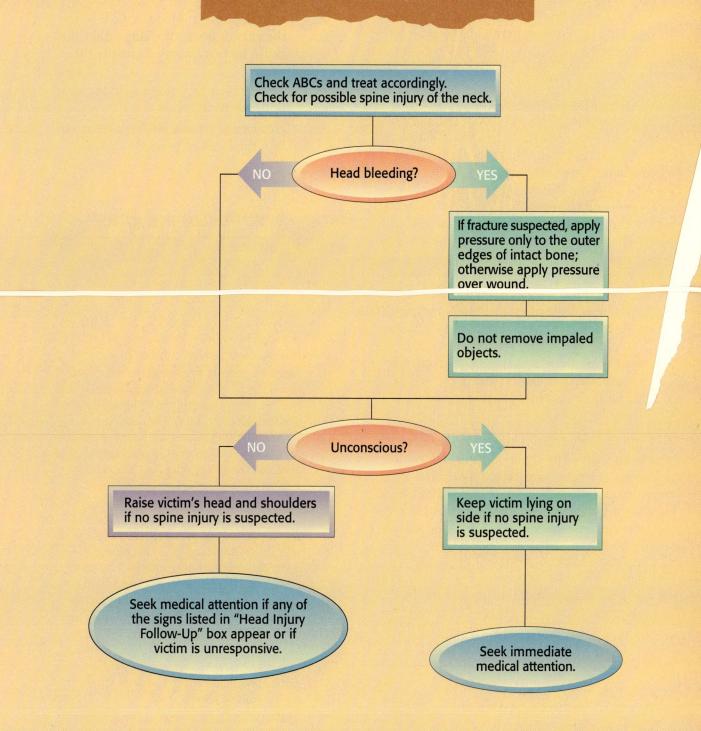

Check ABCs and treat accordingly.
Check for possible spine injury of the neck.

Head bleeding?

NO → ← YES

If fracture suspected, apply pressure only to the outer edges of intact bone; otherwise apply pressure over wound.

Do not remove impaled objects.

Unconscious?

NO → ← YES

Raise victim's head and shoulders if no spine injury is suspected.

Keep victim lying on side if no spine injury is suspected.

Seek medical attention if any of the signs listed in "Head Injury Follow-Up" box appear or if victim is unresponsive.

Seek immediate medical attention.

6. Keep the victim in a slightly head-elevated position to prevent increased blood pressure. If the victim is unconscious, positioning on the side is best for possible vomiting and to keep the airway open.

7. The victim's level of responsiveness or mental status is one of the best indicators of neurologic function. Observations over the first 24 hours may offer clues to problems. Use the mnemonic AVPU to assess and describe a victim's mental status. It is especially helpful with small children who don't talk.

A: The victim is **alert** and can recognize and respond to people.

V: The victim responds to **verbal** stimuli. The victim may appear sleepy or drowsy but responds to verbal questions by opening the eyes, moving, or waking up.

P: The victim responds to **painful** stimuli. The victim is not awake and does not respond to verbal stimuli but does respond to painful stimuli by moving, opening the eyes, or groaning. To stimulate pain, pinch the victim's skin over the clavicle.

U: The victim is **unresponsive** to voices or to painful stimulus.

Unfortunately, there is little a first aider can do for a brain injury. The victim must be transported to the care of a neurosurgeon to relieve pressure and stop intracranial bleeding. If the victim is wearing a helmet (e.g., motorcycle, football), only a few instances call for helmet removal by a first aider:

- A suspected obstructed airway.
- Signs of a severe head injury.
- A helmet so loose that the spine cannot be stabilized.

FIRST AID TIPS

"Halo Sign" for Cerebrospinal Fluid

When evaluating a head injury, it is often difficult to distinguish a simple nosebleed from a nosebleed with accompanying cerebrospinal fluid. Blood or fluid coming from the ear or nose may indicate a skull fracture. The "halo sign" is a test for cerebrospinal fluid.

On a pillowcase, cerebrospinal fluid will often look like a slightly blood-tinged center spot surrounded by a ring of lighter color. Save a head-injury victim's stained pillowcases for a physician to examine.

CAUTION: DO NOT

- stop the flow of blood or CSF from the ears or nose. Blocking either flow could increase pressure inside the skull.
- elevate the legs—that might increase pressure in the skull.
- clean an open skull injury—infection into the brain may result.

Head Injury Follow-Up

If any of the following signs appear within 48 hours of a head injury, seek medical attention:

- *Headache.* Expect a headache. If it lasts more than one or two days or increases in severity, however, seek medical advice.

- *Nausea, vomiting.* If nausea lasts more than two hours, seek medical advice. Vomiting once or twice, especially in children, may be expected after a head injury. Vomiting does not tell anything about the severity of the injury. However, if vomiting begins again hours after one or two episodes have ceased, consult a physician.

- *Drowsiness.* Allow a victim to sleep, but wake the victim at least every two hours to check the state of consciousness and sense of orientation by asking his or her name, address, telephone number, and an information-processing question (e.g., adding or multiplying numbers). If the victim cannot answer correctly or appears confused or disoriented, call a physician.

- *Vision problems.* If the victim "sees double," if the eyes fail to move together, or if one pupil appears to be larger than the other, seek medical advice.

- *Mobility.* If the victim cannot use his or her arms or legs as well as previously or is unsteady in walking, medical care should be sought.

- *Speech.* If the victim has slurred speech or is unable to talk, a doctor should be consulted.

- *Seizures or convulsions.* If the victim has a violent involuntary contraction (spasm) or series of contractions of the skeletal muscles, seek medical assistance.

Eye Injuries

Of all the parts of the human body, an injured eye probably causes the most anxiety and concern in a victim. Eye injuries account for up to 10 percent of all bodily injuries.

The eyes—arguably the most important human sense organs—are easily damaged by trauma. A very small penetration by a metal fragment, for example, means hospitalization. Medical treatment may include hazardous surgery that can lead to blindness or loss of both eyes. Significant eye injuries should be treated in the hospital by ophthalmic surgeons who are experienced at handling eye injuries.

CAUTION: DO NOT
- assume that any eye injury is innocent. When in doubt, seek medical attention immediately.

Penetrating Injuries

Penetrating eye injuries are relatively common, severe injuries that result when a sharp object, such as a knife or a needle, penetrates the eye and then is withdrawn or when pieces from a tool enter the eye and lodge there as foreign bodies.

Any foreign body is hazardous but especially so when it contains iron or copper. Those metals often dissociate, and their atoms or ions can destroy the eye gradually over days or years.

Most penetrating injuries are obvious. Suspect penetration any time you see a lid laceration or cut.

What to Do

1. Seek immediate medical attention. Any penetrating eye injury should be managed in the hospital by an experienced ophthalmic surgeon who is equipped with a microsurgical unit.
2. Protect the injured eye with a paper cup, cardboard folded into a cone, or a doughnut-shaped pad made from a roller gauze bandage or a cravat bandage to prevent the object from being driven deeper into the eye. See page 141 on how to stabilize an impaled object.
3. Cover the undamaged eye to stop movement of the damaged eye (known as sympathetic eye movement).

Blows to the Eye

Blunt trauma varies in severity from negligible to sight threatening. One such injury is the common

CAUTION: DO NOT
- remove an object stuck in the eye or try to wash out an object with water.
- exert pressure on an injured eyeball or a penetrating object.

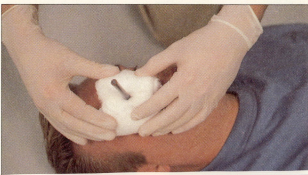

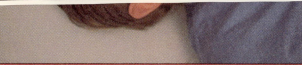

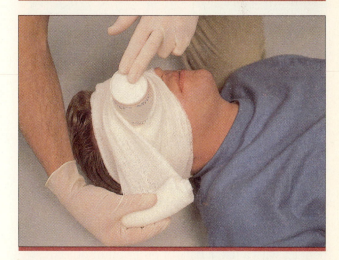

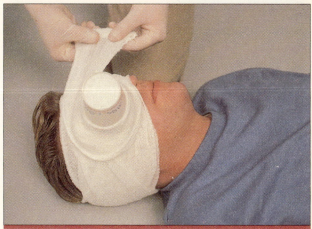

Protecting a long penetrating object against movement (using paper cup)

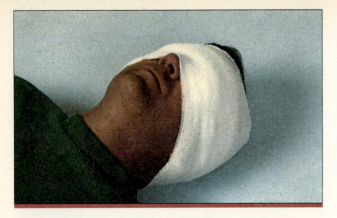
Bandaging both eyes stops sympathetic eye movement.

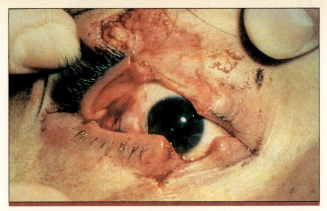
Lacerated eyelid

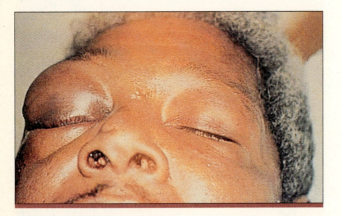
Blow to the eye

"shiner" or "black eye," which occurs when some of the many delicate blood vessels around the eye rupture. The bleeding itself is insignificant and will disappear, but it may hide damage to the eyeball.

Bone around the eyeball can be broken from contact with a fist, a ball, or other blunt object. Symptoms that indicate such a break are double vision and the inability to look upward.

What to Do

1. Apply an ice pack immediately for about 15 minutes to reduce pain and swelling. Do not exert any pressure on the eye.
2. Seek medical attention immediately in cases of pain, reduced vision, or discoloration (a black eye). Every victim should be examined by an ophthalmologist. An eyeball could be ruptured.

Cuts of the Eye and Lid
1. Bandage both eyes lightly.
2. Seek medical attention immediately.

Chemical Burns
Chemical burns of the eyes are extremely sight threatening. In such cases, first aid can determine the fate of the eye and vision.

Alkalies cause greater damage than acids because they penetrate deeper and continue to burn longer. Common alkalies include drain cleaners, cleaning agents, ammonia, cement, plaster, and caustic soda. Common acids include hydrochloric acid, nitric acid, sulfuric (battery) acid, and acetic acid.

Damage can happen in one to five minutes, so speed in removing the chemical is vital.

What to Do

1. Use your fingers to keep the eye open as wide as possible.
2. Flush the eye with water immediately. If possible, use warm water. If water is not available, use milk or other nonirritating liquid.
   • Hold the victim's head under a faucet or pour water into the eye from any clean container for at least 20 minutes, continuously and

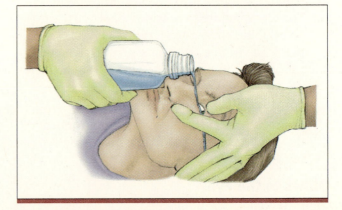
Flushing eye for chemical burn

gently. You cannot use too much water on these injuries.

- Irrigate from the nose side of the eye toward the outside, to avoid flushing material into the other eye.
- Tell the victim to roll the eyeball as much as possible to help wash out the eye.

3. Loosely bandage both eyes with cold, wet dressings.
4. Seek immediate medical attention.

▶ **CAUTION: DO NOT**

- try to neutralize the chemical. Water usually is readily available and better for eye irrigation.
- use an eye cup for a chemical burn.

Eye Avulsion

A blow to the eye can avulse it (knock it out) from its socket.

What to Do

1. Cover the eye loosely with a sterile dressing that has been moistened with clean water. Do *not* try to push the eyeball back into the socket.
2. Protect the injured eye with a paper cup, cardboard folded into a cone, or a doughnut-shaped pad made from a roller gauze bandage or a cravat bandage.
3. Cover the undamaged eye with a patch to stop movement of the damaged eye (known as sympathetic eye movement).
4. Seek medical attention immediately.

Foreign Objects

Foreign objects in the eye are the most frequent eye injury and can be very painful. Tearing is common as the body's way of trying to remove the object. Try one or more of the following, starting with number 1.

What to Do

1. Lift the upper lid over the lower lid, allowing the lashes to brush the object off the inside of the upper lid. Have the victim blink a few times and let the eye move the object out. If the object remains, keep the eye closed.
2. Try flushing the object out by rinsing the eye gently with warm water. Hold the eyelid open and tell the victim to move the eye as it is rinsed.
3. Examine the lower lid by pulling it down gently. If you can see the object, remove it with a moistened sterile gauze or clean cloth.
4. Many foreign bodies lodge under the upper eyelid, requiring some expertise in everting the

a. If tears or gentle flushing do not remove object, gently pull lower lid down. Remove an object by gently flushing with lukewarm water or a wet sterile gauze.

b. Tell the person to look down. Pull gently downward on upper eyelashes. Lay a swab or match stick across the top of the lid.

c. Fold the lid over the swab or matchstick. Remove an object by gently flushing with lukewarm water or a wet sterile gauze.

Removing foreign object from the eye

EYE INJURIES

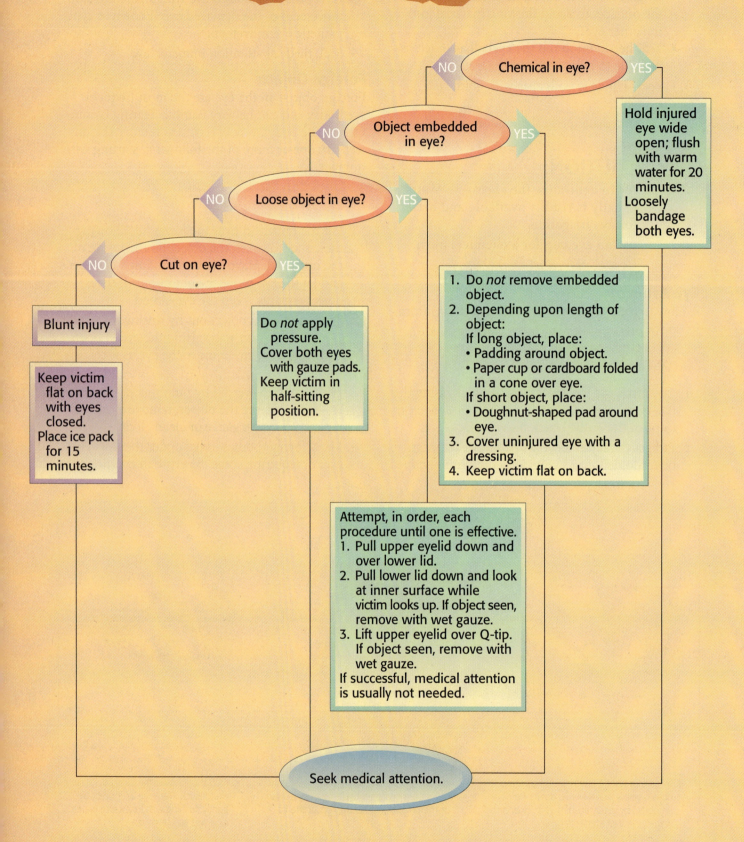

Chemical in eye? — NO / YES

YES → Hold injured eye wide open; flush with warm water for 20 minutes. Loosely bandage both eyes.

Object embedded in eye? — NO / YES

YES →
1. Do *not* remove embedded object.
2. Depending upon length of object:
   If long object, place:
   • Padding around object.
   • Paper cup or cardboard folded in a cone over eye.
   If short object, place:
   • Doughnut-shaped pad around eye.
3. Cover uninjured eye with a dressing.
4. Keep victim flat on back.

Loose object in eye? — NO / YES

YES →
Attempt, in order, each procedure until one is effective.
1. Pull upper eyelid down and over lower lid.
2. Pull lower lid down and look at inner surface while victim looks up. If object seen, remove with wet gauze.
3. Lift upper eyelid over Q-tip. If object seen, remove with wet gauze.
If successful, medical attention is usually not needed.

Cut on eye? — NO / YES

YES → Do *not* apply pressure. Cover both eyes with gauze pads. Keep victim in half-sitting position.

NO → Blunt injury

Keep victim flat on back with eyes closed. Place ice pack for 15 minutes.

Seek medical attention.

lid and removing the object. Examine the upper lid by grasping the lashes of the upper lid, placing a match stick or cotton-tipped swab across the upper lid and roll the lid upward over the stick or swab. If you can see the object, remove it with a moistened sterile gauze or clean cloth.

CAUTION: DO NOT
- allow the victim to rub the eye.
- try to remove an embedded foreign object.
- use dry cotton (cotton balls or cotton-tipped swabs) or instruments (e.g., tweezers) on an eye.

The only eye injuries that should be handled outside the well-equipped ophthalmology department are small foreign bodies, such as grains of sand.

Eye Burns from Light
Burns can result if a person looks at a source of ultraviolet light (e.g., sunlight, arc welding, bright snow, tanning lamps). Severe pain happens one to six hours after exposure.

1. Cover both eyes with cold, wet packs. Tell the victim not to rub the eyes.
2. Have the victim rest in a darkened room. Do not allow light to reach the victim's eyes.
3. Give an analgesic for pain, if needed.
4. Call an ophthalmologist for advice.

An Unconscious Victim's Eyes
An unconscious victim may lose the reflexes that protect the eye (i.e., blinking). Therefore, keep the victim's eyes closed either by taping them closed (use nonallergenic tape) or by covering them with moist dressings.

Contact Lenses
Determine if a victim is wearing contact lenses by asking, by checking a driver's license, or by looking for them on the eyeball, using a light shining on the eye from the side. In cases of chemical burns, lenses should be removed immediately. Usually the victim can remove the lenses.

Ear Injuries
Most ear problems are not life threatening. Fast action may be needed, however, to relieve pain and to prevent or reverse any hearing loss. Head trauma may involve the ear. In those cases, assess the ABCs and treat accordingly.

Foreign bodies in the ear canal usually produce overzealous removal attempts. Except for disk batteries (which damage moist tissue by creating a current) and live insects, few foreign bodies must be extracted immediately. First aiders should elect to seek medical attention for the victim since attempts to remove a foreign body from the ear can result in eardrum (membrane) rupture or ear canal laceration.

A live insect crawling around in the ear canal can be very uncomfortable for the victim. Shine a small light into the ear. Sometimes the insect will crawl out toward the light. If it will not leave the ear, drown the insect by placing several drops of light mineral oil or vegetable oil (not motor oil) into the ear. Often the insect will crawl out before it dies. When it stops moving, and if the eardrum is intact and the insect is near the opening, carefully irrigate the ear with warm water. The insect should wash out. If that is unsuccessful, use a bulb syringe to suck the insect out.

Children insert all sorts of things into their ears that may be impossible for you to remove safely. If the object is near the ear canal opening and you feel it is safe, cautiously try removing the object with tweezers. Small objects can sometimes be removed by irrigating the ear with warm water. Do not try irrigation if the object is near the eardrum, if it blocks the entire ear canal, if the eardrum has a hole in it, or if the object is vegetable matter (e.g., kernel of corn, bean), which will swell when wet.

FIRST AID TIPS

Insect in an Ear
Do not try to kill a lodged insect by poking something into the victim's ear. Insects are attracted to light, so it may be coaxed out with light. Outdoors, pull the ear lobe gently to straighten the canal and turn the ear toward the sun. Indoors, turn off all lights, then shine a flashlight into the ear while pulling gently on the ear lobe. This may induce the insect to crawl out toward the light.

   If the light method fails, a little mineral oil may cause the insect to float out. Do not use this method if you are not *absolutely* sure that the foreign body in the ear is an insect. If the object is vegetable matter (e.g., a bean, popcorn), the object may swell and be difficult to remove. Do not use mineral oil if there is any sign of eardrum rupture.

   Do not go into the ear canal to remove foreign objects.

Nose Injuries

Nosebleeds

A severe nosebleed frightens the victim and often challenges the first aider's skill. Most nosebleeds are self-limited and seldom require medical attention. In cases of accompanying head or neck injuries, stabilize the head and neck for protection. In some cases, loss of blood could cause shock. There are two types of nosebleeds:

- *Anterior (front of nose)* is the most common type (90 percent). Blood comes out of the nose through one nostril.
- *Posterior (back of nose)* type involves massive bleeding backward into the mouth or down the back of the throat. A posterior nosebleed is serious and requires medical attention.

What to Do

1. Keep the victim in a sitting-up position to reduce blood pressure.
2. Keep the victim's head tilted slightly forward so blood can run out the front of the nose, not down the back of the throat, which can cause

CAUTION: DO NOT

- allow the victim to tilt the head backward.
- probe the nose with a cotton-tipped swab.
- move the victim's head and neck if a spine injury is suspected.

choking, nausea, or vomiting. Vomit could be inhaled into the lungs.

3. Pinch (or have the victim pinch) both nostrils with steady pressure for five minutes. Remind the victim to breathe through the mouth and to spit out any accumulated blood.
4. If bleeding persists, have the victim gently blow the nose to remove any irregular clots and excess blood and to minimize sneezing. This allows new clots to form. Then pinch the nostrils again for five minutes.
5. You might try one of the following methods in conjunction with nose pinching:
   - Place a roll of gauze (the diameter of a pencil) between the upper lip and the teeth. Press

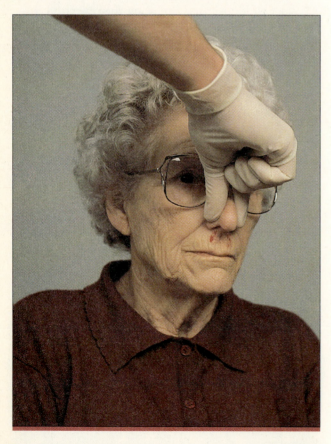

To control a nosebleed, have the victim lean forward and pinch both nostrils together . . .

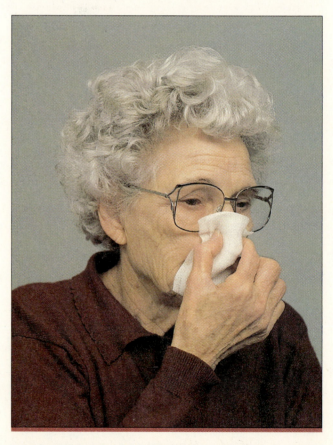

. . . or have the victim pinch his or her own nostrils.

NOSEBLEEDS

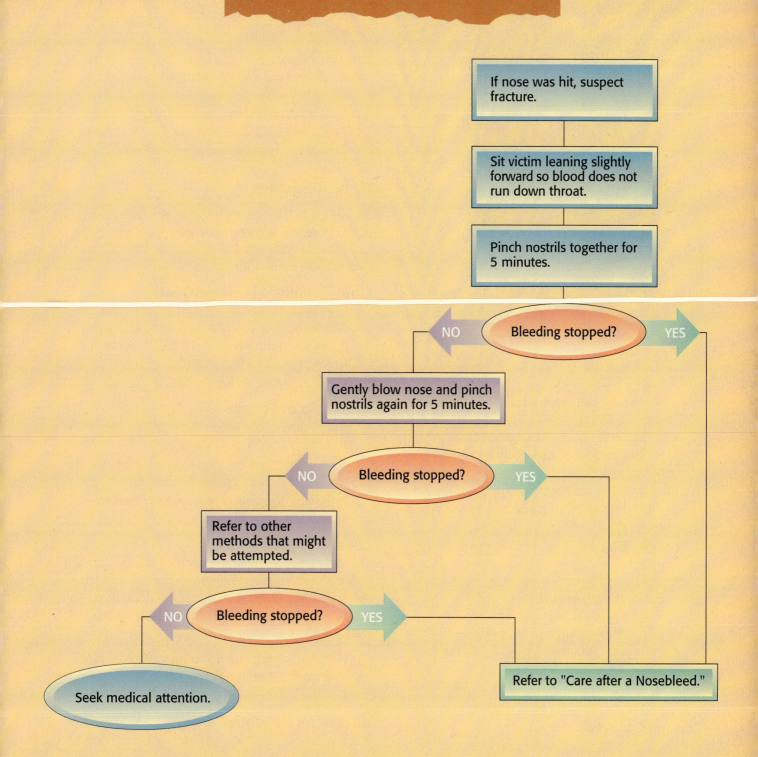

If nose was hit, suspect fracture.

Sit victim leaning slightly forward so blood does not run down throat.

Pinch nostrils together for 5 minutes.

Bleeding stopped?

NO → Gently blow nose and pinch nostrils again for 5 minutes.

YES

Bleeding stopped?

NO → Refer to other methods that might be attempted.

YES

Bleeding stopped?

NO → Seek medical attention.

YES → Refer to "Care after a Nosebleed."

against the gauze roll with your fingers to stop the blood flow.
- Apply an ice pack over the nose area to help control bleeding—especially if caused by a blow to the nose.

6. Place an unconscious victim on his or her side to prevent inhaling of blood and try the procedures listed above.
7. Seek medical attention if any of the following applies:
   - The nostril pinching and other methods do not stop the bleeding.
   - You suspect a posterior nosebleed.
   - The victim has high blood pressure or is taking anticoagulants (blood thinners) or large doses of aspirin.
   - Bleeding happens after a blow to the nose, and you suspect a broken nose.

Foreign Objects

A foreign object in the nose is a problem mainly among small children, who seem to gain some satisfaction from putting peanuts, beans, raisins, and similar objects into their nostrils.

1. Induce sneezing by having the victim sniff pepper or by tickling the opposite nostril.
2. Have the victim blow gently as the opposite nostril is compressed.

3. Use tweezers to pull out an object that is visible. Do not probe or push an object deeper.
4. Seek medical attention if the object cannot be removed.

Broken Nose

1. If you suspect a spine injury, seek medical attention.
2. Treat a nosebleed as described above.
3. Apply an ice pack to the nose for 15 minutes. Do not try to straighten a crooked nose.

Dental Injuries

Because dental emergencies generally cause considerable pain and anxiety, managing them promptly can provide great relief to the victim. Dental emergencies take many forms.

Objects Caught between Teeth

1. Try to remove the object with dental floss. Guide the floss carefully to avoid cutting the gums. Do not try to remove the object with a sharp or pointed instrument.
2. If unsuccessful, seek a dentist's attention.

Bitten Lip or Tongue

1. Apply direct pressure to the bleeding area with sterile gauze or a clean cloth.
2. If swelling is present, apply an ice pack or have victim suck on a Popsicle or ice chips.
3. If the bleeding does not stop, seek medical attention.

Loosened Tooth

Trauma can cause teeth to become loosened in their sockets. Applying pressure on either side of each tooth with the fingers can determine looseness. Any tooth movement, even if it is barely felt, indicates a possibly loose tooth.

1. Have the victim bite down on a piece of gauze to keep the tooth in place.
2. Consult a dentist or an oral surgeon.

Knocked-Out Tooth

A knocked-out tooth is a true dental emergency. It is also a common one. More than 90 percent of the two million teeth knocked out each year in the United States could be saved with proper treatment. Have the victim rinse his or her mouth and put a rolled gauze pad in the socket to control bleeding.

Emergency care for knocked-out teeth has changed dramatically in recent years. The first question you want to ask when a tooth has been knocked out is, "Where is the tooth?" Time is crucial for successful reimplantation. Ligament fiber fragments attached to the tooth and the bone in the socket are left after the tooth has been knocked out. The ligament fibers begin to die soon after the injury. Therefore, it is important to prevent the tooth from drying. Moisture alone is not sufficient since it must also preserve the tooth's ligament fibers. Steps must be taken both to prevent the tooth from becoming dehydrated and to protect the ligament fibers from damage.

1. Find the tooth and handle it by the crown, never the root, to minimize damage to the ligament fibers.

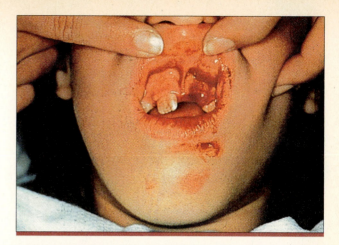

Tooth knocked out

Dental Emergency Procedures

Toothache	Rinse the mouth vigorously with warm water to clean out debris. Use dental floss to remove any food that might be trapped between the teeth. *(Do not place aspirin on the aching tooth or gum tissues.)* See your dentist as soon as possible.
Orthodontic Problems (braces and retainers)	If a wire is causing irritation, cover end of the wire with a small cotton ball, beeswax, or a piece of gauze until you can get to the dentist.
	If a wire is embedded in the cheek, tongue, or gum tissue, do not attempt to remove it. Go to your dentist immediately.
	If an appliance becomes loose or a piece of it breaks off, take the appliance and the piece and go to the dentist.
Knocked-Out Tooth	If the tooth is dirty, rinse it gently in running water. *Do not scrub it.*
	Gently insert and hold the tooth in its socket. If this is not possible, place the tooth in a container of milk or a special tooth preserving solution.
	Go immediately to your dentist (within 30 minutes, if possible). Don't forget to bring the tooth.
Broken Tooth	Gently clean dirt or debris from the injured area with warm water. Place cold compresses on the face, in the area of the injured tooth, to minimize swelling. Go to the dentist immediately.
Bitten Tongue or Lip	Apply direct pressure to the bleeding area with a clean cloth. If swelling is present, apply cold compresses. If bleeding does not stop, go to a hospital emergency room.
Object Wedged between Teeth	Try to remove the object with dental floss. Guide the floss carefully to avoid cutting the gums. If not successful in removing the object, go to the dentist.
	Do not try to remove the object with a sharp or pointed instrument.
Possible Fractured Jaw	Immobilize the jaw by any means (necktie, dish towel). If swelling is present, apply cold compresses. Call your dentist or go immediately to a hospital emergency room.

Source: Copyright by the American Dental Association; reprinted with permission.

2. The best place for a knocked-out tooth is its socket. A tooth often can be successfully reimplanted if it has been put back in its sockets within 30 minutes after the injury; the odds of successful reimplantation decrease about 1 percent for every minute the tooth is absent from the socket.

Try to replace the tooth into the socket, using adjacent teeth as a guide. Push down on the tooth so the top is even with the adjacent teeth. Biting down gently on gauze is helpful.

Immediate reinsertion is not always possible, however. The victim may be reluctant to put the knocked-out tooth back into its socket, especially if it has fallen on the ground and is covered with debris. Or the tooth may repeatedly fall out, putting the victim at risk of inhaling or swallowing it. In victims with multiple trauma, reinsertion may be prevented by the presence of more serious injuries.

When immediate reinsertion is not feasible, one of the worst things you can do to a knocked-out tooth is to transport it dry. Consider using saliva for the short term (less than one hour). Milk is much better because of its calcium and magnesium concentrations. Ideally, the milk should be whole milk and kept cold to minimize bacterial growth. Do not use reconstituted powdered milk or milk by-products such as yogurt; they are damaging to the ligaments.

The best transport medium is Hank's solution, a balanced-pH cell-culture medium that helps restore the ligament fibers. The use of Hank's solution extends the viability of the ligament fibers for 6 to 12 hours. The solution, which is available commercially as the Save-a-Tooth™ kit, has been approved by the FDA for use up to 24 hours after an injury, and there is some evidence that its use enables successful reimplantation, even after 96 hours. The Save-a-Tooth™ kit is available in drugstores and deserves consideration as a standard item in the home medicine chest.

In the case of a young child, the tooth can be stored in the parent's mouth. Some experts recommend that the tooth be placed in the victim's mouth to keep it moist until dental treatment is available. This method, though convenient, presents the risk, especially in children, of the tooth's being accidentally swallowed.

3. Take the victim and the tooth to a dentist immediately.

CAUTION: DO NOT

- handle a knocked-out tooth roughly.
- put a knocked-out tooth in water, mouthwash, alcohol, or Betadine.
- put a knocked-out tooth in skim milk, reconstituted powdered milk, or milk by-products such as yogurt.
- rinse a knocked-out tooth unless you are reinserting it in the socket.
- place a knocked-out tooth in anything that can dry or crush the outside of the tooth.
- scrub a knocked-out tooth or remove any attached tissue fragments.
- remove a partially extracted tooth. Push it back into place and seek a dentist so the loose tooth can be stabilized.

Just getting the avulsed (knocked-out) tooth back into the socket, even if it is improperly placed, puts the tooth in a good physiologic environment that will only increase its viability.

Broken Tooth

The front teeth are frequently broken by falls or direct blows. Such damage is not unusual in the victims of violent acts or automobile accidents. It is also common in children, especially those with an overbite.

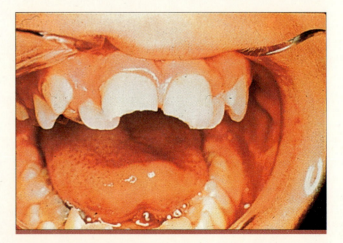

Broken teeth

DENTAL INJURIES

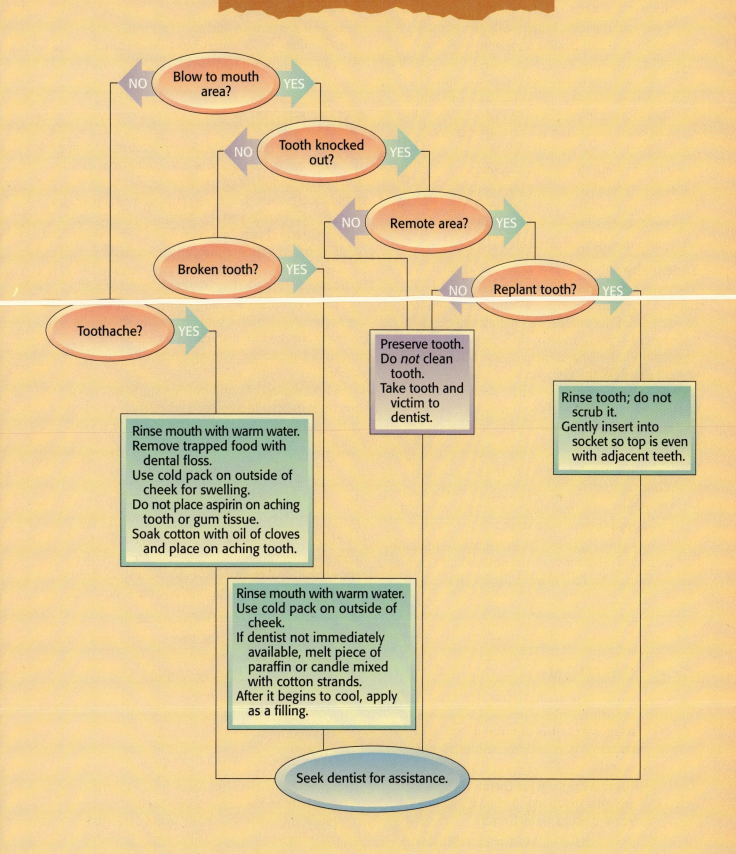

Blow to mouth area? NO / YES

Tooth knocked out? NO / YES

Remote area? NO / YES

Broken tooth? YES

Replant tooth? NO / YES

Toothache? YES

Preserve tooth.
Do *not* clean tooth.
Take tooth and victim to dentist.

Rinse tooth; do not scrub it.
Gently insert into socket so top is even with adjacent teeth.

Rinse mouth with warm water.
Remove trapped food with dental floss.
Use cold pack on outside of cheek for swelling.
Do not place aspirin on aching tooth or gum tissue.
Soak cotton with oil of cloves and place on aching tooth.

Rinse mouth with warm water.
Use cold pack on outside of cheek.
If dentist not immediately available, melt piece of paraffin or candle mixed with cotton strands.
After it begins to cool, apply as a filling.

Seek dentist for assistance.

1. Gently clean dirt and blood from the injured area with a sterile gauze pad or a clean cloth and warm water.

2. If you are in a remote area with no dentist nearby, you can make a temporary cap from melted candle wax or paraffin and a few strands of cotton. When the wax begins to harden but can still be molded, press a wad of it onto the tooth. Other improvisations include using ski wax or chewing gum (preferably sugarless).

3. Apply an ice pack on the face in the area of the injured tooth, to decrease swelling.

4. If you suspect a jaw fracture, stabilize the jaw by tying a bandage wrapped under the chin and over the top of the head.

5. Seek a dentist immediately.

Toothache

The most common reason for toothaches is dental decay. Victims frequently complain of pain limited to one area of the mouth, although it can be more widespread—pain can also affect the ear, eye, neck, or even opposite side of the jaw. The tooth will be sensitive to heat and cold. Identify the diseased tooth by tapping the area with a spoon handle or similar object. A diseased tooth will hurt.

Emergency care for toothaches focuses on reducing the pain:

1. Rinse the mouth with warm water to clean it out.

2. Use dental floss to remove any food that might be trapped between the teeth.

3. If you suspect a cavity, insert a small cotton ball soaked in oil of cloves (eugenol) to help depress the pain. Take care to keep the oil off the gums,

CAUTION: DO NOT

- place aspirin, acetaminophen, or ibuprofen on the aching tooth or gum tissues or allow them to dissolve in the mouth. A serious acid burn can result.

- cover a cavity with cotton if there is any pus discharge or facial swelling. See a dentist immediately.

- stick anything into the exposed cavity or into the softened exposed root.

lips, and inside surfaces of the cheeks. If applicable, follow the same procedures as for a broken tooth.

4. Give the victim an analgesic (aspirin, acetaminophen, or ibuprofen) to reduce pain.

5. Seek a dentist immediately.

Spine Injuries

The spine is a column of vertebrae stacked one on the next from the skull's base to the tailbone. Each vertebra has a hollow center through which the spinal cord passes. The spinal cord consists of long tracts of nerves that join the brain with all the other body organs and parts.

If a broken vertebra pinches spinal nerves, paralysis can result. All unconscious victims should be treated as though they have a spine injury. All conscious victims sustaining injuries from falls, diving accidents, or motor vehicle crashes should be carefully checked for a spine injury before being moved. Suspect a spine injury in all head-injury victims.

A mistake in the handling of a spine-injury victim could mean a lifetime in a wheelchair or a bed for the victim. Suspect a spine injury in *all* severe accidents.

What to Look For

Head injuries serve as a clue since the head may have been snapped suddenly in one or more directions, endangering the spine. About 15 to 20 percent of head-injury victims also have a spine injury. Other signs and symptoms include the following:

- Painful movement of the arms or legs
- Numbness, tingling, weakness, or burning sensation in the arms or legs
- Loss of bowel or bladder control
- Paralysis of the arms or legs
- Deformity (odd-looking angle of the victim's head and neck)

Ask a responsive victim these questions:

- *Is there pain?* Neck (cervical spine) injuries radiate pain to the arms; upper-back (thoracic spine) injuries radiate pain around the ribs; lower-back injuries usually radiate pain down the legs. Often, the victim will describe the pain as "electric."

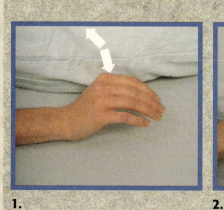

1.

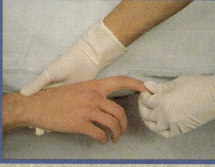

2.

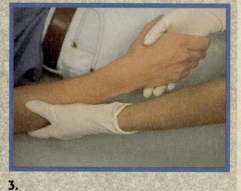

3.

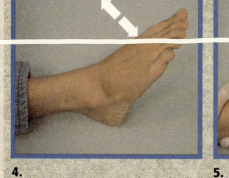

4.

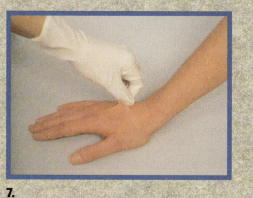

5.

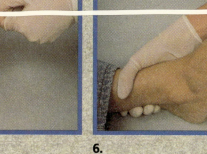

6.

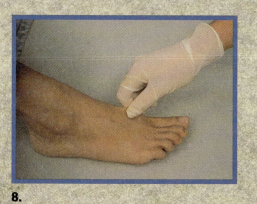

7.

8.

Conscious Victim— Upper Extremity Checks

1. Victim wiggles fingers.
2. Rescuer touches fingers.
3. Victim squeezes rescuer's hand.

Conscious Victim— Lower-Extremity Checks

4. Victim wiggles toes.
5. Rescuer touches toes.
6. Victim pushes foot against rescuer's hand.

Victim's failure to perform may mean spine injury!

Unconscious Victim

7. Pinch hand.
8. Pinch foot.

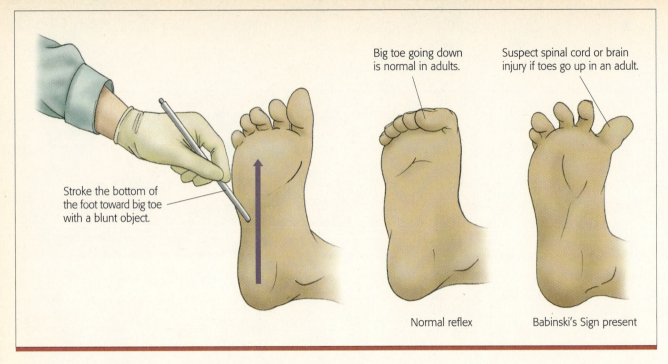

Stroke the bottom of the foot toward big toe with a blunt object.

Big toe going down is normal in adults.

Suspect spinal cord or brain injury if toes go up in an adult.

Normal reflex

Babinski's Sign present

Babinski test checks the nervous system (spinal cord and brain) for injury

- *Can you move your feet?* Ask the victim to press a foot against your hand. If the victim cannot perform this movement or if the movement is extremely weak against your hand, the victim may have injured the spine.
- *Can you move your fingers?* Moving the fingers is a sign that nerve pathways are intact. Ask the victim to grip your hand. A strong grip indicates that a spine injury is unlikely.

If the victim is unresponsive, do the following:

- Look for cuts, bruises, and deformities.
- Test responses by pinching the victim's hand (either palm or back of the hand) and bare foot (sole or top of the foot). No reaction could mean spine damage.
- Test the nervous system (spinal cord) by using the Babinski test: Stroke the bottom of the foot firmly toward the big toe with a key or similar sharp object. The normal response is an involuntary reflex that makes the big toe go down (except in infants). If the spinal cord or brain is injured, an adult's and child's toe will flex upward.
- Ask bystanders what happened. If you still are not sure about a possible spine injury, assume the victim has one until it is proved otherwise.

What to Do

1. Check and monitor the ABCs. For an unresponsive victim, use the procedures described on page 70 for opening the airway.
2. Stabilize the victim against any movement, using one of the following methods. Whatever method you use, tell the victim not to move.
   - Grasp the victim's clavicle and trapezius muscle (shoulder) and cradle the head between the inside of your forearms. Hold the victim's head and neck still until the EMS responds.
   - Grasp the victim's head over the ears and hold the head and neck still until the EMS responds.
   - If a long wait for the EMS to respond is anticipated or if you are tired from holding the victim's head in place, kneel with the victim's head between your knees or place objects on each side of the victim's head to prevent it from rolling from side to side.

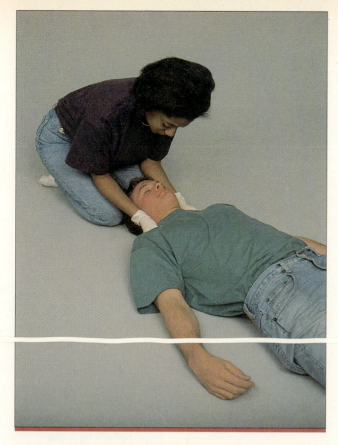

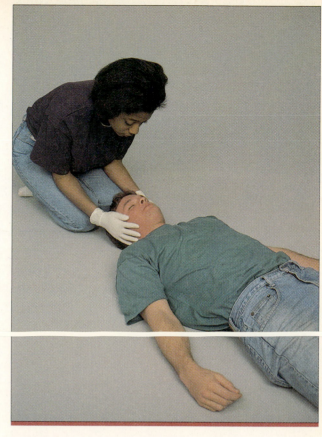

Stabilize against movement by holding onto shoulders and gently squeeze head between arms.

Stabilize against movement by holding the head.

 CAUTION: DO NOT

- move the victim, even if the victim is in water. Wait for the EMS to arrive—they have the proper training and equipment. Victims with suspected spine injury require cervical collars and stabilization on a spine board. It is better to do nothing than to mishandle a victim with a spine injury.

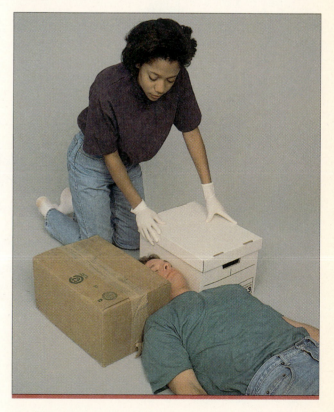

Stabilize against movement by placing objects on each side of the head.

SPINE INJURIES

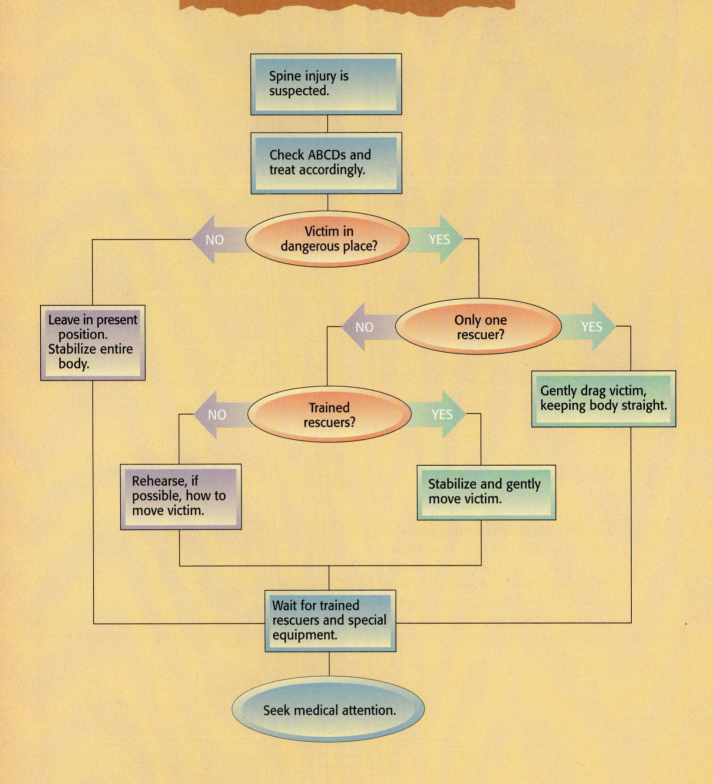

Spine injury is suspected.

Check ABCDs and treat accordingly.

Victim in dangerous place?

NO → Leave in present position. Stabilize entire body.

YES → Only one rescuer?

YES → Gently drag victim, keeping body straight.

NO → Trained rescuers?

NO → Rehearse, if possible, how to move victim.

YES → Stabilize and gently move victim.

Wait for trained rescuers and special equipment.

Seek medical attention.

STUDY QUESTIONS 10

Name _____ Course _____ Date _____

Activities

Activity 1

Check (✔) the signs and symptoms of a skull fracture.

_____ 1. pain at the injury site

_____ 2. deformed skull

_____ 3. fluid leaking from the ears or nose

_____ 4. discoloration around the eye(s) (raccoon eyes)

_____ 5. pupil of one eye larger than pupil of the other eye.

Mark each sign yes (Y) or no (N).

After a head injury, which signs indicate a need for medical attention?

_____ 6. Headache lasting more than a day or increased severity

_____ 7. Vomiting beginning hours after the initial injury

_____ 8. One pupil appearing larger than the other

_____ 9. Convulsions or seizures

_____ 10. "Seeing double"

Mark each statement as true (T) or false (F).

T F 11. A nosebleed victim should sit up with the head tilted back.

T F 12. A "halo sign" or "ring sign" results from a cerebrospinal fluid leak.

T F 13. Preserve a knocked-out tooth in mouthwash or rubbing alcohol.

T F 14. If it is necessary to bandage one eye, it is advisable to cover both eyes.

T F 15. If pupils are unequal in size, brain damage may exist.

T F 16. The first aider should not remove foreign objects embedded in an eyeball.

T F 17. To remove a foreign body from the surface of an eyeball, it is best to use cotton wrapped around a matchstick.

T F 18. Scalp wounds tend to bleed freely.

T F 19. Clear or blood-tinged fluid draining from the ears is a good indicator of a skull fracture.

T F 20. For a skull fracture, good first aid involves placing the victim's head lower than the rest of the body.

Check (✔) the signs and symptoms that indicate a possible spine injury.

_____ 21. description by the victim of pain down the arms or legs

_____ 22. ability to strongly grip your hand and move a foot against your hand pressure

_____ 23. a severe head injury

_____ 24. inability of the victim to move fingers and toes when asked to do so

Mark each statement as true (T) or false (F).

T F 25. Do not move a victim unless extreme hazards exist (e.g., burning building or car).

T F 26. Careless moving of a victim may permanently confine him or her to a wheelchair.

T F 27. Move a spine-injury victim as quickly as possible to a medical facility.

Activity 2

Mark each action yes (Y) or no (N).

Which is proper first aid for an embedded object in the eye?

_____ 1. Use a damp and sterile or clean cloth to remove the object from the eyeball's surface.

_____ 2. Use a toothpick or a matchstick to remove the foreign object.

_____ 3. Use a paper cup or similar item over the eye but not touching the object.

_____ 4. Allow the victim to see by leaving the uninjured eye uncovered.

Mark each statement as true (T) or false (F).

T F 5. Hitting the eye may cause a black eye.

T F 6. A victim with blurred vision should consult an ophthalmologist.

T F 7. For an eyeball knocked out of socket, gently and carefully replace the eyeball in the socket and cover with a dressing.

T F 8. After a blow to the eye, apply a cold compress immediately for about 15 minutes to reduce pain and swelling.

Mark each action yes (Y) or no (N).
If a tree limb scrapes against an eye and cuts the eyeball, first aid, besides seeking medical help for the victim, would include:

_____ 9. applying a dressing tightly over the injured eye

_____ 10. holding the eyelids of the injured eye open

_____ 11. applying direct pressure to the cut eyeball to control the bleeding

_____ 12. loosely applying dressings over both eyes

_____ 13. tightly applying a dressing over both eyes

Choose the best answer.

_____ 14. Corrosive acid has spilled into your co-worker's eyes, resulting in severe pain. What should you do first?
   a. Cover both eyes with dressings and immediately obtain medical aid.
   b. Hold the eyes open and flood them with water for 15 minutes.
   c. Allow tears to flush out the chemicals.
   d. Pour water into the eyes for about 20 minutes.

_____ 15. Following your initial actions, what should you do?
   a. Place wet dressings over both eyes.
   b. Leave both eyes uncovered and seek medical attention.

   c. Allow the victim to rest for at least 30 minutes.
   d. Apply dressings over both eyes and seek medical attention.

Activity 3
Choose the best techniques for controlling most nosebleeds.

_____ 1. a. Position victim in a sitting position.
         b. Position victim lying down.

_____ 2. a. Keep the head tilted slightly backward.
         b. Keep the head tilted slightly forward.

_____ 3. a. Pinch both nostrils for 5 minutes.
         b. Pinch only one nostril for 60 seconds.

_____ 4. a. Always seek medical attention.
         b. Seek medical attention for victims taking blood thinners or large doses of aspirin and those with high blood pressure.

Case Situations

Case 1
During a football game, a player is knocked out for 10 minutes.
1. Define the term *concussion*._____
_____

2. List four signs of a concussion.
   a._____
   b._____
   c._____
   d._____

3. Give an example of a mental test you could use on a conscious victim. _____
_____
_____

4. When should the victim be allowed to return to activity?
_____
_____

STUDY QUESTIONS 10

Name _____ Course _____ Date _____

Case 2
Several children are playing on a swing set. One child is hit on the forehead by another child coming back on a swing. The child is knocked several feet behind the swing set by the impact and appears dizzy, confused, and very weak. There is no bleeding. The child's pupils react slowly to light.

1. You would most likely suspect
   ____ a. a skull fracture
   ____ b. a brain concussion
   ____ c. both, since the signs and symptoms are almost identical

2. First aid care for the child would include
   a. _____
   _____
   b. _____
   _____
   c. _____
   _____
   d. _____
   _____

3. With any head injury, always suspect:
   ____ a. The worst. Inform the parents the child may die.
   ____ b. Neck and spine injury.
   ____ c. The best. No real emergency care is needed if there is no bleeding or other major sign of injury.

Case 3
During an automobile accident, a young woman passenger is thrown from the back seat into the windshield. Her left eyelid is bleeding profusely, and the left eyeball appears to be bulging. Other injuries include a laceration of the forehead and bruises on her arms and legs.

1. What first aid should you provide to this victim?
   a. _____
   _____
   b. _____
   _____
   c. _____
   _____
   d. _____
   _____

2. Should both eyes be bandaged? (Explain why or why not.)
   _____
   _____
   _____
   _____

3. What special precautions should you take in caring for the avulsed eyeball?
   a. _____
   _____
   b. _____
   _____

Case 4
The victim of a motorcycle accident complains of loss of sensation in both lower extremities. You found him lying on his back with no other obvious injury. He is still wearing a helmet.

1. What should you suspect in this case?
   _____
   _____

2. What leads you to suspect this?
   _____
   _____

3. What is the correct first aid for this victim?
   _____
   _____

4. Should you move this victim?
   _____
   _____

5. When would you be justified in moving this victim?
   _____
   _____

Case 5

A child falls off a bike and knocks out a permanent tooth. The victim's dentist is minutes away. Which are the proper procedures in this situation?

_____ 1. Rinse the child's mouth out with water and put a gauze pad on the socket to control bleeding.

_____ 2. Stick the tooth back in the child's tooth socket.

_____ 3. Scrub the dirt off the tooth in water and call your dentist.

_____ 4. Put the tooth in a glass of whole milk and take the child immediately to a dentist.

_____ 5. Depending on the child, have the child hold the tooth in his or her mouth with instructions not to swallow.

_____ 6. Place the tooth in a glass of mouthwash and take the child to a dentist.

_____ 7. Do not worry about the tooth, but take the child to a dentist.

Case 6

You and a friend have been cross-country skiing. Due to the sunlight reflection off the snow and not wearing dark goggles or glasses, your friend suffers light injuries to her eyes.

_____ 1. What other sources of light can produce this type of eye injury?

    a. looking at a welder's arc

    b. watching an eclipse of the sun

    c. reflection off large bodies of water

    d. all the above

_____ 2. Treatment for this injury would consist of

    a. applying moist dressings or eye patches to the closed eyes

    b. irrigating the eyes with a steady stream of water

    c. keeping both the victim's eyes closed

    d. irrigating the eyes with a saline solution

NOTES

11

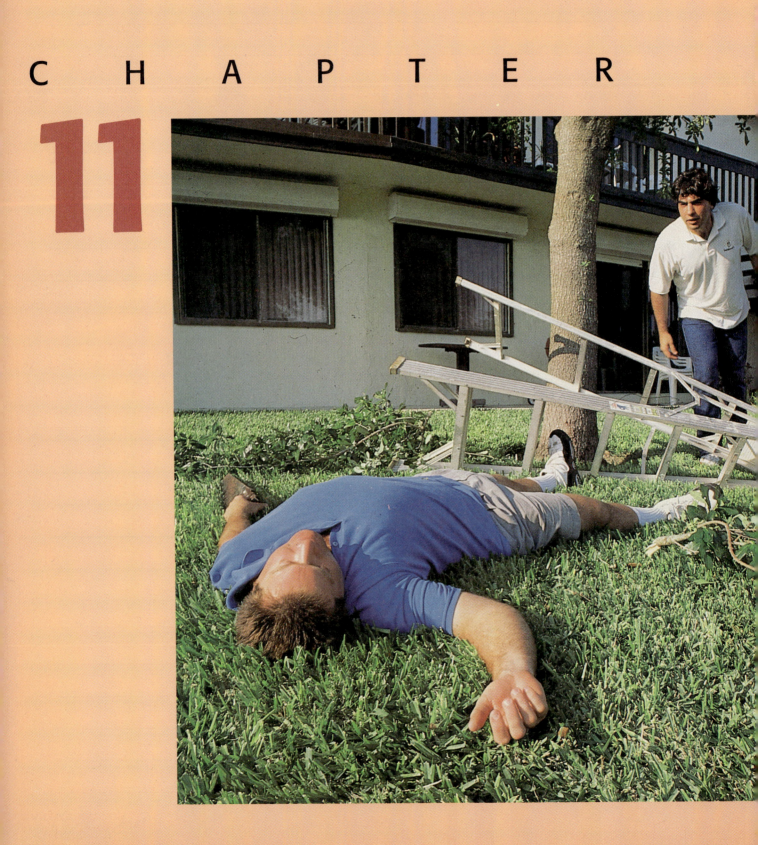

CHEST, ABDOMINAL, AND PELVIS INJURIES

Chest Injuries

Chest injuries fall into two categories: those to the chest wall and those to the lungs. Injuries to the chest wall (the ribs) include:

- rib fracture
- flail chest

In a lung injury, one of the following conditions occurs:

- Blood fills up the chest, causing incomplete lung expansion (**hemothorax**).
- Air fills a portion of chest cavity (**pneumothorax**).
- Air in the chest cavity moves in and out; the lung does not expand (**open pneumothorax**, or "sucking chest wound").
- Air is pulled into the chest cavity but cannot exit, causing tension or pressures that reduce heart and lung function (**tension pneumothorax**).

All chest-injury victims should have their ABCs checked and rechecked. A conscious chest-injury victim usually should be sitting up or place the victim with the injured side down. That position protects the uninjured side from blood inside the chest cavity and allows the good lung to expand.

To prevent pneumonia, encourage or force victims with chest-wall injuries to clear their lungs at least hourly by coughing, despite the pain.

Rib Fractures

The upper four ribs are rarely fractured because they are protected by the collarbone and the shoulder blades. Those ribs are so enmeshed by muscles that they rarely need to be splinted or realigned like other broken bones. The lower two ribs are hard to fracture because they are attached on only one end and have the freedom to move (which is why they are called "floating ribs"). The main symptom of a fractured rib is pain when the victim breathes, coughs, or moves.

What to Do

1. Stabilize the ribs by having the victim hold a pillow or other similar soft object against the injured area. Or you can use bandages to hold the pillow in place or tie an arm over the injured area.

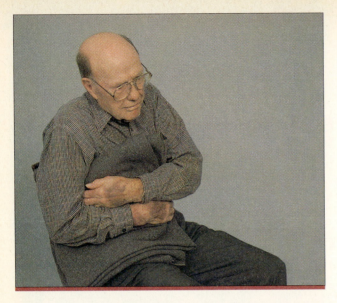

What to Do

1. Stabilize the chest by one of several methods:
   - Apply hand pressure. This is useful for a short time.
   - Place the victim on the injured side with a blanket or clothing underneath.
   - Apply a sand- or dirt-filled bag to the injured area.
2. Seek medical attention.

Impaled Object in Chest

What to Do

1. Stabilize the object in place with bulky dressings. *Do not try to remove an impaled object—bleeding and air in the chest cavity can result.* See page 213.
2. Seek medical attention.

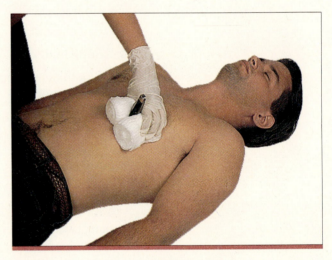

Stabilize penetrating object with bulky padding.

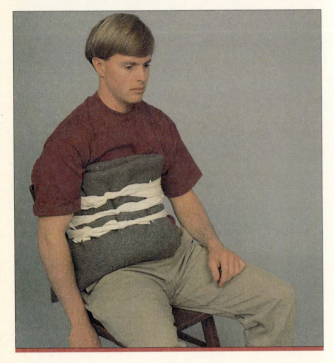

Stabilize chest with soft object such as pillow, coat, or blanket (hold or tie). Tell victim to occasionally take a deep breath and to cough.

2. Tell the victim to take deep breaths and to cough at least once each hour to prevent pneumonia.
3. Seek medical attention.

Flail Chest

A **flail chest** is a serious injury that involves several adjacent ribs fractured in two or more places. The victim's chest wall may move in a direction opposite that of the rest of the chest wall during breathing (known as "paradoxical breathing").

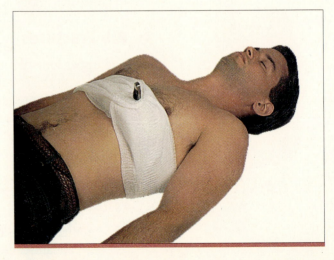

Secure padding and object.

CHEST INJURIES

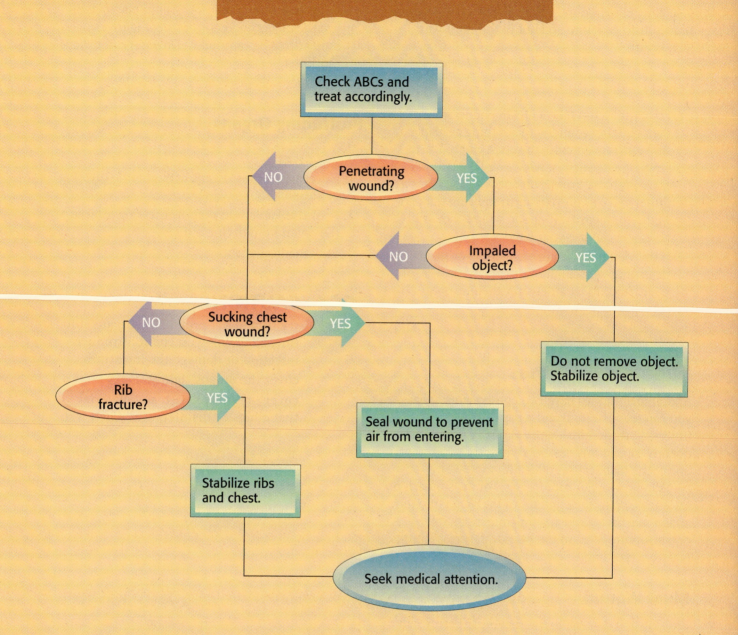

Check ABCs and treat accordingly.

Penetrating wound?

NO   YES

Impaled object?

NO   YES

Sucking chest wound?

NO   YES

Do not remove object. Stabilize object.

Rib fracture?

YES

Seal wound to prevent air from entering.

Stabilize ribs and chest.

Seek medical attention.

Sucking Chest Wound

A sucking chest wound results when a chest wound allows air to pass into and out of the chest with each breath.

What to Do

1. Have the victim take a breath and let it out; then seal the wound with anything available to stop air from entering the chest cavity. Plastic wrap or a plastic bag works well. Tape it in place with one corner untaped. That creates a flutter valve to prevent air from being trapped in the chest cavity. If plastic wrap is not available, you can use your hand.
2. If the victim has trouble breathing or seems to be getting worse, remove the plastic cover (or your hand) to let air escape, then reapply.
3. Seek medical attention.

Abdominal Injuries

Abdominal injuries have two components: what you can see (external) and what you cannot see (internal). Abdominal injury is one of the most frequently missed injuries; when missed, it becomes one of the main causes of death.

A hollow-organ rupture (e.g., of the stomach or intestines) spills the contents of the organ into the abdominal cavity, causing inflammation. Solid-organ rupture (e.g., of the liver or pancreas) results in severe bleeding.

Blunt Wound

Bruising and damage to internal organs can result from a severe blow to the abdomen.

What to Do

1. Place the victim on one side in a comfortable position and expect vomiting. Do not give the victim any food or drink. If you are hours from a medical facility, allow the victim to suck on a clean cloth soaked in water to relieve a dry mouth.
2. Seek medical attention.

Penetrating Wound

Expect internal organs to be damaged.

What to Do

1. If the penetrating object is still in place, stabilize the object and control bleeding by using bulky dressings around it. *Do not try to remove the object.*
2. Seek medical attention.

Protruding Organs
What to Do

1. Cover protruding organs with a sterile dressing or clean cloth.
2. Pour drinkable water on the dressing to keep the organ from drying out.
3. Seek medical attention.

 CAUTION: DO NOT
- try to reinsert protruding organs into the abdomen—you could introduce infection or damage the intestines.
- cover the organs tightly.
- cover the organs with any material that clings or disintegrates when wet.

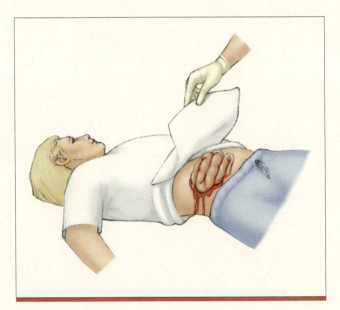

Do not reinsert protruding organs. Cover them with a moist, sterile dressing.

Pelvis Injuries

Pelvic fractures are usually caused by falls, crushing accidents, and sharp blows. Severe pain, shock, in-

ABDOMINAL INJURIES

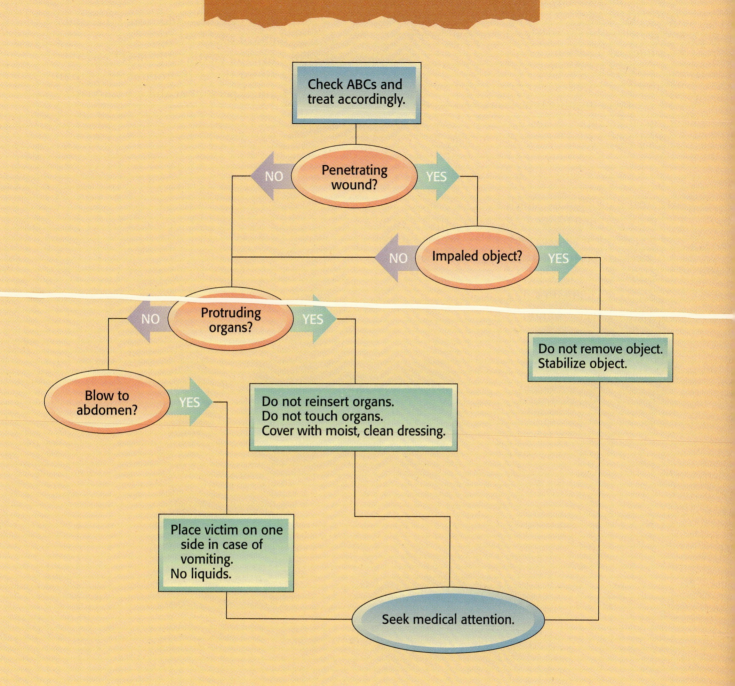

Check ABCs and treat accordingly.

Penetrating wound?

NO

YES

Impaled object?

NO

YES

Protruding organs?

NO

YES

Do not remove object.
Stabilize object.

Blow to abdomen?

YES

Do not reinsert organs.
Do not touch organs.
Cover with moist, clean dressing.

Place victim on one side in case of vomiting.
No liquids.

Seek medical attention.

ternal bleeding, and loss of the ability to use the lower extremities may be present. The bladder may be injured or ruptured, as well as other organs that are protected by the pelvis. Victims will have massive internal bleeding.

To determine if a victim's pelvis is fractured, gently press the sides of the pelvis downward and squeeze them inward at the iliac crests (upper points of the hips). A fractured pelvis will be painful. See Figures 6a and 6b, on page 59.

What to Do

1. Treat the victim for shock.
2. Place padding between the victim's thighs, then tie the victim's knees and ankles together. If the knees are bent, place padding under them for support.
3. Keep the victim on a firm surface.
4. Seek medical attention.

CAUTION: DO NOT

- roll the victim—additional internal damage could result.
- move the victim. Whenever possible, wait for the EMS ambulance, with its trained personnel and a backboard.

STUDY QUESTIONS 11

Name _____ Course _____ Date _____

Activities

Activity 1

Check (✔) the appropriate action(s).

1. Which of the following actions serve(s) as effective immediate first aid for a sucking chest wound?

   _____ a. Remove a penetrating object from the chest.

   _____ b. Apply a sterile or clean dressing loosely over the wound.

   _____ c. Leave the wound uncovered.

   _____ d. Tape a piece of plastic over the wound.

2. If the victim has trouble breathing after you have taped a piece of plastic over a sucking chest wound, you should:

   _____ a. apply a second piece of plastic over the first.

   _____ b. remove the plastic covering from the wound to allow air to escape from the chest cavity and then reapply.

   _____ c. leave the plastic in place and check breathing.

   _____ 3. The aim of first aid for a sucking chest wound is to

   a. not cover the wound

   b. cover the hole immediately to prevent air from entering the chest

   _____ 4. The aim of first aid for a flail chest is to

   a. stabilize the injured chest wall

   b. not bind the injured chest since binding interferes with breathing

   _____ 5. Which of the following materials, when taped at the edges, would make an effective covering for a sucking chest wound?

   a. clear plastic wrap

   b. a large gauze dressing

   c. a wash cloth

   d. a pillow case

   _____ 6. Signs and symptoms of flail chest include

   a. blood oozing from the injury site

   b. pain when breathing

   c. neck injury

   d. abnormal movement of part of the chest wall during breathing

Activity 2

Which is proper first aid for a blow to the abdomen if you suspect internal injuries?

   _____ 1. a. Place the victim on his or her back with a support on the abdomen.

   b. Place the victim on his or her side.

   _____ 2. a. Give the victim ice chips or sips of water to drink.

   b. Give the victim nothing to eat or drink.

Select the best first aid choice for a victim's abdominal open wound resulting from a penetrating object.

   _____ 3. a. Remove the penetrating object.

   b. Leave the object in place and stabilize it.

When protruding organs appear through an abdominal wound, you should

   _____ 4. a. gently push the organs back into the abdomen

   b. not attempt to push them back into the abdomen

   _____ 5. a. cover the wound with a clean, moist dressing

   b. cover the wound with a cotton dressing

T   F   6. Reinsert any protruding intestines or organs into open wounds of the abdomen

T   F   7. A dressing for exposed intestines should be kept dry if possible.

T   F   8. In a penetrating wound of the chest, the object should be left in place.

Activity 3

1. List two procedures you would use to check for a pelvic fracture.

   a._____

   b._____

2. Name two things you can do for a person with a fractured pelvis.

   a._____

   b._____

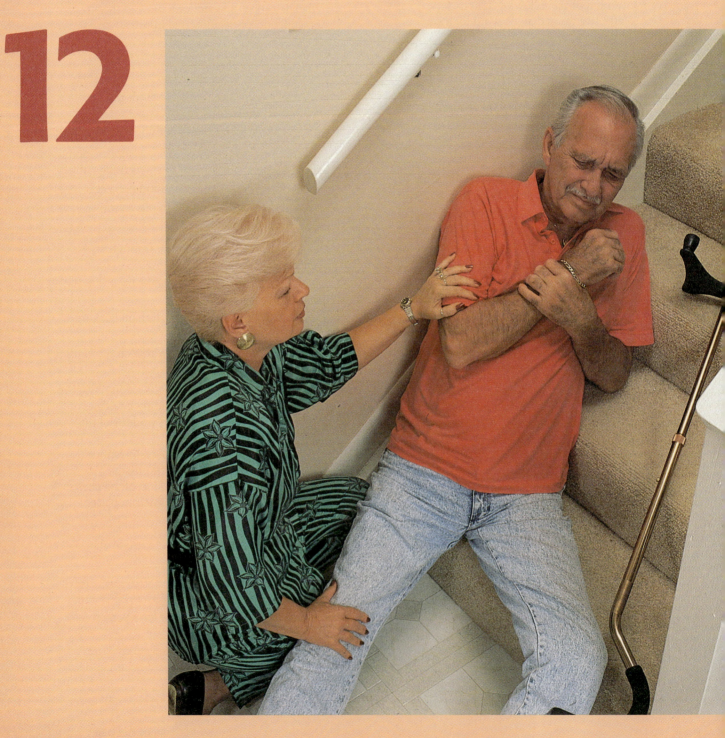

Bone, Joint, and Muscle Injuries

Fractures

The terms **fracture** and **broken bone** have the same meaning: a break or crack in a bone. There are two categories of fractures:

- **Closed (simple) fracture.** The skin is intact and no wound exists anywhere near the fracture site.
- **Open (compound) fracture.** The overlying skin has been damaged or broken. The wound may be the result of the bone protruding through the skin or of a direct blow that cuts the skin at the time of the fracture. The bone may not always be visible in the wound.

> *"The broken bone, once set together, is stronger than ever."*
>
> John Lyly Euphues

It is not possible outside a medical facility to determine the exact nature of a broken bone. It is helpful, however, for first aiders to be familiar with the terminology that physicians use to describe fractures. A **transverse fracture** cuts across the bone at right angles to its long axis and is often caused by direct injury. **Greenstick fractures** are incomplete fractures that commonly occur in children, whose bones (like green sticks) are pliable. A **spiral fracture** usually results from a twisting injury, and the fracture line has the appearance of a spring. The fracture line of an **oblique fracture** crosses the bone at an oblique angle, or in a slanting direction. In an **impacted fracture,** the broken ends of the bone are jammed together and may function as if no fracture were present. A **comminuted fracture** is one in which the bone is fragmented into more than two pieces (i.e., splintered or crushed).

What to Look For

It may be difficult to tell if a bone is fractured. When in doubt, treat the injury as a fracture. Signs and symptoms of a fracture include the following and can be remembered by using the mnemonic DOTS (deformity, open wound, tenderness, swelling):

- *Deformity* is not always obvious. Compare the injured part with the uninjured opposite part.

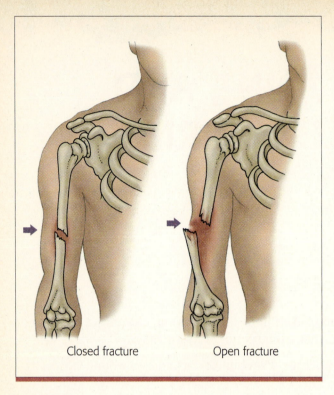

Fractures

- *Open wound* may indicate an underlying fracture.
- *Tenderness* and pain are commonly found only at the injury site. The victim usually will be able to point to the site of the pain. A useful procedure for detecting a fracture is to gently feel along the bones; victim complaints about pain or tenderness serve as a reliable sign of a fracture.
- *Swelling* caused by bleeding happens rapidly after a fracture.

Additional signs and symptoms include:

- *Loss of use* may or may not occur. "Guarding" occurs when motion produces pain; the victim refuses to use the injured part. Sometimes,

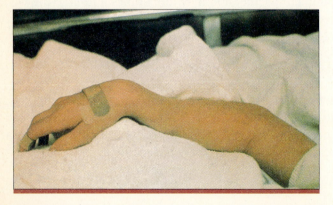

Forearm fracture

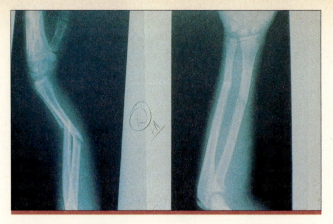

X-rays of victim with forearm fracture before and after setting

however, the victim is able to move a fractured limb with little or no pain.

- A *grating sensation,* called **crepitus,** can be felt and sometimes even heard when the ends of the broken bone rub together. Do *not* move the injured limb in an attempt to detect crepitus.
- *The history of the injury* can lead you to suspect a fracture whenever a serious accident has happened. The victim may have heard or felt the bone snap.

What to Do

1. Check and treat ABCs. Fractures, even open fractures, seldom present an immediate threat to life. Therefore, their treatment should be deferred until life-threatening conditions have been handled, for example, opening an airway or controlling massive bleeding. A tourniquet is practically never necessary to treat an open fracture, even when an extremity has been mangled beyond all possibility of salvage or a limb has been amputated. Only when all life-threatening conditions have been dealt with is it appropriate to identify and stabilize fractures.

2. Treat the victim for shock.

3. Determine what happened and the location of the injury.

4. Gently remove clothing covering the injured area. Do not move the injured area unless necessary. Cut clothing at the seams if necessary.

5. Use the mnemonic LAF (look and feel) as a reminder of how to examine an extremity.
   - Look at the injury site. Swelling and black-and-blue marks, which indicate escape of blood into the tissues, may come from either the bone end or associated muscular and blood vessel damage. Shortening or severe de-

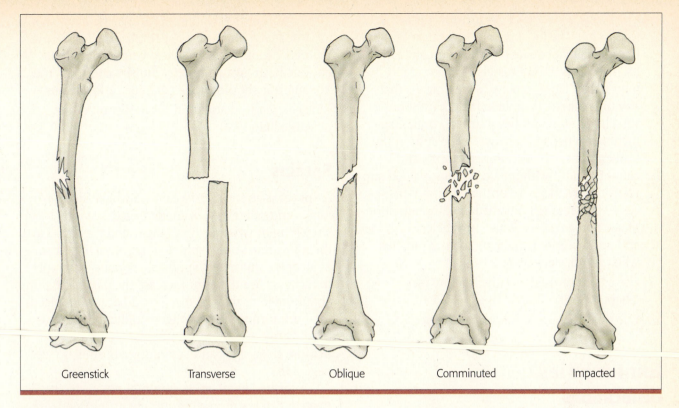

| Greenstick | Transverse | Oblique | Comminuted | Impacted |

Types of fractures

formity (angulation) between the joints or deformity around the joints, shortening of the extremity, and rotation of the extremity when compared with the opposite extremity indicate a bone injury. Lacerations or even small puncture wounds near the site of a bone fracture are considered open fractures.

- **A**nd
- **F**eel the injured area. If a fracture is not obvious, gently press, touch, or feel along the length of the bone for deformities, tenderness, and swelling.

6. Check blood flow and nerves. Use the mnemonic CSM (circulation, sensation, movement) as a way of remembering what to do.

- *Circulation.* Feel for the radial pulse (located on the thumb side of the wrist) for an arm injury and the posterior tibial pulse (located between the inside ankle bone and the Achilles tendon) for a leg injury. A pulseless arm or leg is a significant emergency that requires immediate surgical care. If there is no pulse, gently manipulate the extremity to try to restore the blood flow.

   Some experts recommend the capillary refill test. (Press on a fingernail or toenail, then release it. If circulation is normal, the nail bed should return to its normal color within two

seconds.) Performing the capillary refill test in the dark or the cold may limit its accuracy. The National EMT curriculum does not recommend using the capillary refill test on victims over 6 years of age.

- *Sensation.* Lightly touch or squeeze one of the victim's toes or fingers and ask the victim what he or she feels. Loss of sensation is an early sign of nerve damage or spine damage.
- *Movement.* Check for nerve damage by asking the victim to wiggle his or her toes or fingers. If the toes or fingers are injured, do not have the victim attempt to move them.

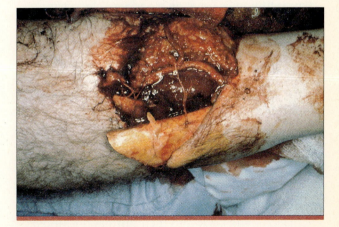

Open tibia, fibula fracture

A quick nerve and circulatory check is very important. The most serious complication of a fracture is inadequate blood flow in an extremity. The major blood vessels of an extremity tend to run close to bone, which means that any time a bone is broken, the adjacent blood vessels are at risk of being torn by bone fragments or pinched off between the ends of the broken bone. The tissues of the arms and legs cannot survive without a continuing blood supply for more than two or three hours. This necessitates seeking immediate medical attention. Major nerve pathways also travel close to bone and are susceptible to being torn or pinched when an adjacent bone is broken.

7. Use a splint to stabilize the fracture (see Chapter 14).
8. Use the RICE procedures (see Chapter 13).

Joint Injuries

Dislocations

A **dislocation** occurs when a joint comes apart and stays apart with the bone ends no longer in contact. The shoulders, elbows, fingers, hips, kneecaps (patellas), and ankles are the joints most frequently affected. Dislocations have signs and symptoms similar to those of a fracture: deformity, severe pain, swelling, and the inability of the victim to move the injured joint. The main sign of a dislocation is deformity—its appearance will be different from that of a comparable uninjured joint.

What to Do

1. Check the CSM (circulation, sensation, movement). If the end of the dislocated bone is pressing on nerves or blood vessels, corresponding functions also may be compromised, that is, numbness or paralysis may exist below the dislocation. When dealing with a fracture or a dislocation, always check the pulses. If there is no pulse in the injured extremity, transport the victim to a medical facility immediately.
2. Use a splint to stabilize the joint in the position in which it was found. (See Chapter 14.)
3. Use the RICE procedures (see Chapter 13).
4. Do not try to **reduce** the joint (put the displaced parts back into their normal positions), since nerve and blood vessel damage could re-

sult. Experts in wilderness medicine have identified easy and safe ways to treat the following dislocations when medical help is more than one hour away: kneecap, fingers and toes, and anterior shoulder. See Chapter 22 for details.

5. Seek medical attention for reduction of the dislocation.

Sprains

A **sprain** is an injury to a joint in which the ligaments and other tissues are damaged by violent stretching or twisting. The ankles and the knees are the joints most often sprained. Eighty-five percent of all ankle injuries in sports are sprains. Attempts to move or use the joint increase the pain. The skin about the joint may be discolored because of bleeding from torn tissues. It often is difficult to distinguish between a severe sprain and a fracture, because their signs and symptoms are similar (see page 236).

A severe lateral ankle sprain, if not correctly treated, can result in a chronically unstable ankle that is prone to sprains. Any ligament or bone injury on the inner side of the ankle usually represents a serious problem and requires medical attention. Ankle sprains most often occur when the foot turns inward and stress is placed on the outside of the ankle.

The goal of sprain care is to prevent further injury to the torn ligaments. Initial treatment consists of rest, ice, compression, and elevation (RICE; see Chapter 13). Swelling is like glue and can lock up a joint in a matter of hours. It is vitally important to keep swelling out of a joint by using cold promptly; it is even more important to make the swelling recede as quickly as possible with a compression (elastic) bandage.

Muscle Injuries

Although muscle injuries pose no real emergency, first aiders have ample opportunities to care for them.

Strains

A normal, warmed-up muscle is much like a rubber band. When stretched, it will not snap. When a cold or tight muscle is stretched, however, there is a likelihood that it will tear. A muscle **strain**, also known as a muscle pull, occurs when a muscle is stretched beyond its normal range of motion, re-

SKILL SCAN: Checking an Extremity's CSM

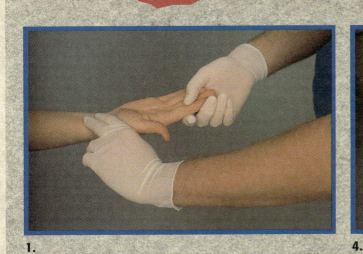

1.

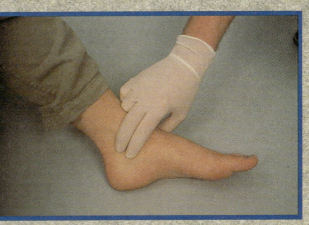

4.

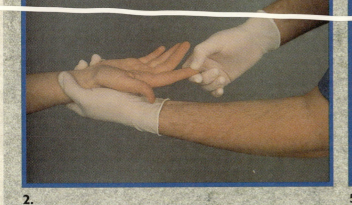

2.

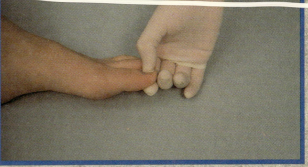

5.

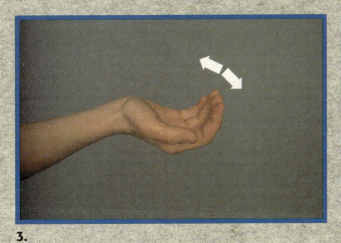

3.

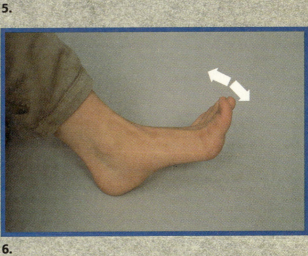

6.

Check an upper extremity for:

1. Circulation—radial pulse
2. Sensation—squeeze fingers
3. Movement—wiggle fingers

Check a lower extremity for:

4. Circulation—posterial tibial pulse
5. Sensation—squeeze toe
6. Movement—wiggle toes

sulting in the muscle tearing. When muscle fibers tear, fluid from nearby tissues leaks out and starts to build up near the injury. The area becomes inflamed, swollen, and tender. Inflammation begins immediately after an injury, but it can take 24–72 hours for enough tissue fluid to build up to cause pain and stiffness.

What to Look For

Any of the following signs and symptoms may indicate a muscle strain:

- sharp pain
- extreme tenderness when the area is touched
- cavity, indentation, or bump that can be felt or seen
- severe weakness and loss of function of the injured part
- a "snap" sound heard
- stiffness and pain when the victim moves the muscle

What to Do

Use the RICE procedures (see Chapter 13).

Contusions

A muscle **contusion** results from a blow to the muscle. Contusions are also known as **bruises.**

What to Look For

Any of the following signs and symptoms may occur in a muscle contusion:

- swelling
- pain and tenderness
- black-and-blue mark appearing hours later

What to Do

Use the RICE procedures (see Chapter 13).

Cramps

A cramp occurs when a muscle goes into an uncontrolled spasm and contraction, resulting in severe

pain and restriction or loss of movement. Although scientific literature has yet to confirm the causes of muscle cramps, several factors are associated with them. For example, muscle cramping is associated with certain diseases (e.g., diabetes, atherosclerosis). Muscle cramps are often, but not always, associated with physical activity and can be roughly divided into two categories: night cramps, which include any cramp occurring while an individual is at rest, and heat cramps, which are related to dehydration and electrolyte imbalance. (The electrolytes potassium and sodium carry an electric charge that helps trigger muscles to contract and relax.)

What to Do

There are many treatments for cramps. Try one or more of the following:

1. Have the victim gently stretch the affected muscle. Because a muscle cramp is an uncontrolled muscle contraction or spasm, a gradual lengthening of the muscle may help lengthen the muscle fibers and relieve the cramp.
2. Relax the muscle by applying pressure to it.
3. Apply ice to the cramped muscle to make it relax. The exception might be in a cold environment.
4. Pinch the upper lip hard (an accupressure technique) to reduce calf-muscle cramping.
5. Drink lightly salted cool (dissolve ¼ teaspoon salt in a quart of water) water or a commercial sports drink.

 CAUTION: DO NOT

- give salt tablets to a person with muscle cramps. They can cause stomach irritation, nausea, and vomiting.
- massage or rub the affected muscle. That only causes more pain and does not relieve the cramping.

EXTREMITY INJURIES

Injuries to the extremities are common because more and more people are involved in active lifestyles that include sports and wilderness activities. This chapter focuses on bone, joint, and muscle injuries of the extremities; bleeding, wounds, and other soft-tissue injuries are covered elsewhere. Most of the conditions discussed here result from sudden trauma, although some chronic injuries incurred over a period of time, such as tennis elbow, are included.

Assessment

Use these guidelines to assess injuries to the extremities:

- Look for signs and symptoms of fractures and dislocations (see Chapter 12).
- Examine the extremities, keeping in mind the mnemonic DOTS (Deformity, Open wound, Tenderness, Swelling). Look at and gently feel the extremity, starting at the distal end (fingers or toes) and working upward.
- Compare one extremity with the other to determine size and shape differences.
- Use the "rule of thirds" for extremity injuries. Imagine each long bone as being divided into thirds. If deformity, tenderness, or swelling is located in the upper or lower third of a long bone, assume that the nearest joint is injured.
- Consider the mechanism of injury (MOI) in evaluating the possibility of a fracture and its location. Forces that cause musculoskeletal injuries are direct forces (e.g., car bumper striking a pedestrian's tibia), indirect forces along the long axis of bones (e.g., a person falling onto his or her outstretched hand, resulting in a clavicle fracture), and twisting forces (e.g., while a person's foot is fixed in one spot, the leg is suddenly twisted).
- Use the mnemonic CSM as a reminder to check the extremity for circulation, sensation, and movement of fingers or toes. Without adequate blood flow into an extremity, amputation may result.

Types of Injuries

There are many types of injuries to the extremities, ranging from simple contusions to complex open fractures:

- **contusions,** or bruising of the tissue
- **strains,** in which muscles are stretched or torn
- **sprains,** which involve tearing or stretching of the joints, causing mild to severe damage to the ligaments and joint capsules
- **dislocations,** in which bones are displaced from their normal joint alignment, out of their sockets, or out of their normal positions
- **fractures,** which are breaks in bones and which may or may not be accompanied by open wounds
- **tendinitis,** which is inflammation of a tendon from overuse

First Aid

- Use the RICE procedures (see page 243) for injuries described in this chapter.
- Apply a splint to stabilize fractures and dislocations (see Chapter 14 for specific techniques).

Shoulder Injuries

Shoulder Dislocation (Separation)

Three bones come together at the shoulder: the scapula, the clavicle, and the humerus. The shoulder is the most freely movable joint in the body. The extreme range of all its possible movements makes the shoulder joint highly susceptible to dislocation. A dislocation of the shoulder occurs when the different bones of the shoulder come apart as a result of a blow or a particular movement. Shoulder dislocation is second in frequency only to finger dislocations.

What to Look For

- In about 95 percent of shoulder dislocations, the victim holds the upper arm away from the body, supported by the uninjured arm. This position differentiates a dislocation from a fracture of the humerus (upper arm), in which the victim holds the arm against the chest.
- The dislocated arm cannot be brought across the chest wall to touch the opposite shoulder (i.e., in the sling position).
- The victim has extreme pain in the shoulder area.
- In a dislocation, the shoulder is squared off, rather than rounded.

- An injury to the shoulder resulting in complete loss of function is more apt to be a dislocation than a fracture.
- The victim may describe a history of previous dislocations.

Clavicle Fracture

Fractures of the clavicle (collarbone) are common and usually are the result of falling with the arm and hand outstretched. The victim falls onto his or her hand, and the force from the fall is transmitted to the shoulder. Eighty percent of clavicle fractures occur in the middle third of the bone. Usually the fracture is easy to detect because the clavicle lies immediately under the skin and a deformity can be seen. You generally can feel a clavicle fracture by running a finger along the bone and noting a deformed, tender, or swollen area.

With a clavicle fracture, the victim usually holds the injured arm against the chest to stabilize the injury. The shoulder on the injured side may droop forward.

Contusions

Blows that cause contusions, or bruises, about the shoulder result in pain, swelling, sometimes black-and-blue marks, and restricted arm movement. Often called "shoulder pointers," contusions of this type may cause the victim severe discomfort.

Tendinitis (Painful Shoulder)

The cause of tendinitis in the shoulder generally is continuous overuse. Repeated arm movement, as in many of the throwing sports (e.g., baseball) and other sports in which the shoulder is used extensively (e.g., swimming), often results in painful shoulders.

Humerus (Upper-Arm) Fracture

The shaft of the humerus can be felt throughout its entire length along the inner side of the upper arm. Pain and tenderness at the fracture site and an obvious deformity may be present. The deformity may be hidden by swelling or by the large muscles surrounding the upper part of the arm. The victim may be unable to move the arm. The victim will be holding the upper arm against the chest for comfort.

Elbow Injuries

A deformity is obvious when a seriously injured elbow is compared with the other one. Restricted, painful motion also is present.

All elbow injuries should be considered serious and treated with extreme care. Inappropriate care can result in injury to the nearby nerves and blood vessels.

Tennis Elbow

Tennis elbow results from sharp, quick twists of the wrist (not just from playing tennis). The muscles that bend the wrist back and straighten the fingers all begin in one spot, no bigger than a dime, on the outside bony protrusion, or bump, of the elbow. Tennis elbow, which is an inflammation of the tendons on this outer side of the elbow, can be very painful whenever the wrist and the elbow are used.

Little Leaguer's Elbow

This injury is the equivalent of the more common tennis elbow but with pain on the inside of the elbow. It is a tendinitis (inflammation) of the tendons attached to the bony protrusion, or bump, on the inside of the elbow.

Radius and Ulna (Forearm) Fractures

There are two large bones (radius and ulna) in the forearm, and either one or both bones may be broken. When only one bone is broken, the other acts as a splint and there may be little or no deformity. However, a marked deformity may be present in a fracture near the wrist. When both bones are broken, the arm usually appears deformed. In any fracture of the forearm, pain, tenderness, swelling, and inability to use the forearm may be present. Suspect a fracture if pain occurs when the victim rotates the palm up and down.

Wrist Fracture

The wrist usually is broken when the victim falls with the arm and hand outstretched. Generally, a lumplike deformity occurs on the back of the wrist, along with pain, tenderness, and swelling.

Hand Injuries

Crushed Hand

The hand may be fractured by a direct blow or by a crushing injury. There may be pain, swelling, loss of motion, open wounds, and broken bones.

Finger Injuries

The three bones that make up each finger are the most commonly broken bones in the body. Many of the tendons attached to the finger bones can tear with or without a fracture, and the three joints—the distal interphalangeal (DIP), the proximal interphalangeal (PIP), and the metacarpal phalangeal (MCP)—can also suffer injury. A so-called "finger sprain" may turn out to be a complicated fracture or dislocation.

Finger Fracture

Contrary to popular belief, broken bones—especially the fingers—can move when they are broken. When a finger is fractured, there is immediate pain, and the finger hurts with or without movement. Swelling occurs, and the finger has a twisted look.

Gently feel each bone of the injured finger. Pinpointed tenderness usually indicates a fracture. Ask the victim to make a half-fist with each hand and compare nail alignments for malrotation of the fingers, which could indicate a fracture.

Finger Dislocation

Finger dislocations are common. Motion of the joint usually is impossible, and there may be some loss of circulation and sensation. In a dislocation, the abnormal position of the two adjoining bones looks like a lump at the joint. There is pain, swelling, and shortening of the finger, and the victim may be unable to bend the finger in the injured area.

Sprained Finger

The upper joints of the fingers have a ligament on each side of the joint. A sprain can cause severe pain and swelling over a joint.

Feel both sides of the joints for tenderness. Pain will be directly over the side of the injured joint rather than above or below it.

Nail Avulsion

An injury in which a nail is partly or completely torn loose is known as a nail **avulsion.**

1. Secure the damaged nail in place with an adhesive bandage.
2. If part or all of the nail has been completely torn away, apply antibiotic ointment and secure a partly torn loose nail with an adhesive bandage. Do not trim away the loose nail. Consult a physician for further advice.

Splinters

Remove a splinter in the skin by teasing it out with a sterile needle until the end can be grasped with tweezers or fingers.

If a splinter enters the skin under a nail and breaks off flush, cut a V-shaped notch in the nail to gain access to the splinter. Remove the embedded splinter by grasping its end with tweezers.

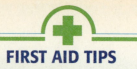

FIRST AID TIPS

Paper Cuts and Hangnails

Keeping a minor wound such as a paper cut or torn hangnail clean and dry can be difficult. Use one of these methods:

- Apply two thin coats of a flexible, waterproof, and durable clear nail polish to the surface of the wound, or
- Place a drop of "super glue" on the hangnail or paper cut and pinch the skin together. Avoid putting the glue inside the cut.

Blood under a Nail

When a fingernail has been crushed, blood collects under the nail. This condition usually is very painful because of the pressure of the blood pressing against the nail.

1. Immerse the finger in ice water or apply an ice pack with the hand elevated.
2. Relieve the pressure under the injured nail by one of the following methods:
   - Using a rotary action, drill through the nail with the sharp point of a knife. This method may be painful.
   - Straighten the end of a metal (noncoated) paper clip or use the eye end of a sewing needle. Hold the paper clip or needle with pliers and use a match or cigarette lighter to heat it until the metal is red hot. Press the glowing end of the paper clip or needle against the nail so it melts through. Little pressure is needed. The nail has no nerves, so it is painless.
3. Apply a dressing to absorb the draining blood and to protect the injured nail.

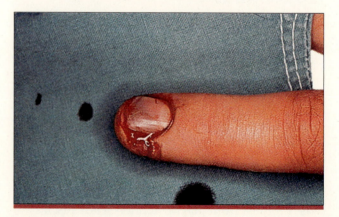

Relieve pain by releasing blood under a nail.

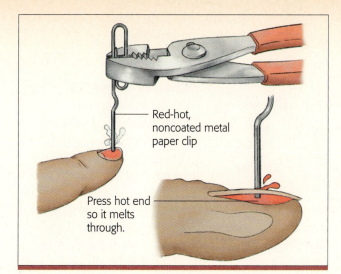

Red-hot,
noncoated metal
paper clip

Press hot end
so it melts
through.

Making a hole in a fingernail.

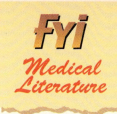

FYi

Medical Literature

Ring Removal from an Extremely Swollen Finger

Rings on swollen fingers are not uncommon, but they must be removed or serious problems can result. Generally, the removal method is simply to cut the ring off the finger or use one of several nondestructive methods of removal using string or a rubber band. A new yet simple method that eliminates the swelling and permits the removal of a ring involves the entire finger distal to the ring being wrapped with a tight, elastic band, which reduces the swelling and frees the ring.

Source: C. R. Cresap, "Removal of a Hardened Steel Ring from an Extremely Swollen Finger," *American Journal of Emergency Medicine* 13(3):318–320 (May 1995).

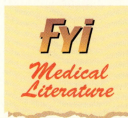

FYi

Medical Literature

Blood Clot under a Fingernail

Blood clots are common problems. Relieving the pressure of blood under nails in 45 victims was successfully done using a heated object (first aiders could use a heated paperclip). All victims reported relief of pain after this procedure. No complications of infection or major nail deformities occurred. This method is preferred over removing the nail.

Source: D. C. Seaberg et al., "Treatment of Subungual Hematomas with Nail Trephination," *American Journal of Emergency Medicine* 9(3):209–210 (May 1991).

Ring Strangulation

Sometimes a finger is so swollen that a ring cannot be removed. Ring strangulation can be a serious problem if it cuts off circulation long enough. Gangrene may result within four or five hours. Try one or more of the following methods to remove a ring:

- Lubricate the finger with grease, oil, butter, petroleum jelly, or some other slippery substance, then try to remove the ring.
- Immerse the finger in cold water or apply an ice pack for several minutes to reduce the swelling.
- Massage the finger from the tip to the hand to move the swelling; lubricate the finger again and try removing the ring.
- Smoothly wind thread around the finger, starting about an inch from the ring edge and going toward the ring, with each course touching the next. Wind smoothly and tightly right up to the edge of the ring. This action will push the swelling toward the hand. Slip the end of the thread under the ring with a matchstick or toothpick, then slowly unwind the thread on the hand side of the ring. You should be able to gently twist the ring over the thread and off the finger.
- Lubricate the finger well, then pass a rubber band under the ring. Hold both ends of the rubber band and, while maintaining tension on the rubber band toward the end of the finger, pull the rubber band around and around the finger.
- Cut the narrowest part of the ring with a ring saw, jeweler's saw, ring cutter, or fine hacksaw blade. Be sure to protect the exposed portions of the finger.
- Inflate an ordinary balloon (preferably a slender, tube-shaped one) about three-fourths full. Tie the end. Insert the victim's swollen finger into the end of the balloon until the balloon evenly surrounds the entire finger. In about 15 minutes, the air pressure in the balloon should return the finger to its normal size, and the ring can be removed.
- Liberally spray window or glass cleaner onto the finger, then try to slide the ring off.

Amputations

Fingers and toes are the most often amputated body parts. See Chapter 7 for amputation care.

Hip-Joint Injuries

Hip Dislocation

A hip can be dislocated by a fall, a blow to the thigh, or direct force to the foot or knee. The hip joint is a stable ball-and-socket joint that requires great force to dislocate. Often a hip is dislocated when the knee strikes the dashboard during a motor vehicle collision. There will be severe pain and loss of motion, and marked deformity may be present. The most common deformity has the victim's hip flexed and the knee bent and rotated inward toward the opposite hip. The foot may hang loose, and the victim is unable to flex the foot or lift the toes. It is difficult to differentiate a hip dislocation from a fracture.

Hip Fracture

A hip fracture is a fracture of the upper end of the femur, not the pelvis. A fractured hip usually is caused by a fall. Elderly people, especially women, are susceptible to this type of injury because of brittle bones (osteoporosis). There is severe pain in the groin area, and the victim may not be able to lift the injured leg. The leg may appear shortened and be rotated with the toes pointing abnormally outward.

Thigh Injuries

Femur (Thighbone) Fracture

Because the femur is the largest bone in the body, considerable force is required to break it. Femur injuries can occur in any part of the femur, from the hip to just above the knee joint. A fracture of the femur usually is caused by a fall or a direct blow. There is severe pain, a shortening of the leg, deformity, and a grating sensation. The limb has a wobbly appearance. Below the fracture there is a complete loss of control. Severe damage to the nerves and blood vessels may occur, resulting in swelling. Because fractures often include open wounds, internal bleeding may be severe. If the blood vessels are severed, the victim may lose one or two liters of blood into the thigh. There may be damage down to the lower part of the extremity. Check especially with lower-

[...] thigh muscle, [...] for tenderness,

swelling, and possibly black-and-blue marks. It results from a direct blow to the thigh.

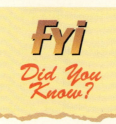

Charley Horse The term *charley horse* was derived from baseball players who experienced blows to muscles in the early twentieth century. At that time, the outfield grass of some major league ballparks was mowed by horses pulling lawn mowers. At Ebbit's Field in New York, the horse that did this chore—"Charley"—had a continual limp. When a baseball player was hit in the leg with a ball or, while sliding into base, received a blow to his leg muscle that subsequently caused him to limp, it was said that he was walking like Charley the horse. Consequently, the muscle blow and the contusion that caused an athlete's pain and limping were referred to as a charley horse injury. The term is still popular in America today.

Muscle Strain

The hamstring muscles (back of thigh) tear most commonly from the upper center of the muscle, but occasionally from the pelvic bone under the buttocks. Hamstring tears are mildly to severely disabling. The injury occurs most often in sports, especially track and field.

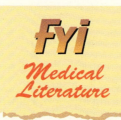

Thigh Muscle Injuries: Strain or Contusion? Athletes often injure the large quadriceps muscles of their thighs. According to one report, strains (pulling of the muscle, which causes tears) should be treated first with ice, compression, elevation of the limb, nonsteroidal anti-inflammatory drugs, and use of crutches. After several days, start gentle stretching and knee extension but avoid straight leg raises. For thigh contusions (direct blow, causing bruising), immediately flex the knee and immobilize it in that position for 24 hours. Apply ice for the first half hour and intermittently thereafter, to slow bleeding and prevent swelling.

Source: C. C. Kaeding et al., "Quadriceps Strains and Contusions," *Physician and Sportsmedicine* 23:59 (Jan. 1995).

Knee Injuries

Knee injuries, of which there are many types, can be serious. You probably have seen a physician or an athletic trainer performing stress tests on a player's knee on the sidelines at a football game. Controversy exists as to the exact meaning and interpretation of many of the ligament stress tests. First aiders should not perform such testing unless they have the training and experience to do so.

Knee Fracture

A fracture of the knee generally occurs as a result of a fall or a direct blow. Besides the usual signs of a fracture, a groove in the kneecap may be felt. The victim will be unable to kick the leg forward, and the leg will drag if the victim tries to walk.

Knee Dislocation

A knee dislocation is a serious injury. Deformity will be grotesque. A first aider should be more concerned about possible injury to the popliteal artery (just behind the knee joint) than about any ligament damage. This major artery, which supplies the leg below the knee, can be lacerated or compressed by a displaced tibia.

For a knee dislocation, always check the ankle pulse. If an ankle pulse is absent, make one attempt to realign the leg to restore blood circulation. Try to gently straighten the knee *only once*. Then stabilize the knee in the position of deformity. Do not attempt to straighten any knee injury when an ankle pulse is present or when any attempt to realign the knee produces severe pain. In those cases, stabilize the knee in the position found. *Seek medical attention immediately*. Waiting longer than eight hours to reduce a knee dislocation can result in loss of the leg.

Do not confuse a knee dislocation with a patella dislocation. A knee dislocation is a much more serious injury.

Patella Dislocation

A dislocated patella (kneecap) can be a very painful injury and must be treated immediately. Some people have repeated kneecap dislocations, just as others have a tendency for shoulder dislocations.

When the patella is dislocated, a significant deformity appears, with the knee semiflexed and the patella on the outside (lateral side) of the joint. Compare it with the other kneecap.

Knee Sprain

Ligament injuries occur most often in sports. The knee is very prone to ligament injury, ranging from mild sprains to complete tearing. The knee will be swollen and painful and usually cannot be used normally.

Contusion

A knee bruise, or contusion, will be tender and swollen and may have black-and-blue marks.

Lower-Leg Injuries

Tibia and Fibula Fractures

Tibia and fibula injuries can occur at any place between the knee joint and the ankle joint. When both bones are broken, there is a marked deformity of the leg. When only one bone is broken, the other acts as a splint, and little deformity may be present. Some victims with a fibula fracture can walk on the injured leg. When the tibia (bone in the front of the leg) is broken, an open fracture and severe deformity are likely to exist. Injuries to the blood vessels, caused by the extreme deformity, are common with injuries of the tibia and the fibula, and the pain usually is severe.

Contusion

Many contusions simply cause a black-and-blue mark and some soreness, then clear up with little attention.

Muscle Cramp

Muscle spasm or cramping usually occurs in the calf, sometimes in the thigh or hamstring. It is a temporary condition of little consequence. Refer to the section on heat cramps in Chapter 19 for more information.

What to Do

There are many treatments for cramps. Try one or more of the following:

1. Have the victim gently stretch the affected muscle. Because a muscle cramp is an uncontrolled muscle contraction or spasm, a gradual lengthening of the muscle may help lengthen the muscle fibers and relieve the cramp.
2. Relax the muscle by applying pressure to it.

3. Apply ice to the cramped muscle to make it relax. The exception might be in a cold environment.

4. Pinch the upper lip hard (an accupressure technique) to reduce calf-muscle cramping.

5. Drink lightly salted cool (dissolve ¼ teaspoon salt in a quart of water) water or a commercial sports drink.

> ### ⚠ CAUTION: DO NOT
>
> - give salt tablets to a person with muscle cramps. They can cause stomach irritation, nausea, and vomiting.
> - massage or rub the affected muscle. That only causes more pain and does not relieve the cramping.

Shin Splints

Experts disagree just what shin splints are other than that they are pain in the shins and are caused by running and extensive walking. Pain and tenderness occur along the front edge of the shin where the muscles are attached.

Ankle and Foot Injuries

The ankle and the foot frequently get injured, mainly by twisting, which stretches or tears the supporting ligaments. Careless treatment can have consequences that include lifelong disability. In some cases, the damage requires surgical correction.

Most ankle injuries are sprains; about 85 percent of sprains involve the ankle's outside (lateral) ligaments and are caused by the ankle having turned or twisted outward.

What to Look For

It is difficult to tell the difference between a severely sprained ankle and a fractured ankle. A useful two-part test can help determine whether the ankle or the midfoot needs to be x-rayed:

1. Press along the bones. Pain and tenderness over (a) the back edge or the tip of either of the ankle knob bones (malleolus bones) or (b) the midfoot's outside bone (fifth metatarsal) or inside bone (navicular) may indicate a broken bone.

2. Ask the victim, "Have you tried standing on it?" Putting some weight on the foot may hurt a little, but if the victim is able to do that and take four or more steps, most likely the ankle or foot is sprained. If it is broken, the victim will not want to put any weight on it and will not be able to take more than four steps.

A few additional signs and symptoms may help you determine whether an injured ankle is sprained or fractured. These indicators are not hard-and-fast rules but rather useful guidelines to help you treat foot and ankle injuries.

- If the victim hops on the good foot and the injured ankle cannot tolerate the jarring, suspect a fracture.

- Some experts say that nausea right after an ankle injury indicates a fracture rather than a sprain.

- Foot injuries often are quite swollen. It has been observed that ankle sprains tend to swell on only one side of the foot (usually the lateral, or outer, side), whereas swelling on both sides of the foot usually accompanies fractures.

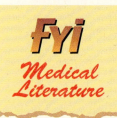

Ankle and Foot Injuries: Is Something Broken?

In a study of 1,500 people with ankle injuries, two symptoms were 100 percent accurate in predicting if a bone was broken: (1) inability to bear weight and take four steps immediately after the injury; and (2) tenderness at the back edge or tip of either malleolus bones (the projections on each side of the ankle). Similar symptoms predicted whether a foot bone was broken: (1) pain in the midfoot or tenderness at the base of the fifth metatarsal bone at the outer edge of the foot or at the navicular bone at the inner edge, plus (2) inability to take four steps.

Source: I. G. Stiell et al., "Decision Rules for the Use of Radiography in Acute Ankle Injuries," *Journal of the American Medical Association* 269:1127 (March 1993).

What to Do

Controversy exists about whether to remove a shoe from an injured foot. Those favoring leaving the shoe on believe it acts as a splint and helps retard

FRACTURES

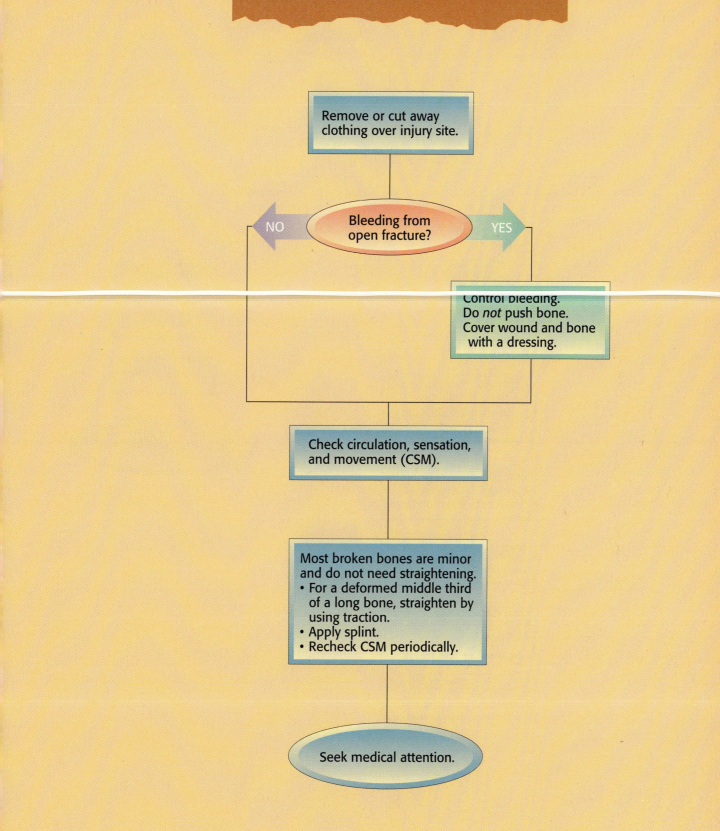

Remove or cut away clothing over injury site.

Bleeding from open fracture?

NO | YES

Control bleeding. Do *not* push bone. Cover wound and bone with a dressing.

Check circulation, sensation, and movement (CSM).

Most broken bones are minor and do not need straightening.
• For a deformed middle third of a long bone, straighten by using traction.
• Apply splint.
• Recheck CSM periodically.

Seek medical attention.

SPRAINS, STRAINS, CONTUSIONS, DISLOCATIONS

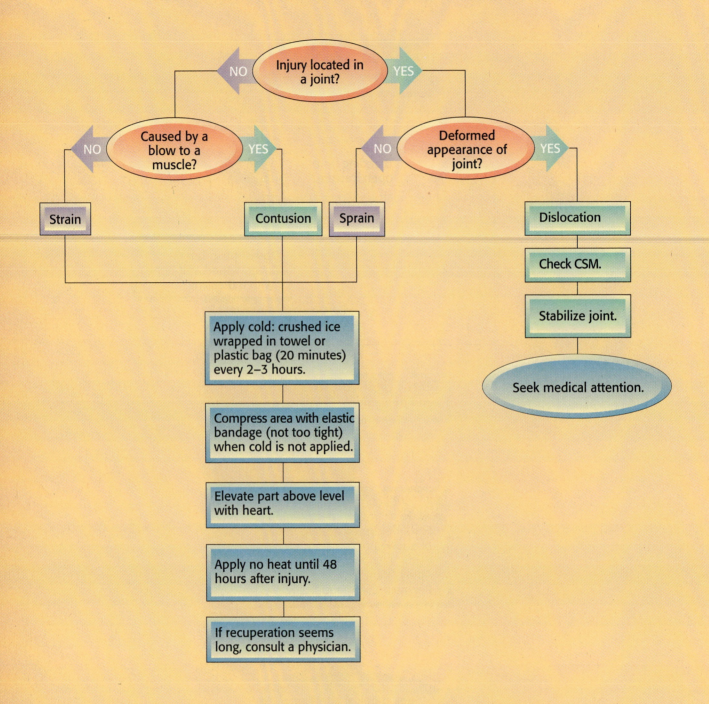

Injury located in a joint?

NO → Caused by a blow to a muscle?

YES → Deformed appearance of joint?

Caused by a blow to a muscle?
- NO → Strain
- YES → Contusion

Deformed appearance of joint?
- NO → Sprain
- YES → Dislocation

Strain

Contusion

Sprain

Dislocation

Check CSM.

Stabilize joint.

Seek medical attention.

Apply cold: crushed ice wrapped in towel or plastic bag (20 minutes) every 2–3 hours.

Compress area with elastic bandage (not too tight) when cold is not applied.

Elevate part above level with heart.

Apply no heat until 48 hours after injury.

If recuperation seems long, consult a physician.

MUSCLE INJURIES

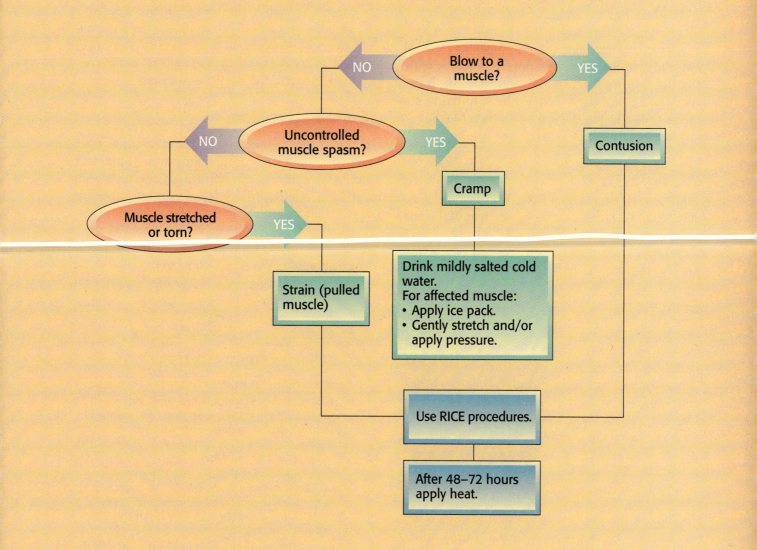

Blow to a muscle? — NO

Blow to a muscle? — YES → Contusion

Uncontrolled muscle spasm? — NO

Uncontrolled muscle spasm? — YES → Cramp

Muscle stretched or torn? — YES → Strain (pulled muscle)

Cramp → Drink mildly salted cold water.
For affected muscle:
• Apply ice pack.
• Gently stretch and/or apply pressure.

Use RICE procedures.

After 48–72 hours apply heat.

RICE Procedure for Bone, Joint, and Muscle Injuries

RICE is the acronym for the first aid procedures—rest, ice, compression, elevation—for bone, joint, and muscle injuries. What is done in the first 48–72 hours following such an injury can do a lot to relieve, even prevent, aches and pains. **Treat all extremity bone, joint, and muscle injuries with the RICE procedure. In addition to RICE, fractures and dislocations should be splinted to stabilize the injured area. (See Chapter 14 for splinting techniques.)**

R = Rest

Injuries heal faster if rested. Rest means the victim stays off the injured part. Using any part of the body increases the blood circulation to that area, which can cause more swelling to an injured part. For the lower extremities, crutches may be considered.

I = Ice

An ice pack should be applied to the injured area for 20 to 30 minutes every 2 or 3 hours during the first 24 to 48 hours. Skin being treated with cold passes through four stages: cold, burning, aching, and numbness. When the skin becomes numb, usually in 20 to 30 minutes, remove the ice pack. After removing the ice pack, compress the injured part with an elastic bandage and keep it elevated (the "C" and "E" of RICE).

Cold constricts the blood vessels to and in the injured area, which helps reduce the swelling and inflammation and at the same time dulls the pain and relieves muscle spasms. Cold should be applied as soon as possible after the injury—healing time often is directly related to the amount of swelling that occurs. One minute delayed means an additional hour needed for healing. Heat has the opposite effect when applied to fresh injuries: it increases circulation to the area and greatly increases both the swelling and the pain.

Use either of the following methods to apply cold to an injury:

- Put crushed ice (or cubes) into a double plastic bag, hot water bottle, or wet towel. Apply one layer of a wet cloth over the injury, place the ice pack on the cloth, and then use an elastic bandage to hold the ice pack in place. Ice bags can conform to the body's contours.

- Use a chemical "snap pack," a sealed pouch that contains two chemical envelopes. Squeezing the pack mixes the chemicals, producing a chemical reaction that has a cooling effect. Although they do not cool as well as other methods, snap packs are convenient to use when ice is not readily available. They lose their cooling power quickly, however, and can be used only once. Also, they may be impractical because of their expense and the danger of breakage.

C = Compression

Compression of the injured area may squeeze some fluid and debris out of the injury site. Compression limits the ability of the skin and of other tissues to expand. To try to limit internal bleeding, apply an elastic bandage to the injured area, especially the foot, ankle, knee, thigh, hand, or elbow. Fill the hollow areas with padding (e.g., sock, washcloth) before applying the elastic bandage.

Elastic bandages come in various sizes, for different body areas:

FIRST AID TIPS

Homemade Ice Packs

- Ice bags kept in a freezer freeze solid and cannot be shaped to fit the injured area. One part isopropyl (rubbing) alcohol to three parts water prevents freezing, and the ice bag can be easily molded. Bags can be reused for months.

- An unopened bag of frozen vegetables is inexpensive; keeps its basic shape (unlike ice chips, which melt); molds to the shape of the injured area; is reusable; and is packaged in a fairly puncture-resistant, watertight bag.

- For cold therapy over a fairly large area, soak a face towel in cold water, wring it out, fold it, and place it in a large self-sealing plastic bag. Store the bag in the freezer. To use the cold pack, wrap it in a light cotton towel and apply for 20 minutes, after which it can be refrozen. A washcloth in a smaller bag can be used to treat a smaller area.

- Fill a plastic bag with snow.

- Fill a polystyrene plastic cup with water and freeze it. When you need an ice pack, peel the cup to below ice level; the remaining part of the cup forms a cold-resistant handle. Rub the ice over the injured area (movement is necessary to prevent skin damage). These ice "packs" are inexpensive and convenient and take up little space.

- To fashion a funnel for filling an ice bag, push out the bottom of a paper cup and fit it into the neck of the ice bag. The ice will slide through the cup and into the bag.

SKILL SCAN: RICE Procedures for an Ankle

1.

R = Rest
Stop using the injured part. Continued use could cause further injury, delay healing, increase pain, and stimulate bleeding. Get the victim into a comfortable position, either sitting or lying down. This slows blood flow to the injured area.

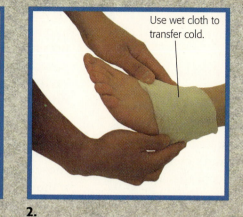

2.

Use wet cloth to transfer cold.

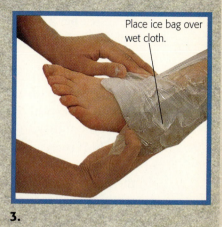

3.

Place ice bag over wet cloth.

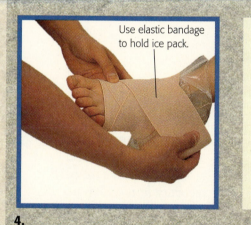

4.

Use elastic bandage to hold ice pack.

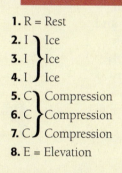

1. R = Rest
2. I ⎫
3. I ⎬ Ice
4. I ⎭
5. C ⎫
6. C ⎬ Compression
7. C ⎭
8. E = Elevation

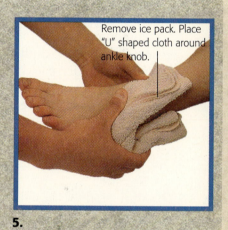

5.

Remove ice pack. Place "U" shaped cloth around ankle knob.

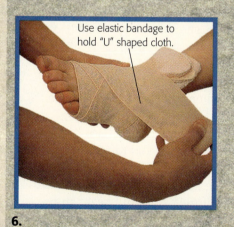

6.

Use elastic bandage to hold "U" shaped cloth.

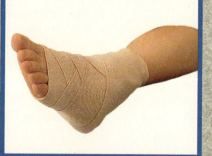

7.

Cover heel and close to the toes.

8.

E = Elevation
Elevating the injured part is another way to decrease swelling and pain. While icing or compressing, elevate the part in whatever way is most convenient. The aim of this step is to get the injured part higher than the heart, if possible.

CAUTION: DO NOT

- apply an ice pack for more than 20 to 30 minutes at a time. Frostbite or nerve damage can result.
- apply an ice pack on the back outside part of the knee. Nerve damage can occur.
- place an ice pack directly on the skin. Protect the skin with a wet cloth, which conducts cold better (a dry cloth insulates the injury from the cold).
- apply cold if the victim has a history of circulatory disease, Raynaud's syndrome (spasms in the arteries of the extremities that reduce circulation), or abnormal sensitivity to cold, or if the injured part has been frostbitten previously.
- stop using an ice pack too soon. A common mistake is too early use of heat, which will result in swelling and pain. Use an ice pack 3 to 4 times a day for the first 24 hours, preferably up to 48 hours, before applying any heat. For severe injuries, 72 hours is recommended.

- 2-inch width, used for the wrist and hand
- 3-inch width, used for the ankle, elbow, and arm
- 4-inch width, used for the knee and leg

Start the elastic bandage several inches below the injury and wrap in an upward, overlapping (about one-half the bandage's width) spiral, starting with even and somewhat tight pressure, then gradually wrapping more loosely above the injury.

Applying compression may be the most important step in preventing swelling. The victim should wear the elastic bandage continuously for 18 to 24 hours (except when cold is applied). At night, have the victim loosen but not remove the elastic bandage.

For an ankle injury, place a horseshoe-shaped pad around the ankle knob and under the elastic bandage. The pad will permit compression of the soft tissues rather than just the bones. Wrap the bandage tightest nearest the toes and loosest above the ankle. It should be tight enough to decrease swelling but not tight enough to inhibit blood flow.

For a contusion or a strain, place a pad between the injury and the elastic bandage.

CAUTION: DO NOT

- apply an elastic bandage too tightly. If applied too tightly, elastic bandages will restrict circulation. Stretch a new elastic bandage to about one-third its maximum length for adequate compression. Leave fingers and toes exposed so possible color change can be easily observed. Compare the toes or fingers of the injured extremity with the uninjured one. Pale skin, pain, numbness, and tingling are signs of a too tight elastic bandage. If any of these symptoms appears, immediately remove the elastic bandage. Leave the elastic bandage off until all the symptoms disappear, then rewrap the area, but less tightly. Always wrap from below the injury and move toward the heart.

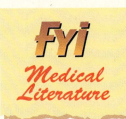

Heat and Cold: When to Use Which?

Many people use heat devices or ice packs to speed recovery from sports injuries. But what's the right time to use each technique? Cold usually should be applied immediately after an acute injury, such as an ankle sprain. Putting ice chips in a plastic bag is a good way to apply cold. To avoid cold injury, ice should be applied for no more than 15 to 20 minutes at a time. At the same time, compression and elevation of the limb also should be used. Icing reduces pain, swelling, and muscle spasm immediately after injury, but its use should be discontinued after two or three days. Application of heat with heat packs, radiant heat, or whirlpool baths then can be used to reduce muscle spasms and pain. In addition, heat increases blood flow and joint flexibility. Vigorous heating is used to treat chronic injuries, but mild heat can reduce muscle spasm. Heating is also effective for acute back pain, but ice massage is preferred if back pain persists for two weeks or more.

Source: M. P. Kaul and S. A. Herring, "Superficial Heat and Cold," *Physician and Sportsmedicine* 22:65 (Dec. 1994).

STUDY QUESTIONS 13

Name _____ Course _____ Date _____

Activities

Activity 1

Mark each answer as true (T) or false (F).

T   F   1. A horseshoe-shaped pad under an elastic bandage is recommended for ankle sprains.

T   F   2. Dislocations happen only in joints.

T   F   3. After suffering a sprain or strain, you should immediately apply heat to the affected joint.

T   F   4. Sprains are muscle injuries.

T   F   5. Splint a fracture before moving a victim.

T   F   6. The "rule of thirds" applies to the assessment of muscle injuries.

Activity 2

Check the appropriate answer(s).
Relieve the painful pressure caused by the accumulation of blood under a fingernail or toenail by

_____ 1. placing the finger in hot water for several minutes

_____ 2. drilling a hold through the nail with the point of a knife

_____ 3. melting a hole through the nail to the site of the blood with a red-hot paper clip

Mark each technique yes (Y) or no (N).
Which techniques can be useful in removing a stuck ring?

_____ 4. Lubricate the finger with oil, butter, or other slippery substance.

_____ 5. Place the finger in hot water for several minutes.

_____ 6. Use thread wrapped tightly around the finger.

_____ 7. Cut the ring with a fine-toothed hacksaw.

_____ 8. Cut the skin along the ring to relieve pressure.

Activity 3

Mark each statement as true (T) or false (F).

T   F   1. The letters RICE represent the treatment for an ankle injury.

T   F   2. When using ice, place it directly on the skin.

T   F   3. A common mistake is the application of heat too soon.

T   F   4. An elastic bandage, if used correctly, can help control swelling.

T   F   5. Using an elastic bandage alone provides adequate compression.

T   F   6. Controversy exists about whether to take a shoe off an injured ankle.

Activity 4

Those engaging in various types of sports may experience one of three different muscle injuries.
Match the lettered types of muscle injury with the numbered definitions.

_____ 1. strain   a. result of a blow

_____ 2. contusion   b. uncontrolled spasm

_____ 3. cramp   c. a tear

4. All muscle injuries can benefit from the RICE procedures. What do the letters represent?

R = _____

I = _____

C = _____

E = _____

5. How can compression be applied?

_____

_____

6. Give two sources of ice or cold.

a. _____

b. _____

7. How long and how often should cold be applied?

_____ minutes every _____ hours for the first _____ hours.

8. Cold will decrease swelling and relieve

_____

9. It is best not to apply heat for _____ to _____ hours after an injury.

Case Situations

Case 1

A neighbor falls from a ladder. You find him lying down complaining about the pain. His lower leg looks deformed.

____ 1. How would you assess the leg?

    a. See whether he can stand on the leg.

    b. Ask him to wiggle his toes.

    c. Gently rotate the leg to check for a broken bone.

    d. With your fingers gently probe the leg for pain or tenderness and check for feeling and a pulse below the affected area.

____ 2. Which bones compose the lower leg?

    a. tibia, fibula

    b. radius, ulna

    c. radius, tibia

    d. fibula, ulna

____ 3. Proper splinting includes stabilizing the joint above and the joint below the fracture. In your neighbor's case, the joints to be stabilized would be the:

    a. hip, knee

    b. shoulder, elbow

    c. knee, ankle

    d. hip, ankle

Case 2

At an ice skating rink, an 18-year-old male crashes through a gate and tumbles down a flight of stairs. You note that he is conscious but obviously intoxicated. You find deformity and swelling in the upper right leg. No other injuries are obvious.

____ 1. This victim is suffering from a fractured:

    a. tibia

    b. humerus

    c. femur

    d. pelvis

____ 2. Which of the following pulse sites is used to assess blood flow into a lower extremity?

    a. posterior tibial

    b. femoral

    c. radial

    d. brachial

____ 3. Treatment for this victim would include

    a. placing him in a sitting position

    b. stabilizing the injured extremity by tying the legs together

    c. stabilizing the injured extremity by having a bystander hold the legs together

    d. raising the leg up to treat for shock

Case 3

During a pick-up basketball game, one of the players turns his ankle.

____ 1. What indicates a possible fractured ankle?

    a. Victim has pain over the ankle-knob bone when you press on it.

    b. Victim cannot take four steps.

    c. Victim refuses to stand on the injured ankle.

    d. All the above.

____ 2. For a suspected fracture, should you use the RICE procedures?

    a. yes

    b. no

____ 3. In which direction do most injured ankles turn?

    a. inward

    b. outward

Case 4

A 10-year-old boy suffers an injury to his forearm while riding double on a bicycle with his brother.

____ 1. What would indicate a fracture?

    a. deformity

    b. tenderness

    c. swelling

    d. all of these

____ 2. Which pulse would you check for blood flow in an arm?

    a. radial artery

    b. carotid artery

    c. femoral artery

Case 5

A 20-year-old softball player tips a ball off the end of her index finger.

_____ 1. What test might indicate a broken finger?

    a. percussion test

    b. rule of nines

    c. rule of the palm

    d. rule of 50s

_____ 2. Suspect a fracture if the test involves pain.

    a. true

    b. false

Case 6

A 20-year-old male is struck by a thrown baseball bat. A physical exam reveals deformity to the forearm with the bone ends protruding through the wound.

_____ 1. This type of injury is known as a(n) _____ fracture.

    a. closed

    b. greenstick

    c. open

    d. impacted

_____ 2. To determine the circulatory effectiveness in the injured arm, which of the following pulses should you check?

    a. carotid

    b. radial

    c. femoral

    d. brachial

_____ 3. What should you apply to control the bleeding?

    a. direct pressure over the bleeding site

    b. pressure around the bleeding site

    c. pressure on the brachial artery

    d. a tourniquet

Case 7

A motorcycle accident victim appears to have a closed fracture of the right femur. No other injuries are evident.

1. How can the circulation of a leg be checked?

_____

_____

_____

_____

2. How much blood could be lost because of a femur fracture?

_____ a. 1 pint

_____ b. 1–2 quarts

_____ c. 1 gallon

Case 8

A mountain biker skids on loose rocks, catapults over the bike's handlebars, and lands on his shoulder.

1. What injuries would you suspect?

    a. _____

    b. _____

    c. _____

2. Which injury involves the victim holding his or her arm away from the body?

_____ a. shoulder dislocation

_____ b. clavicle fracture

CHAPTER

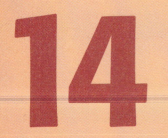

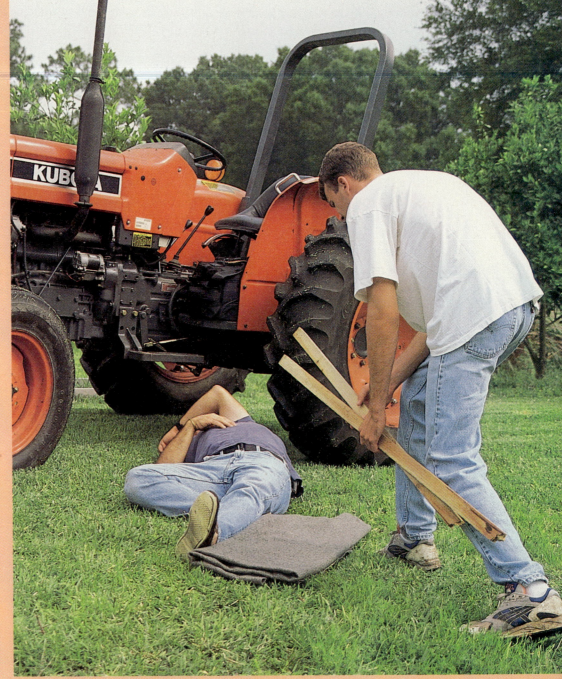

SPLINTING THE EXTREMITIES

Most extremity fractures are minor. The extremity is straight and medical help is nearby, so the injury can be stabilized by splinting the extremity in the position it was found. To *stabilize* means to use any method to hold a body part still and prevent movement. All fractures should be stabilized before a victim is moved. The reasons for splinting to stabilize an injured area are to:

- reduce pain
- prevent damage to muscle, nerves, and blood vessels
- prevent a closed fracture from becoming an open fracture
- reduce bleeding and swelling

All fractures are complicated to some degree by damage to the soft tissue and structures surrounding the bone. The major cause of tissue damage at a fracture site is movement of the end of the broken bone. The end of a broken bone is sharp, and it is important to prevent a fractured bone from moving into soft tissues.

Types of Splints

A **splint** is any device used to stabilize a fracture or a dislocation. Such a device can be improvised (e.g., a folded newspaper), or it can be one of several commercially available splints (e.g., SAM Splint™, air splint). Lack of a commercial splint should never prevent you from properly stabilizing an injured extremity. Many situations require ingenuity in improvisation for a first aider to render adequate care.

A rigid splint is an inflexible device attached to an extremity to maintain stability. It may be a padded board, a piece of heavy cardboard, or a SAM Splint™ molded to fit the extremity. Whatever its construction, a rigid splint must be long enough to be secured well above and below the fracture site. A soft splint, such as an air splint, is useful mainly for stabilizing fractures of the lower leg or the forearm.

A self, or anatomic, splint is almost always available. A self splint is one in which the injured body part is tied to an uninjured part (e.g., injured finger to adjacent finger, legs together, injured arm to chest).

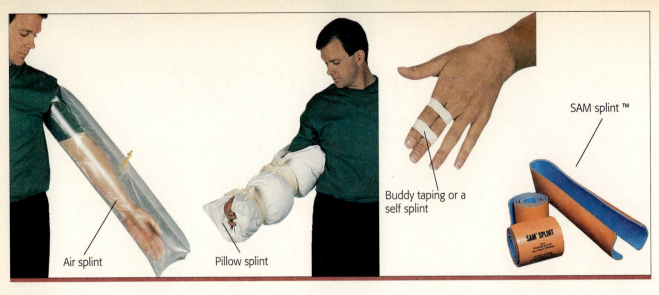

Air splint   Pillow splint   Buddy taping or a self splint   SAM splint ™

Examples of splints

A traction splint should be used only on a broken femur (thigh bone). Since traction splints normally are found only on ambulances and require two trained people (EMTs), the application of this type of splint is not a first aid–level skill.

Splinting Guidelines

All fractures and dislocations should be stabilized before the victim is moved. When in doubt, apply a splint.

You should attempt to straighten a fracture only if you are in a remote location (more than one hour from medical care) *and* one of the following situations exists: (1) the extremity is deformed (angulated) from its normal anatomical position, or (2) the circulation-sensation-movement (CSM) check is negative. Use **traction**—a firm and steady pull to improve the position of a badly deformed, shortened, or angulated extremity—to achieve a more normal alignment. If you are not sure what the extremity should look like, check the corresponding undamaged part. Traction is not an attempt to pull the limb back in perfect alignment. That process, called **reduction** of a fracture, is done in a hospital with x-rays to assist medical personnel in visualizing the exact positions of the broken-bone ends. For first aid purposes, traction should be applied only for midshaft (use rule of thirds) long-bone fractures to help prevent further soft-tissue injury, improve circulation, and relieve pain. If the victim

shows increased pain or the extremity is resistant to traction, splint the extremity in the deformed position.

To apply traction, follow these steps:

1. Explain to the victim that straightening the fracture may cause a momentary increase in pain, but that the pain will be relieved once the fracture is straightened and splinted.

2. For an injured arm, grasp the arm firmly with one hand above and the other below the injury site. Exert steady, gentle traction in a line with the bone. Do not use excessive force. For an injured leg, with both hands pull on the leg below the injury while the victim's body acts as an anchor or another person holds the upper leg in place.

CAUTION: DO NOT

- straighten dislocations or fractures of the spine, elbow, wrist, hip, or knee because of the proximity of major nerves and arteries. Instead, if the CSM is all right, splint joint injuries in the position found.
- apply traction on open fractures. Instead, cover the wound with a sterile dressing and apply a splint.

If the victim shows increased pain or you feel resistance, stop applying traction and splint the extremity as it is.

Medical experts disagree whether an open fracture should be straightened. Traction usually is not recommended because dirt and bacteria can be pulled deeper into the wound. Instead, simply cover the open wound with a sterile dressing and splint the extremity. If, however, an open fracture has no CSM, you should attempt to straighten the extremity to restore blood flow.

1. Cover all open wounds, if any, with a dry, sterile dressing before applying a splint.

2. Check CSM in the extremity. If pulses are absent, manipulate the fracture or dislocation to restore blood flow. Do *not* straighten dislocations or fractures involving the spine, elbow, hip, wrist, or knee. According to wilderness experts, if you are more than one hour from medical care, you can safely reduce three types of dislocations: anterior shoulder, patella (kneecap—not to be confused with the knee joint), and finger.

3. Determine what to splint by using the **"rule of thirds."** Imagine each long bone as being divided into thirds. If the injury is located in the upper or lower third of a bone, assume that the nearest joint is injured. Therefore, the splint should extend to stabilize the bones above and below the unstable joint; for example, for a fracture of the upper third of the tibia (shinbone), the splint must extend to include the upper leg, as well as the lower leg, because the knee is unstable.

   For a fracture of the middle third of a bone stabilize the joints above and below the fracture (e.g., wrist and elbow for fractured radius or ulna; shoulder and elbow for fractured humerus; knee and ankle for fractured tibia or fibula). An upper extremity fracture in addition to being splinted should be placed in an arm sling and a swathe (binder).

4. If two first aiders are present, one should support the injury site and minimize movement of the extremity until splinting is completed.

5. When possible, place splint materials on both sides of the injured part, especially when two bones are involved (e.g., radius/ulna or tibia/fibula). This "sandwich splint" prevents rotation of the injured extremity and keeps the two bones from touching. With rigid splints, use extra padding in natural body hollows and around any deformities.

6. Apply splints firmly but not so tight that blood flow into an extremity is affected. Check CSM before and periodically after the splint is applied. If the pulse disappears, loosen the splint enough so you can feel the pulse. Leave the fingers or toes exposed so CSM can be checked easily.

7. Use RICE on the injured part. Elevation of the injured extremity after stabilization promotes drainage from the limb by gravity and reduces swelling. *Do not, however, apply ice packs if a pulse is absent.*

If the victim has a possible spine injury as well as an extremity injury, the spine injury takes precedence. Splinting the spine is always a problem. Tell the victim not to move. Then stabilize the spine with rolled blankets or similar objects placed on each side of the neck and torso. In most cases, it is best to wait until the EMS arrives with trained personnel and proper equipment to handle spine injuries.

Most fractures do not require rapid transportation. An exception is an arm or a leg without a pulse, which means insufficient blood flow to that extremity. In that case, *immediate* medical attention is necessary.

Seek medical attention for the following injuries or situations:

- Any open fracture.
- Any dislocation (injury that causes joint deformity).
- Any joint injury with moderate to severe swelling.
- Any injury in which there is deformity, tenderness, or swelling over the bone.
- The victim is unable to walk or bear weight after an ankle or knee injury.
- A "snap, crackle, or pop" was heard at the time of injury.
- The injured area, especially a joint, becomes hot, tender, swollen, or painful.
- There is doubt about whether or not a bone was broken.
- The injury does not improve after two weeks of treatment.

Slings

Slings support and protect the upper extremities. The sling is not a bandage but is used as a support for any injury to the shoulder or arm.

Arm Slings

An arm sling supports the forearm and the hand when there are injuries to an upper extremity or the ribs. To apply an arm sling, follow these steps:

1. Support the injured arm slightly away from the chest, with the wrist and hand slightly higher than the elbow.
2. Place an open triangular bandage between the forearm and the chest, with the point of the bandage stretching well beyond the elbow.
3. Pull the upper end over the shoulder on the uninjured side and around the neck to rest on the collarbone of the injured side.
4. Bring the lower end of the bandage over the hand and the forearm and tie it to the other end at the hollow above the collarbone.
5. Bring the point around to the front of the elbow and secure it to the sling with a safety pin or twist it into a "pigtail," which can be tied into a knot or tucked away.
6. Check the pulse and fingernail color for signs of circulation loss. The hand should be in a thumb-up position in the sling and above the level of the elbow.

Splinting Specific Areas
Shoulder

Shoulder injuries involve the clavicle (collarbone), the scapula (shoulder blade), or the head of the humerus (upper arm). To stabilize the shoulder and upper arm against movement, follow these steps to apply a shoulder sling:

1. Support the injured arm slightly away from the chest, with the wrist and hand higher than the elbow.
2. Place an open triangular bandage between the forearm and the chest, with the point stretching well beyond the elbow.
3. Pull the upper end of the bandage over the shoulder on the uninjured side.
4. Bring the lower end of the bandage over the forearm, under the armpit on the injured side, and around the victim's back.

5. Tie the upper and lower ends of the triangular bandage.
6. Check the pulse and fingernail color for signs of circulation loss.

The hand should be in a thumb-up position in the sling and slightly above the level of the elbow.

To further stabilize the arm, fold another triangular bandage to make a 3- to 4-inch-wide swathe. Tie one or two swathes (binders) around the upper arm and chest of the victim. This stabilizes the clavicle (collarbone) and most shoulder injuries, as well as upper-humerus (upper arm) fractures.

If triangular bandages are not available, loop gauze or a belt around the victim's wrist and suspend the arm from the neck. Secure the arm gently, but firmly, to the chest wall with another length of gauze or belt. You can make a temporary splint by pinning a shirt or coat sleeve to the front of the coat or shirt.

Most shoulder dislocations (95 percent) are anterior (top of the humerus pops out in front of the shoulder joint). The victim will hold the arm in a fixed position away from the chest wall. Probably the most comfortable splinting method is to place a pillow or rolled blanket between the involved arm and the chest to fill the space created and then to use cravats or a roller bandage to secure the arm against the chest. For remote settings (more than one hour from medical attention), there are several

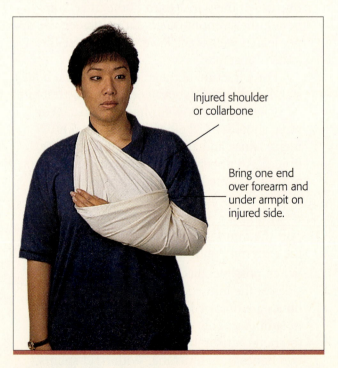

Injured shoulder or collarbone

Bring one end over forearm and under armpit on injured side.

Splinting a clavicle or shoulder injury

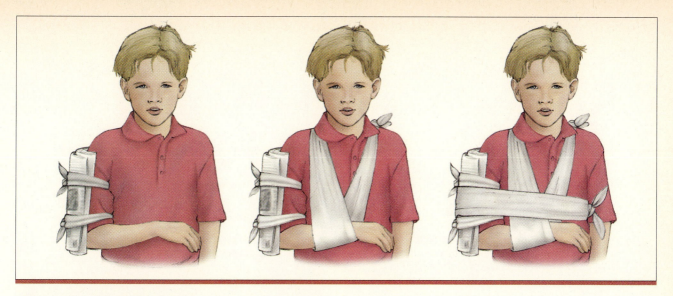

Splinting a humerus fracture

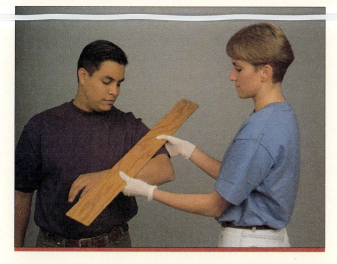

Splint elbow in position found. If bent, splint it bent.

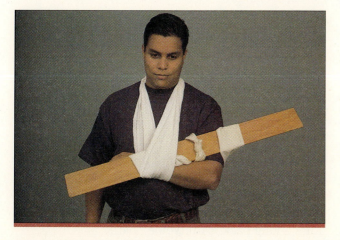

Completed splint for a bent elbow

methods of reducing an anterior shoulder dislocation; those methods are described in Chapter 22.

Humerus (Upper Arm)

Fractures of the humerus (upper arm) should be
stabilized with a rigid splint. Extend the splint
along the outside of the humerus. Place padding
between the arm and the chest. Then apply a sling
and a swathe over the rigid splint, using the chest
wall as an additional splint.

Elbow

An elbow must be stabilized in the position it is
found: if bent, splint it bent; if straight, splint it
straight. If the injured elbow is straight, place a
rigid splint along the inside of the arm from hand
to armpit. Secure the splint with a roller bandage or
several cravat bandages. For a bent elbow, apply a

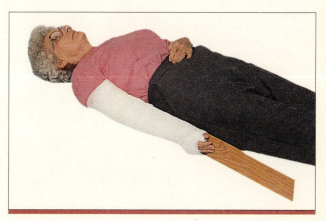

Splint elbow in position found. If straight, splint it straight.
Rigid splint extends from hand to armpit.

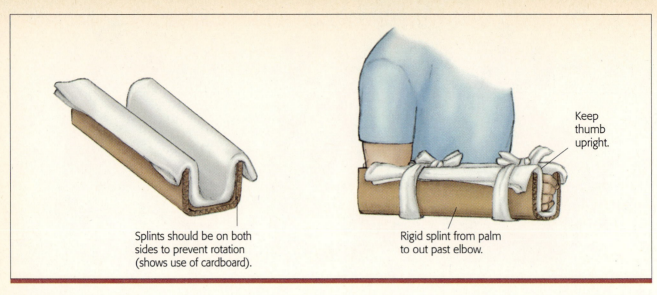

Splints should be on both sides to prevent rotation (shows use of cardboard).

Keep thumb upright.

Rigid splint from palm to out past elbow.

Splinting a forearm fracture

rigid splint extending from the humerus (near the armpit) to the wrist, to prevent motion of the elbow. Depending on the angle of the elbow, sometimes a sling and a swathe (binder) are sufficient.

Forearm

To stabilize a forearm fracture, use one rigid splint extending from the palm of the hand out past the elbow, and a second one on the opposite side of the arm. Placing splints on both sides of the injured part ("sandwich splint") prevents rotation of the forearm. Keep the victim's thumb in an upright position to prevent the two bones in the forearm (radius and ulna) from touching each other. Secure the

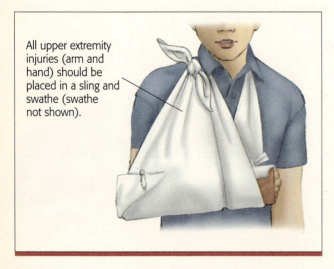

All upper extremity injuries (arm and hand) should be placed in a sling and swathe (swathe not shown).

An arm sling can help stabilize upper-extremity injuries.

splint with either a roller bandage or several cravats. A pillow or a rolled, folded blanket also can be secured onto the arm. Put the arm in a sling and secure it with a swathe (binder) around the body.

Wrist, Hand, and Fingers

To stabilize the wrist, hand, and fingers, use either of two methods:

- Place the injured hand in the "position of function" (hand looks like it is holding a baseball) by placing a rolled pair of socks or a roller bandage in the palm. Then attach a rigid splint that extends past the tips of the fingers along the forearm, or

- Place the hand into its position of function, mold a pillow around the hand and forearm, and tie the pillow in place with cravats or a roller bandage.

Then place the arm in a sling and a swathe (binder), with the thumb in an upright position.

Another way to splint fingers is to tape them together ("buddy taping"), with gauze separating the fingers.

Pelvis and Hip

If you suspect a pelvic or hip fracture, stabilize the victim as she or he is found. Treat the victim for shock (do not lift the legs) and wait for the EMS ambulance to arrive. Pelvic and hip fractures require a long backboard (spine board).

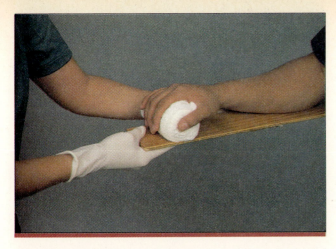

Splinting a wrist, hand, or finger fracture

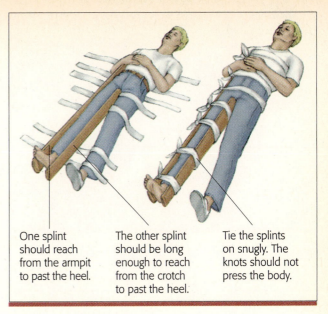

One splint should reach from the armpit to past the heel.

The other splint should be long enough to reach from the crotch to past the heel.

Tie the splints on snugly. The knots should not press the body.

Splinting a femur fracture

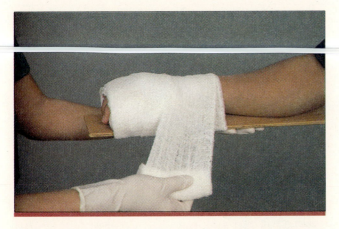

Use gauze roller bandage. Apply roller working up the elbow.

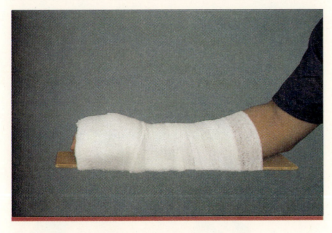

Overlap previous layer by one-half to three-quarters.

Femur (Thigh)

A fractured femur is best splinted with a traction splint, the use of which requires special training. Traction splints are seldom available except on ambulances.

First aiders can use one of two methods:

- Place a folded blanket or pillows between the victim's legs for padding, then tie the injured leg to the uninjured leg with several cravats or bandages, or
- Secure two boards, one placed between the victim's legs and extending from the groin to the foot and the other placed along the victim's side extending from the armpit to the foot. The boards must be well padded along their entire length. Stabilize the hip and the knee against movement.

Knee

Always stabilize an injured knee in the position in which it is found. If the knee is straight, splint it straight; if it is bent, splint it bent. For a straight knee, tie one long, padded board extending from the hip to the ankle underneath the leg. An alternative for a straight knee is to tie two boards, one placed between the victim's legs and extending from the groin to the foot and the other extending from the hip to the foot. Another alternative is to tie the injured leg to the uninjured one.

For a bent knee, tie a long board extending from just below the hip to just above the ankle, to prevent motion of the knee. An alternative for a bent knee is to place a pillow or a rolled blanket beneath the knee and then tie the injured leg to the uninjured leg.

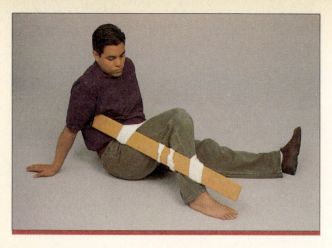
Splint knee in position found. If bent, splint it bent.

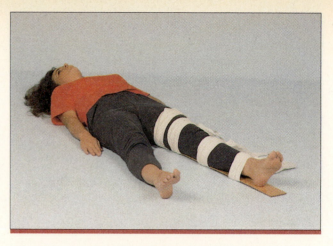
Splint knee in position found. If straight, splint it straight.

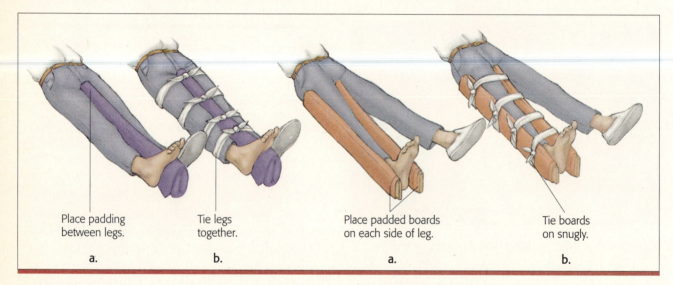

Place padding between legs.

a.

Tie legs together.

b.

Place padded boards on each side of leg.

a.

Tie boards on snugly.

b.

Two methods of splinting tibia and fibula fractures: self-splint (left) and two boards (right)

Lower Leg

Stabilize the lower leg with two boards extending from the upper thigh to the bottom of the foot. Another method is to place a folded blanket between the victim's legs for padding and then tie the injured leg to the uninjured leg with several swathes, cravats, or bandages.

Ankle and Foot

Treat ankle and foot injuries with the RICE procedures (see page 242). To further stabilize an ankle, wrap a pillow or folded blanket around the ankle and foot and tie with cravats.

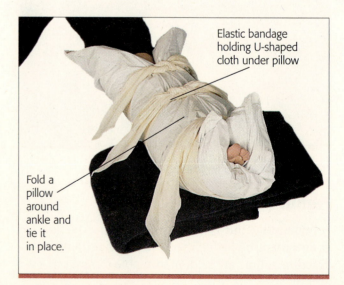

Elastic bandage holding U-shaped cloth under pillow

Fold a pillow around ankle and tie it in place.

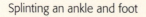
Splinting an ankle and foot

SKILL SCAN: Splinting—Upper Extremities

Arm Sling: Shoulder and Clavicle Injuries

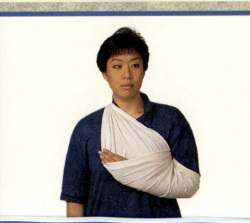

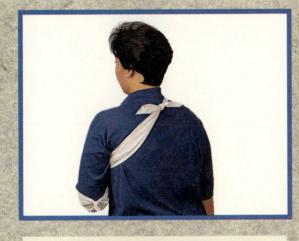

Arm Sling and Swathe for Upper Extremity Injuries

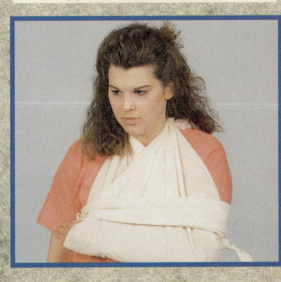

Upper Arm (Humerus)

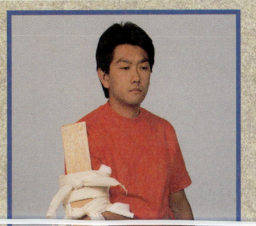

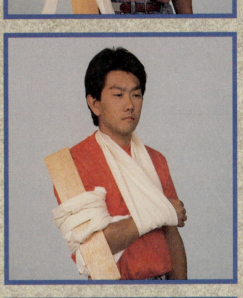

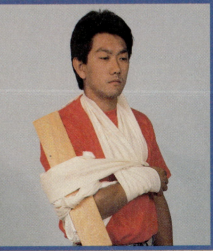

Forearm (Radius/Ulna)

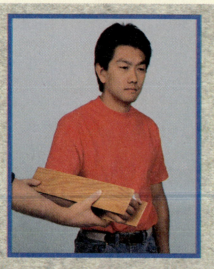

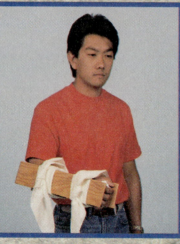

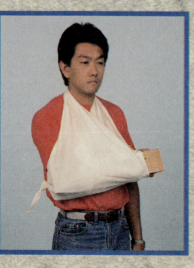

Fingers and Hand (Position of Function)

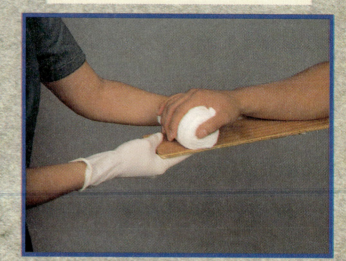

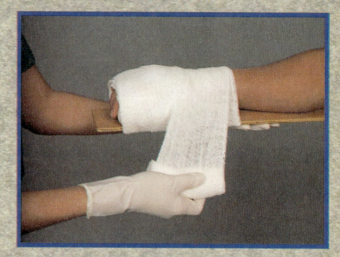

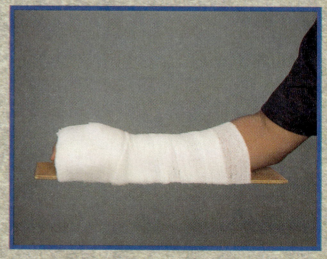

SKILL SCAN: Splinting—Lower Extremities

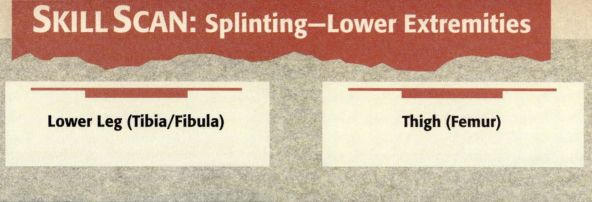

Lower Leg (Tibia/Fibula)	Thigh (Femur)

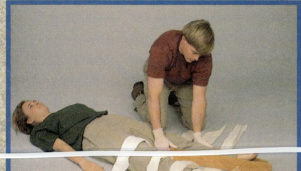

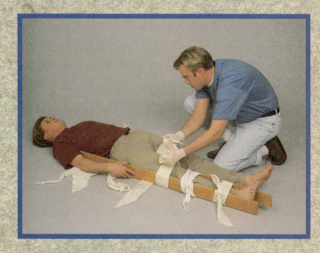

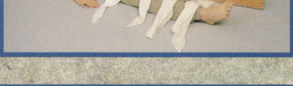

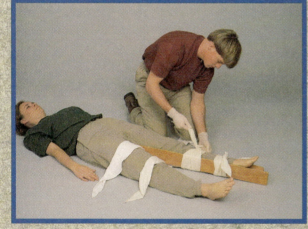

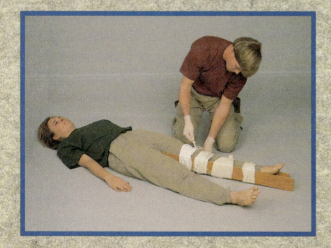

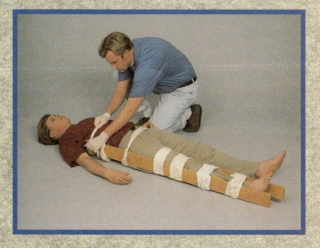

Splinting Specific Areas   **263**

SKILL SCAN: Splinting—Lower Extremities

Ankle/Foot

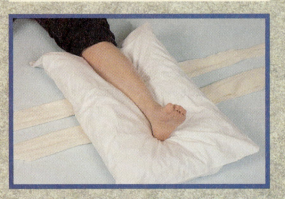

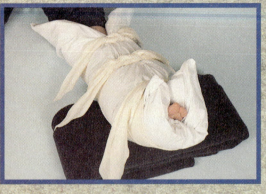

Self-Splint: Fingers/Toes

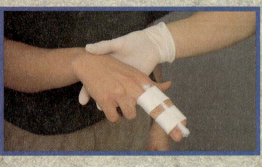

Self-Splint: Leg

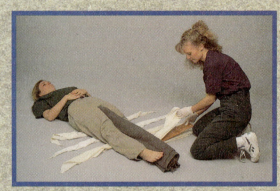

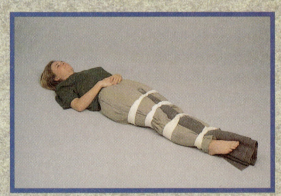

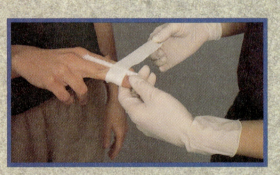

Notes

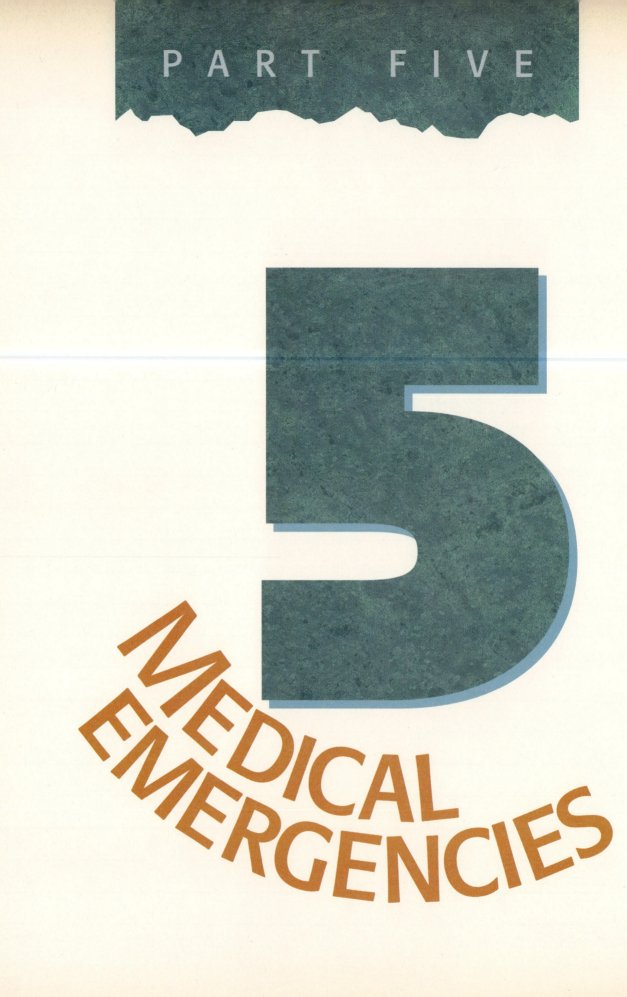

PART FIVE

5

MEDICAL EMERGENCIES

Sudden Illnesses

Heart Attack

A heart attack, or **acute myocardial infarction (AMI),** occurs when the blood supply to part of the heart muscle is severely reduced or stopped. That happens when one of the coronary arteries (the arteries that supply blood to the heart muscle) is blocked by an obstruction or a spasm.

" A man is as old as his arteries. "

—Pierre J. G. Cabanis

What to Look For

Heart attacks are difficult to determine. Because medical care at the onset of a heart attack is vital to survival and the quality of recovery, if you suspect a heart attack for any reason, seek medical attention *at once*.

The American Heart Association lists the following as possible signs and symptoms of a heart attack:

- uncomfortable pressure, fullness, squeezing, or pain in the center of the chest that lasts more than a few minutes or that goes away and comes back
- pain spreading to the shoulders, neck, or arms
- chest discomfort with lightheadedness, fainting, sweating, nausea, or shortness of breath

Not all these warning signs occur in every heart attack. It is difficult to determine if someone is having a heart attack. Many victims will deny that they might be experiencing something as serious as a heart attack. Don't take "no" for an answer. Delay can seriously increase the risk of major damage. Insist on taking prompt action.

Victims with heart attack symptoms who are brought to a hospital by ambulance receive clot-dissolving drugs (thrombolytics) sooner than those arriving by other means. It is clear that reducing the time from the onset of a heart attack to the receiving of thrombolytic drugs is beneficial and decreases the amount of heart damage.

What to Do

1. Call the EMS or get to the nearest hospital emergency department that offers 24-hour emergency cardiac care.

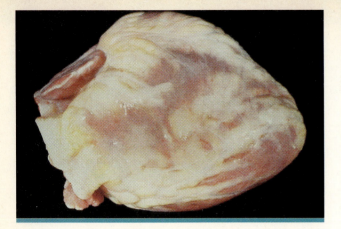
Healthy heart

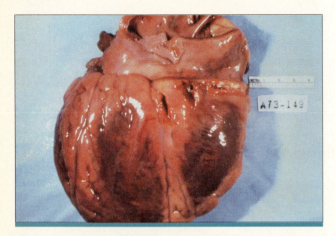
Heart with artery clot after heart attack

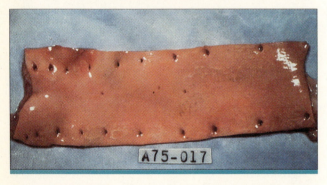
Normal artery (aorta)

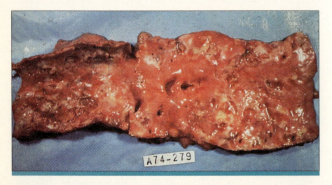
Inside of atherosclerotic artery (aorta)

Risk Factors of Heart Disease

According to the American Heart Association, several factors contribute to an increase risk of heart attack and stroke. The more risk factors present, the greater the chance a person will develop heart disease.

Risk factors you cannot change:
- Heredity. Tendencies appear in family lines.
- Male sex. Men have a greater risk, although heart attack is still the leading cause of death among women.
- Age. Most heart attack victims are 65 or older.

Risk factors you can change:
- Cigarette smoking. Smokers have more than twice the risk of heart attack as nonsmokers.
- High blood pressure. This condition adds to the heart's workload.
- High blood cholesterol level. Too much cholesterol in the blood can cause a buildup on the walls of the arteries.

Other risk factors you can change or control:
- Diabetes. This condition affects the blood's cholesterol and triglyceride levels.
- Obesity. Being overweight influences blood pressure and blood cholesterol, can result in diabetes, and can put an added strain on the heart.
- Physical inactivity. Inactive people have twice the risk of heart attack as active people.
- Stress. All people feel stress but react in different ways. Excessive, long-term stress may create problems in some people.

2. Monitor the ABCs. Give CPR if necessary and if you are properly trained.
3. Help the victim to the least painful position, usually sitting with legs up and bent at the knees (**Rothberg position**). Loosen clothing around the neck and midriff. Be calm and reassuring.
4. Determine if the victim is known to have coronary heart disease and is using nitroglycerin. Nitroglycerin tablets or spray under the tongue or nitroglycerin ointment on the skin may relieve chest pain. Nitroglycerin dilates the coronary arteries, which increases blood flow to the heart muscle, and lowers blood pressure and dilates

Table 15-1: Chest Pain

Cause of Pain	Characteristics	Care
Muscle or rib pain from exercise or injury	Reproduced by movement Tender spot when pressed	Rest Aspirin or ibuprofen
Respiratory infection (pneumonia, bronchitis, pleuritis)	Cough Fever Sore throat Production of sputum	Antibiotics
Indigestion	Belching Heartburn Nausea Sour taste	Antacids
Angina pectoris	Lasts <10 minutes	Rest Victim's nitroglycerin
Heart attack (myocardial infarction)	Lasts >10 minutes Pressure, squeezing, or pain in center of chest Pain spreads to shoulders, neck, or arms Lightheadedness, fainting, sweating, nausea, shortness of breath	Call EMS Check ABCs Rothberg position Victim's nitroglycerin

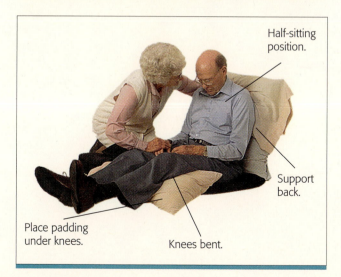

Half-sitting position.

Support back.

Place padding under knees.

Knees bent.

Help the victim into a relaxed position to ease strain on heart.

the veins, which decreases the work of the heart and the heart muscle's need for oxygen.

Caution: Because nitroglycerin lowers blood pressure, the victim should be sitting or lying down. Nitroglycerin normally may be repeated for a total of three doses in 10 minutes if the first dose does not relieve the pain. Keep in mind, though, that the victim may have already taken some nitroglycerin. Also, nitroglycerin is prescribed in different strengths—three tablets of one strength may be a mild dose, while three tablets of another strength may be a very high dose.

5. If the victim is unresponsive, check the ABCs and start CPR if needed.

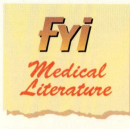

Why Don't They Call? A study of heart attack victims who waited for more than 20 minutes before getting help were asked why they delayed. Their answers included the following:

- They thought the symptoms would go away.
- The symptoms were "not severe enough."
- They thought it was a different illness.
- They were worried about medical costs.
- They were afraid of hospitals.
- They feared being embarrassed.
- They wanted to wait for a better time.
- They did not want to find out what was wrong.

The average time that elapsed between symptom onset and hospital arrival was two hours; 28 percent waited at least one hour, 33 percent one to three hours, 15 percent three to six hours, and 23 percent more than six hours. The researchers noted that the main reason for victim delay appeared to be uncertainty in interpreting heart attack symptoms. Most victims reported they were not sure their symptoms were severe enough to merit such drastic action as calling 911.

The same study concluded that one way to shorten out-of-hospital delay is to encourage victims with heart-related symptoms to use the emergency medical service rather than slower transportation methods.

Source: H. Meischke et al., "Reasons Patients with Chest Pain Delay or Do Not Call 911," *Annals of Emergency Medicine* 25:193–197 (February 1995).

HEART ATTACK

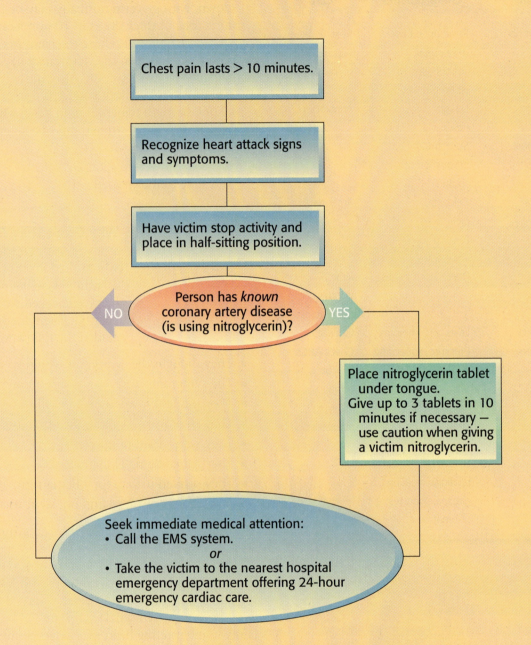

Chest pain lasts > 10 minutes.

Recognize heart attack signs and symptoms.

Have victim stop activity and place in half-sitting position.

Person has *known* coronary artery disease (is using nitroglycerin)?

NO   YES

Place nitroglycerin tablet under tongue.
Give up to 3 tablets in 10 minutes if necessary — use caution when giving a victim nitroglycerin.

Seek immediate medical attention:
• Call the EMS system.
or
• Take the victim to the nearest hospital emergency department offering 24-hour emergency cardiac care.

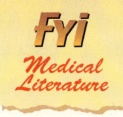

Dangerous Morning Hours The chances of suffering cardiac arrest are higher in the morning hours than at any other time of day. A study of 1,019 consecutive cardiac arrest cases that occurred in Houston during a one-year period found that out-of-hospital cardiac arrest was more common among—and more likely to be survived by—men. Women victims, however, tended to be older than the men.

The study revealed that cardiac arrest events were least common during the night hours, and their occurrence began to increase at around 6 A.M. The incidence of cardiac arrest peaked in the late morning (around 10 or 11) and then declined for the rest of the day. Cardiac arrest may be tied to the circadian rhythm cycle, changes in blood pressure, ability of platelets to aggregate, or fluctuations in epinephrine levels.

Source: R. L. Levine et al., "Prospective Evidence of a Circadian Rhythm for Out-of-Hospital Cardiac Arrests," *Journal of the American Medical Association* 267:2935–2937 (June 3, 1992).

Angina

Chest pain called **angina pectoris** can result from coronary heart disease just as a heart attack does. Angina happens when the heart muscle does not get as much blood as it needs (which means a lack of oxygen).

Angina is brought on by physical exertion, exposure to cold, emotional stress, or the ingestion of food. It seldom lasts longer than 10 minutes and almost always is relieved by nitroglycerin. (In contrast, chest pain from a heart attack is as likely to happen at rest as during activity; the pain lasts longer than 10 minutes and is not relieved by nitroglycerin.)

Nitroglycerin is the drug most often used to dilate coronary arteries to increase the blood supply to the heart. It also relaxes the veins to reduce the amount of blood returning to the heart, thus lessening the work involved in pumping.

1. Determine if the victim is known to have coronary heart disease and is using nitroglycerin. Nitroglycerin tablets or spray under the tongue or nitroglycerin ointment on the skin may relieve chest pain. Nitroglycerin dilates the coronary arteries, which increases blood flow to the heart

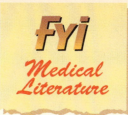

Monday Morning Heart Attacks Studies show that heart attacks occur most frequently in the morning and during the winter months. In one study, 5,596 heart attacks and sudden cardiac deaths were recorded in Augsburg, Germany, from 1958 through 1990. The increased heart attack risk was highest among people employed outside the home, especially in blue collar jobs, when heart attack incidence peaked on Mondays. Sundays had the lowest heart attack rate for all workers. There was no significant daily variation in heart attacks among nonworking people.

Source: S. N. Willich et al., "Weekly Variation of Acute Myocardial Infarction," *Circulation* 90:87 (July 1994).

muscle, and lowers blood pressure and dilates the veins, which decreases the work of the heart and the heart muscle's need for oxygen.

Caution: Because nitroglycerin lowers blood pressure, the victim should be sitting or lying down. Nitroglycerin normally may be repeated for a total of three tablets in 10 minutes if the first dose does not relieve the pain. Keep in mind, though, that the victim may have already taken some nitroglycerin. Also, nitroglycerin is prescribed in different strengths—three tablets of one strength may be a mild dose, while three tablets of another strength may be a high dose.

2. If the pain stops within 10 minutes, suspect angina. If the pain continues for more than 10 minutes, suspect a heart attack and treat the victim accordingly.

Many causes of chest pain have nothing to do with the heart:

- Muscle or rib pain from exercise or injury. The victim can reproduce the pain by movement, and often the area of complaint is tender when pressed. Rest and aspirin or ibuprofen relieve the pain.
- Respiratory infection (e.g., pneumonia, bronchitis, pleuritis) or lung injury. Chest pain from these conditions usually worsens when the victim coughs or breathes deeply. Fever and colored sputum may be present.
- Indigestion, usually accompanied by belching, heartburn, nausea, and a sour taste in the mouth. This type of pain is relieved by antacids.

Stroke (Brain Attack)

A **stroke,** or **cerebrovascular accident (CVA),** occurs when blood vessels that deliver oxygen-rich blood to the brain rupture or become plugged, so part of the brain does not get the blood flow it needs. Deprived of oxygen, nerve cells in the affected area of the brain cannot function and die within minutes. Because dead brain cells are not replaced, the devastating effects of strokes often are permanent. Each year, 550,000 Americans suffer a stroke; 150,000 die, making it the third leading cause of death. Strokes are fatal in 30 percent of cases.

The risk factors for a CVA include the following:

- age (greater than 50 years old)
- taking birth control pills *and* being over 30 years old
- overweight
- hypertension (high blood pressure)
- high blood cholesterol levels
- diabetes

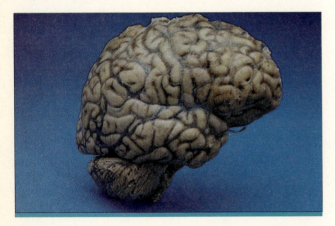

Healthy brain

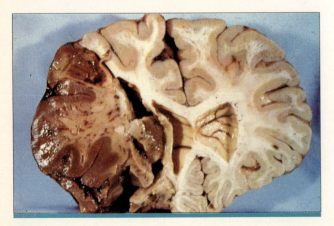

Stroke resulting from a severe hemorrhage

- heart disease
- sickle cell disease
- substance abuse, particularly of crack cocaine
- family history of strokes or transient ischemic attacks

The most common type of stroke (about 80 percent of cases) is *ischemic,* that is, a clot either forms in a brain artery (thrombotic stroke) or travels from the heart to the brain and plugs the artery (embolic stroke). In about 20 percent of cases, a blood vessel ruptures (hemorrhagic stroke). Other causes include tumors pressing on blood vessels, blood vessel spasms, and **aneurysms** (ballooning out of blood vessels).

Transient ischemic attacks (TIAs) are closely associated with CVAs. Because TIAs have many of the same signs and symptoms, they often are confused with strokes. The main difference between a TIA and a stroke is that the symptoms of TIA are transient, lasting from several minutes (75 percent last less than five minutes) to several hours, with a return to normal neurologic function. TIAs are "mini-strokes." A TIA should be considered a serious warning sign of a potential stroke—about one-third of all TIA cases will suffer a CVA two to five years after their first TIA. Any signs and symptoms of a TIA should be reported to a physician.

What to Look For

The next time you think about stroke, think "brain attack." That's the message the American Heart Association and the National Stroke Association want to deliver. The symptoms of stroke should have the same alarming significance in identifying a brain attack that acute chest pain has in identifying a heart attack:

- weakness, numbness, or paralysis of the face, an arm, or a leg on one side of the body
- blurred or decreased vision, especially in one eye
- problems speaking or understanding
- dizziness or loss of balance
- sudden, severe, and unexplained headache
- deviation of the eyes from PEARL (**P**upils **E**qual **A**nd **R**eactive to **L**ight), which may mean the brain is being affected by lack of oxygen

What to Do

First aid for a stroke victim is limited to supportive care:

1. If the victim is unresponsive, check the ABCs: keep the airway open and check the breathing and pulse. If there is no pulse or breathing, give CPR if you are trained. If there is a pulse but no breathing, give rescue breaths every five seconds.
2. Call the EMS. Hospitals staffed with teams trained to treat acute stroke offer the best treatment for stroke. Minimize brain damage by getting the victim to a hospital.
3. Lay the victim down with the head and shoulders slightly elevated, to reduce blood pressure on the brain. Place a victim who is unresponsive but breathing in the recovery position, which is on the left side with the chin extended (to keep the airway open and to permit secretions and vomit to drain from the mouth).

▶ **CAUTION: DO NOT**
- give a stroke victim anything to drink or eat. The throat may be paralyzed, which restricts swallowing.

Asthma

Asthma is a chronic, inflammatory lung disease characterized by recurrent breathing problems. People with asthma have acute episodes (some sufferers call them "attacks" or "flares") when the air passages in their lungs get narrower, and breathing becomes more difficult. The problems are caused by an oversensitivity of the lungs' airways, which overreact to certain triggers and become inflamed and clogged. Asthma affects an estimated 10 million people in the United States and accounts for an annual death toll of 6,000.

The condition is most common in children and young adults and tends to improve or resolve with age. Asthma is the number one prehospital emergency in children. It can happen in infants who are as young as a few weeks; about one-half of all children with asthma experience the condition in their first two years of life. Viral infections are a common cause of acute asthma onset in children younger than six months. Adult-onset asthma tends to be chronic.

Asthma has three components: airway obstruction, airway inflammation, and overly sensitive airways. Some of the known triggers of asthma include the following:

- respiratory tract infection
- exposure to temperature extremes, especially cold air
- strong odors, perfumes, talcum powder, deodorizers, paint
- occupational exposures: dust, fumes, smoke
- certain drugs: aspirin, nonsteroidal anti-inflammatory drugs (NSAIDs), yellow dye #5, beta blockers
- exercise
- emotional stress
- allergens: pollen, mold, dust mites, animal dander, tobacco smoke
- air pollution: ozone, sulfur dioxide

What to Look For

Asthma varies a great deal from one person to another. Symptoms can range from mild to moderate to severe and can be life threatening. The episodes may come occasionally or often. The signs of an asthma attack are

- coughing
- cyanosis (bluish skin color)
- inability to speak in complete sentences without pausing for breath
- nostrils flaring with each breath
- wheezing (high-pitched whistling sound during breathing)

Not all persons with these signs have asthma. Other causes include foreign body aspiration, lung cancer, cystic fibrosis, congestive heart failure, upper-airway obstruction or inflammation, and pneumonia. Some victims of severe asthma may have little or no wheezing.

What to Do

1. Check the ABCs (airway open, breathing, and pulse).
2. Try to determine the onset and possible causes of the shortness of breath, including exposure to possible triggers.
3. Keep the victim in a comfortable upright position. Generally the victim will dictate what position is most tolerable, usually sitting up since that makes it easier to breathe.
4. Ask the victim about any asthma medication he or she may be using. Most asthma sufferers will have some form of asthma medication, usually

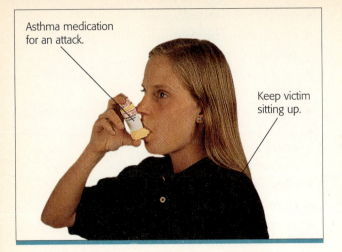
Asthma medication for an attack.

Keep victim sitting up.

Keep an asthma victim comfortable.

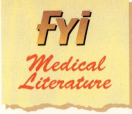

Breathing into a Paper Bag If you are advised to breathe into a paper bag—a popular remedy for anxiety-related hyperventilation (fast breathing)—don't do it. Tests on normal, healthy people show that bag rebreathing rarely restores blood gas balance but often causes dangerous stress to the heart and respiratory system, especially those with a chronic respiratory disease.

Source: M. Callaham, "Hypoxic Hazards of Traditional Paper Bag Rebreathing in Hyperventilating Patients," *Annals of Emergency Medicine* 18:622 (June 1989).

administered through doctor-prescribed, hand-held inhalers.

5. If the victim does not respond well to his or her inhaled medication or is having an extreme asthma attack (known as **status asthmaticus**), seek medical attention immediately.

CAUTION: DO NOT

- **wait too long to get medical help for the victim of a severe asthma attack.**

Asthma is extremely common. As a rule, it also is treated fairly easily. Although asthma is a complex condition that may warrant use of several different medications, the preferred method of initial care for both children and adults is use of their inhaled bronchodilators.

Hyperventilation

Fast, deep breathing is common during psychological stress. The victim may be hysterical or quite calm. Other factors that can cause rapid breathing include untreated diabetes, severe shock, certain poisons, and brain swelling from injury or high altitude.

What to Look For

- dizziness or lightheadedness
- numbness
- tingling of the hands and feet
- shortness of breath
- breathing rates faster than 40 per minute

What to Do

1. Calm and reassure the victim.
2. Encourage the victim to breathe slowly, using the abdominal muscles: inhale through the nose, hold the full inhalation for several seconds, then exhale slowly through pursed lips.

Chronic Obstructive Pulmonary Disease (COPD)

Chronic obstructive pulmonary disease (COPD) is a broad term applied to emphysema, chronic bronchitis, and related lung diseases. The incidence of COPD is very high in North America, and the most common causative factor is cigarette smoking.

Chronic bronchitis is caused by chronic infection and by irritations such as tobacco smoke. The bronchi become thick, unable to stretch, and partially blocked. Early symptoms include a "cigarette cough" or cough due to a cold. Later, more severe symptoms include difficult breathing, increased sputum, and severe coughing.

Emphysema often occurs with chronic bronchitis. The alveoli of the lungs are partially destroyed and the lungs have lost their elasticity, making it difficult for the victim to exhale. Common symptoms include coughing, wheezing, and shortness of breath. Breathing is extremely difficult for emphysema victims.

COPD signs and symptoms are similar to those of asthma. Most victims will wheeze; coughing and shortness of breath may be more prominent in COPD than in asthma. Many COPD victims depend on a constant low level of artificially supplied oxygen to maintain breathing.

FAINTING

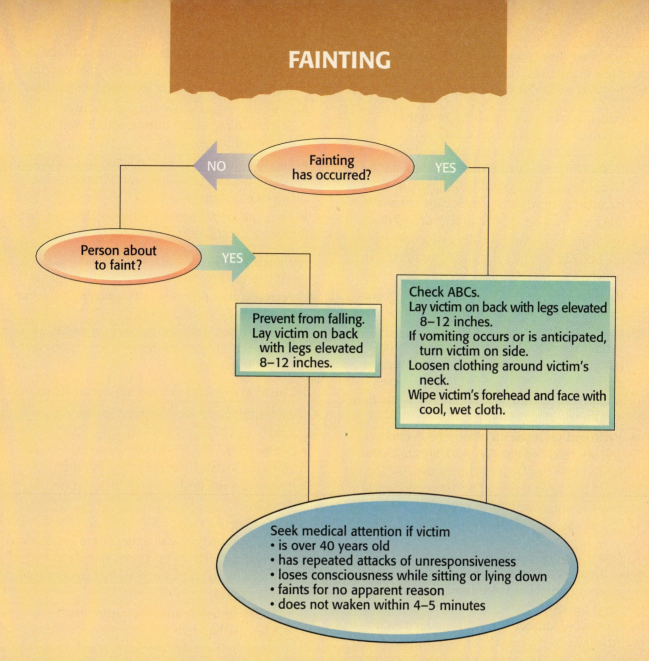

Fainting has occurred?

NO

YES

Person about to faint?

YES

Prevent from falling.
Lay victim on back
with legs elevated
8–12 inches.

Check ABCs.
Lay victim on back with legs elevated
   8–12 inches.
If vomiting occurs or is anticipated,
   turn victim on side.
Loosen clothing around victim's
   neck.
Wipe victim's forehead and face with
   cool, wet cloth.

Seek medical attention if victim
• is over 40 years old
• has repeated attacks of unresponsiveness
• loses consciousness while sitting or lying down
• faints for no apparent reason
• does not waken within 4–5 minutes

There are four types of seizures. Because seizure types are so different, they require different first aid actions, and some require no action at all.

- Generalized motor seizures (**grand mal seizures**) are characterized by loss of consciousness, muscle contraction, and sometimes tongue biting, loss of bladder control, and mental confusion. The grand mal seizure is often frightening to witness. The seizure usually is followed by a period of coma or drowsiness.
- Focal motor seizures usually cause one part of the body (e.g., one side of the face or an arm) to twitch.
- Psychomotor, or temporal-lobe, seizures are characterized by an altered personality state and are often preceded by dizziness or a peculiar metallic taste in the mouth. In some people, temporal-lobe seizures may cause sudden, unexplained attacks of rage; in others, these seizures are manifested by automatic (involuntary) types of behavior.
- **Petit mal seizures** usually occur in children and are rarely an emergency. They are characterized by a brief loss of consciousness. The child suddenly stares off into space for a few seconds and then returns immediately to consciousness.

Because of the nature of the electrical discharge in the brain, grand mal seizures usually follow a typical sequence. Many victims experience an aura, a strange sensation lasting a few seconds. The aura may consist of auditory or visual hallucinations, a peculiar taste in the mouth, or a painful sensation in the abdomen. The victim then loses consciousness and has contractions of the muscles of the extremities, trunk, and head. The attack usually lasts two to five minutes. It may be followed with deep sleep, headache, and muscle soreness.

The following information is important to obtain from the seizure victim, the family, or bystanders:

- Does the victim have a history of seizures? Does the victim take medication for seizures? Has the victim been taking the medication according to instructions?
- What did the seizure look like? How long did the seizure last? Was the seizure preceded by an aura?
- Does the victim have a recent or remote history of head injury? Trauma can irritate parts of the

brain, causing seizures. More than half the victims of acute head injuries will experience a seizure within one year following the injury.

- Does the victim abuse alcohol or drugs? Seizures often occur during withdrawal from alcohol and barbiturates.
- Has the victim recently had a fever, headache, or stiff neck? These signs and symptoms could indicate meningitis.
- Does the victim have a history of diabetes, heart disease, or stroke?

Epilepsy is not a mental illness, and it is not a sign of low intelligence. It also is not contagious. Between seizures, a person with epilepsy can function as normally as a nonepileptic.

The Epilepsy Foundation of America lists the following first aid procedures for convulsions and grand mal seizures:

1. Cushion the victim's head; take away items that could cause injury if the person bumped into them.
2. Loosen any tight neckwear.
3. Turn the victim onto his or her left side.
4. Look for a medical-alert tag (bracelet or necklace).
5. As the seizure ends, offer your help. Most seizures in people with epilepsy are not medical emergencies. They end after a minute or two without harm and usually do not require medical attention.
6. Call EMS if any of the following exists:
   - A seizure happens to someone who is not known to have epilepsy (e.g., there is no "epilepsy" or "seizure disorder" identification). It could be a sign of serious illness.
   - A seizure lasts more than five minutes.
   - The victim is slow to recover, has a second seizure, or has difficulty breathing afterward.

CAUTION: DO NOT

- give the victim anything to eat or drink.
- hold the victim down.
- put anything between the victim's teeth during the seizure.
- throw any liquid on the victim's face or into the mouth.
- move the victim to another place.

SEIZURES

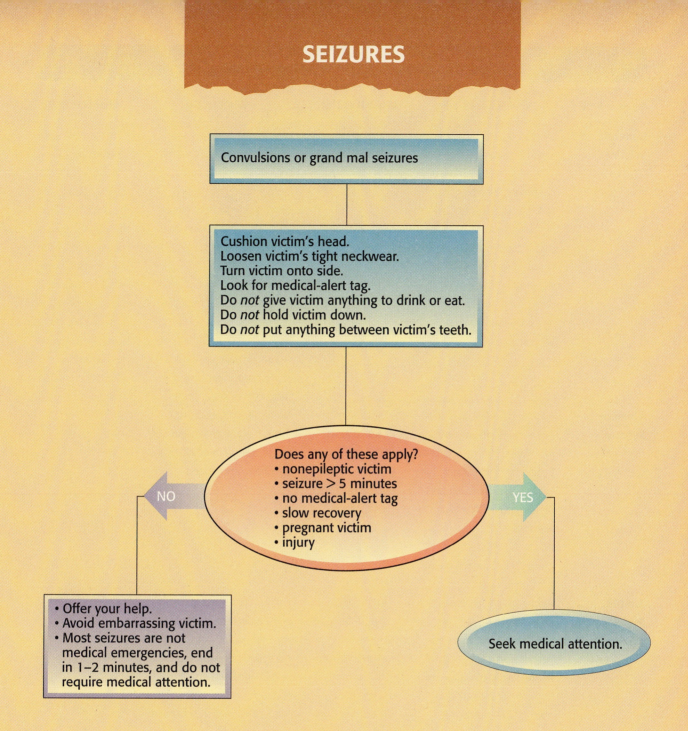

Convulsions or grand mal seizures

Cushion victim's head.
Loosen victim's tight neckwear.
Turn victim onto side.
Look for medical-alert tag.
Do *not* give victim anything to drink or eat.
Do *not* hold victim down.
Do *not* put anything between victim's teeth.

Does any of these apply?
• nonepileptic victim
• seizure > 5 minutes
• no medical-alert tag
• slow recovery
• pregnant victim
• injury

NO

YES

• Offer your help.
• Avoid embarrassing victim.
• Most seizures are not medical emergencies, end in 1–2 minutes, and do not require medical attention.

Seek medical attention.

Table 15-2: Seizures: Recognition and First Aid

Seizure Type	What It Looks Like	What It Is Not	What to Do	What Not to Do
Generalized Seizure (also called grand mal)	Sudden cry, fall, rigidity, followed by muscle jerks, shallow breathing or temporarily suspended breathing, bluish skin, possible loss of bladder or bowel control; usually lasts a couple of minutes. Normal breathing then starts again. There may be some confusion and/or fatigue, followed by return to full consciousness.	• Heart attack • Stroke	Look for medical-alert tag. Protect from nearby hazards. Loosen tie or shirt collars. Protect head from injury. Turn on side to keep airway clear. Reassure when consciousness returns. If single seizure lasted less than 5 minutes, ask if hospital evaluation is wanted. If multiple seizures, or if one seizure lasts longer than 5 minutes, call an ambulance. If person is pregnant, injured, or diabetic, call for aid at once.	Don't put any hard implement in the mouth. Don't try to hold tongue. It can't be swallowed. Don't try to give liquids during or just after seizure. Don't use rescue breathing unless breathing is absent after muscle jerks subside or unless water has been inhaled. Don't restrain.
Absence Seizure (also called petit mal)	A blank stare, lasting only a few seconds; most common in children. May be accompanied by rapid blinking, some chewing movements of the mouth. Child is unaware of what's going on during the seizure but quickly returns to full awareness once it has stopped.	• Daydreaming • Lack of attention • Deliberate ignoring of adult instructions	No first aid necessary, but if this is the first observation of the seizure(s), medical evaluation recommended.	
Simple Partial Seizure	Jerking may begin in one area of the body, arm, leg, or face. Can't be stopped, but patient stays awake and aware. Jerking may proceed from one area of the body to another and sometimes spreads to become a convulsive seizure. Partial sensory seizures may not be obvious to an onlooker. Patient experiences a distorted environment. May see or hear things that aren't there, may feel unexplained fear, sadness, anger, or joy. May have nausea, experience odd smells, and have a generally "funny" feeling in the stomach.	• Acting out, bizarre behavior • Hysteria • Mental Illness • Psychosomatic illness • Parapsychological or mystical experience	No first aid necessary unless seizure becomes convulsive, then first aid as above. No action needed other than reassurance and emotional support. Medical evaluation should be recommended.	

DIABETIC EMERGENCIES

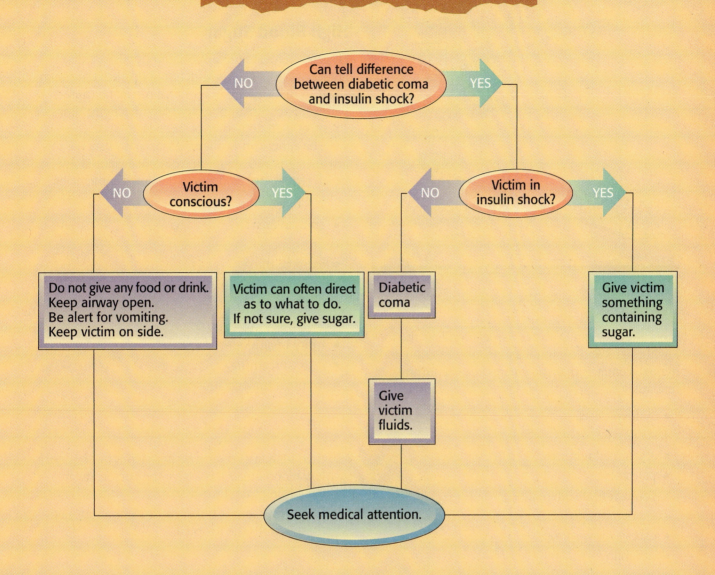

Can tell difference between diabetic coma and insulin shock?

NO → Victim conscious?

YES → Victim in insulin shock?

Victim conscious? — NO:
Do not give any food or drink.
Keep airway open.
Be alert for vomiting.
Keep victim on side.

Victim conscious? — YES:
Victim can often direct as to what to do.
If not sure, give sugar.

Victim in insulin shock? — NO:
Diabetic coma

Give victim fluids.

Victim in insulin shock? — YES:
Give victim something containing sugar.

Seek medical attention.

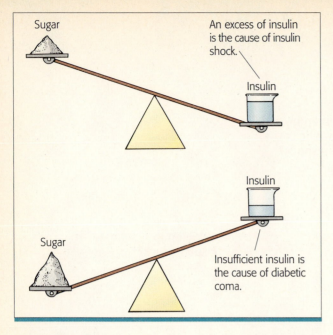

Diabetic emergencies

The American Diabetes Association lists the following signs and symptoms of insulin reaction and hypoglycemia as diabetic emergencies requiring first aid:

- sudden onset
- staggering, poor coordination
- anger, bad temper
- pale color
- confusion, disorientation
- sudden hunger
- excessive sweating
- trembling
- eventual unconsciousness

What to Do

Give sugar if all are present:

- The victim is a known diabetic, and
- The victim's mental status is altered, and
- The victim is awake enough to swallow.

1. Give victim sugar-containing food, such as soda, candy, milk, or fruit juice. Do not use diet drinks—they do not contain sugar.
2. If improvement is not seen in 15 minutes, take the person to a hospital.

An injectible medication called glucagon, available by a physician's prescription, raises blood sugar quickly. A family member or friend should learn when and how to inject glucagon in an emergency.

High Blood Sugar

Hyperglycemia is the opposite of hypoglycemia. Hyperglycemia occurs when the body has too much sugar in the blood. This condition may be caused by insufficient insulin, overeating, inactivity, illness, stress, or a combination of these factors.

The American Diabetes Association lists the following signs and symptoms of diabetic coma, hyperglycemia, and acidosis as diabetic emergencies requiring first aid:

- gradual onset
- drowsiness
- extreme thirst
- very frequent urination
- flushed skin
- vomiting
- fruity breath odor
- heavy breathing
- eventual unconsciousness

What to Do

1. If you are uncertain whether victim has high or low blood-sugar level, give the person sugar-containing food or drink.
2. If improvement is not seen in 15 minutes, take the victim to the hospital.

Abdominal Distress

Persons with gastrointestinal problems usually complain of one or more of the following symptoms:

- *Abdominal pain that is aching, cramping, sharp, or dull.* It may be constant, or it may come and go. The pain may indicate a mild problem or an acute one requiring immediate surgery.
- *Nausea and vomiting.* Vomiting is the ejection of the stomach's contents through the mouth. Nausea is a feeling of the need to vomit.
- *Diarrhea or constipation.* Diarrhea is the frequent passage of loose, watery stools. Constipation is the opposite of diarrhea; stools are infrequent, hard, and difficult to pass.

Abdominal Pain

The abdomen is the area between the nipple line and the groin. Abdominal organs are either hollow or solid. Hollow organs are tubes through which material passes, for example, the stomach and the intestines, which conduct food through the body. Solid organs are solid masses of tissue where much of the chemical work of the body takes place. The liver, spleen, and gallbladder are solid organs. The peritoneum is a thin membrane lining the entire abdominal cavity. Irritation of the peritoneum is called **peritonitis.**

There are many possible causes of abdominal pain, some not so serious and some life threatening. They often can be serious enough to require emergency surgery. Illnesses that affect the abdomen have one thing in common: they are very painful.

Abdominal problems are so difficult to diagnose that even skilled physicians may have trouble pinpointing an exact cause. It is neither feasible nor useful for a first aider to distinguish among the many causes of abdominal pain because first aid usually will be similar regardless of the cause.

What to Look For

- When did the pain start? Where is it located?
- Is the pain constant, or does it come and go? Constant pain may be more serious than a cramping pain. Constant abdominal pain suggests inflammation of an organ; cramping suggests obstruction of a hollow organ.
- Does belching or passing gas relieve the pain? That suggests the intestine is affected.
- Does the victim feel nauseated, or does he or she have a good appetite?
- Is there diarrhea or vomiting?
- Does the victim feel warm (feverish)?
- Does anyone in the group have similar symptoms?
- For a female, is there any chance of pregnancy? Any pain with pregnancy should be treated as an emergency.
- Is the abdomen rigid to touch? That may be a sign of an emergency condition.

What to Do

1. Give the victim only clear fluids (anything you can see through, *except* alcohol and caffeine). Have the victim slowly sip the fluids.
2. Give the victim an antacid.
3. If feasible, place a hot-water bottle against the victim's abdomen or have the victim soak in a warm bath.
4. Recognize the possibility of vomiting and be prepared for it. Keep the victim on the left side to help prevent vomiting.
5. Keep the victim in a comfortable position, usually lying down with knees bent (unless the victim is nauseated).
6. Seek medical care if any of the following applies:
   - Pain is constant for more than six hours.
   - The victim is unable to drink fluids.
   - The victim is or may be pregnant.
   - Abdomen is rigid and painful.
   - Abdomen is swollen.
   - After you press your fingers on the victim's abdomen and suddenly release it, more pain occurs.
   - There is bloody, blood-stained, or black stool.
   - The victim has a fever.
   - Pain began around the belly button and later moved to the lower right abdomen.

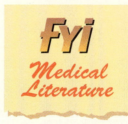

Swallowed Coins: Must They Be Removed? When a child swallows a coin that lodges in the esophagus, it can cause serious injury. That is why an x-ray must be taken to locate the coin, even if it causes no pain or other symptoms. Metal detectors can also be used. A study of 73 children found that a coin is likely to pass into the stomach spontaneously if x-rays show that it is stuck near the bottom of the esophagus. In such cases, it is safe to observe the child for 24 hours to see if the coin passes, before a physician tries to remove it. Coins stuck in the middle or upper esophagus are unlikely to pass and must be removed immediately by a physician.

Source: G. P. Conners et al., "Symptoms and Spontaneous Passage of Esophageal Coins," *Archives of Pediatrics and Adolescent Medicine* 149:36 (January 1995).

Nausea and Vomiting

Nausea (upset stomach) and vomiting (throwing up) often occur with conditions such as mild altitude sickness, motion sickness, brain injury (see page 186), intestinal viruses, eating or drinking too much, and being emotionally upset. In minor illnesses, nausea and vomiting should clear up in a couple of days. Persistent nausea and vomiting may signal more serious illnesses such as appendicitis, food poisoning, or bowel obstruction. In general, if the condition lasts longer than one or two days, the victim may become dehydrated (lose too much fluid). Young children and the elderly may be more seriously affected.

What to Look For

- Is there abdominal pain?
- Is there blood or brown, grainy material in the vomit?
- Is there diarrhea? Vomiting and diarrhea together are *usually* a self-limited viral infection.
- Are there signs of dehydration (i.e., victim is dizzy when standing, has dry, cracked lips, is very thirsty)?
- Does anyone else in the group have similar symptoms?
- Has the victim had a recent head injury?

What to Do

1. Give the victim small amounts of clear fluids (e.g., sports drinks, clear soups, flat soda, apple or cranberry juice), *except* alcohol and caffeine.
2. If the victim is able to keep fluids down, offer carbohydrates (e.g., bread, cereal, pasta) first—they are easier to digest. Avoid milk products and meats for 48 hours.

3. Have the victim rest and avoid exertion until he or she is able to eat solid foods easily.
4. Prevent inhalation of vomit by positioning the victim on his or her side to allow drainage. Inhaled vomit can result in severe pneumonia.
5. Seek medical care if any of the following applies:
   - Blood or brown, grainy material appears in the vomit.
   - There is constant abdominal pain.
   - The victim faints when standing.
   - The victim is unable to keep fluids down for more than 24 hours.
   - The victim has severe, projectile vomiting (vomit shoots out in large quantities).
   - The vomiting follows a recent head injury.

What to Do for Motion Sickness

1. If the victim is prone to motion sickness, he or she should sit near the midsection of a plane, boat, bus, train, or car and close his or her eyes. Those susceptible to motion sickness should not read, should look far ahead to the horizon, not to the sides, and should avoid overeating.
2. Try Dramamine™ (works on the ears) or Bonine™ (works on the stomach) one hour before traveling (follow label directions).

Diarrhea

Diarrhea is the frequent (usually more than four times a day) passage of loose, watery, or unformed stools. Diarrhea may be a symptom of intestinal infection (bacterial, viral, or parasitic), food poisoning, or food sensitivity/allergy, among other ailments. Dehydration can occur if the body loses too much fluid through the stool and the victim cannot drink enough fluid to keep up with the fluid losses from the diarrhea. The elderly and the very young are especially prone to dehydration, which

NOTES

C H A P T E R

16

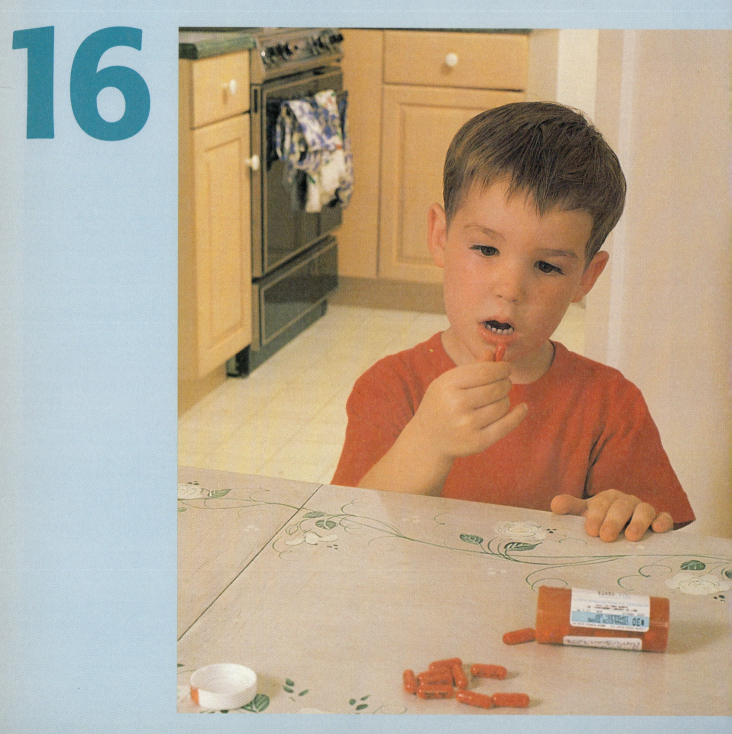

POISONING

Ingested (Swallowed) Poison

Swallowing nonfood substances is so frequent among children that it is unusual for a child to reach the age of five without at least one episode of ingesting a nonfood substance. Hundreds of thousands of poisonings occur in the United States each year. Only a small percentage of episodes, however, progress to severe or life-threatening conditions.

Household cleaning agents account for the largest category of poisoning exposures. Drugs, both prescription and nonprescription, miscellaneous chemicals, and cosmetics also are frequently implicated. Basically, any substance that is accessible to a child is a potential poison. Analgesic products that contain acetaminophen, for example, are involved in poisoning incidents more often than other analgesics, not because acetaminophen is more toxic but because products that contain acetaminophen outsell products that contain other analgesics.

It is important not to confuse poisoning frequency with poisoning severity. Plants and mushrooms, for example, account for about 5.5 percent (over 100,000 cases) of the total poisoning exposures reported each year. However, plant and mushroom ingestion resulted in 0.02 percent of serious poisonings and one death. Therefore, most exposures to plants are minor, with harmless effects. On the other hand, gun-blueing products (agents containing selenious acid that are used to maintain the blue color of gun barrels) were involved in 100 poisoning episodes and resulted in four deaths (death rate of 4 percent).

Fortunately, most poison ingestions happen with products of low toxicity or with amounts so small that severe poisoning rarely occurs. However, the potential for severe or fatal poisoning is always present.

Swallowed poisons usually remain in the stomach only a short time, and the stomach absorbs only small amounts. Most absorption takes place after the poison passes into the small intestine.

What to Look For

- abdominal pain and cramping
- nausea or vomiting
- diarrhea
- burns, odor, stains around and in mouth
- drowsiness or unconsciousness
- poison containers nearby

What to Do

1. Determine critical information:
   - Age and size of the victim?
   - What was swallowed?
   - How much was swallowed (e.g., a "taste," half a bottle, a dozen tablets)?
   - When was it swallowed?
2. If a corrosive or caustic (i.e., acid or alkali) substance was swallowed, immediately dilute it by having the victim drink at least 1–2 eight-ounce glasses of water or milk. (*Cold* milk or water tends to absorb heat better than room-temperature or warmer liquids.)

 CAUTION: DO NOT
- give water or milk to dilute other poisons unless instructed to do so by a poison control center. Fluids may dissolve a dry poison (e.g., tablets or capsules) more rapidly and fill up the stomach, forcing stomach contents (i.e., the poison) into the small intestine, where poisons are absorbed faster.

3. For a responsive victim, call a poison control center *immediately*. Some poisons do not cause harm until hours later, while others damage immediately. More than 70 percent of poisonings can be treated through instructions taken over the telephone from a poison control center. The center also will advise you if medical attention is warranted. Poison control centers routinely follow up calls to check whether additional symptoms or unexpected effects are occurring. The inside front covers of telephone directories contain the poison control center's number.
4. For an unresponsive victim, or if the poison control center number is unknown, call 911 or the local emergency number. Monitor the ABCs often.
5. Place the victim on his or her *left* side to position the end of the stomach where it enters the small intestine (pylorus) straight up. Gravity will delay (by as much as two hours) advancement of the poison into the small intestine, where absorption into the victim's circulatory system is faster. The side position also helps prevent aspiration (inhalation) into the lungs if vomiting begins.

Table 16.1: Toxic Substances in Human Exposures		
Substance	**Annual Number of Exposures**	**Percentage of Total Exposures**
Cleaning substances	203,989	10.6
Analgesics	181,333	9.4
Cosmetics and personal care products	162,807	8.5
Plants	103,616	5.4
Cough and cold preparations	100,347	5.2
Bites, envenomations	82,808	4.3
Pesticides (includes rodenticides)	78,360	4.1
Topicals	71,302	3.7
Foreign bodies	70,891	3.7
Food products, food poisoning	67,421	3.5
Hydrocarbons	64,634	3.4
Antimicrobials	61,322	3.2
Sedatives, hypnotics, antipsychotics	59,532	3.1
Alcohols	50,757	2.6
Antidepressants	49,533	2.6
Chemicals	47,605	2.5
Vitamins	44,238	2.3

Note: Despite a high frequency of involvement, these substances are not necessarily the most toxic but rather may be only the most readily accessible.

Source: American Association of Poison Control Centers.

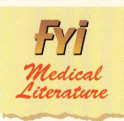

Poisoning: Where Can You Call for Help? If someone swallows poison, do *not* call the hospital emergency room. Call the local poison control center. Researchers who made 156 "test calls" to 52 hospital emergency departments in Illinois found that the advice given was correct only 64 percent of the time. Calls to the same emergency department on different days for the same problem did not consistently produce the same advice. In contrast, poison control centers gave correct advice in 17 out of 18 test calls (94 percent).

Source: H. N. Wigder et al., "Emergency Department Poison Advice Telephone Calls," *Annals of Emergency Medicine* 25:349 (March 1995).

- induce vomiting unless advised to do so by a poison control center or a physician. Reasons for *not* using syrup of ipecac include:
  - Waiting for vomiting to begin may take 20–30 minutes, during which time some poison may pass into the small intestine.
  - Additional treatment will be delayed until vomiting stops.
  - The victim could inhale the vomitus.
  - Removes up to 30–50 percent of the poison from the stomach—leaves 50–70 percent
- induce vomiting in the following instances:
  - The victim is having seizures.
  - The victim is unconscious or drowsy.
  - The victim is in the third trimester (last 3 months) of pregnancy.
  - The victim has a history of advanced heart disease or is likely to suffer a heart attack.
  - The victim swallowed a corrosive or caustic substance (e.g., drain cleaners).
  - The victim swallowed a petroleum product (e.g., lighter fluid, furniture polish, gasoline).
  - The victim swallowed strychnine (rat poison).
  - The victim is less than six months old.
- use saltwater to induce vomiting. It is dangerous and can kill a small child.
- gag or tickle the back of the victim's throat with a finger or a spoon handle. That method is usually ineffective in causing vomiting, and any vomiting produced is not very forceful.
- give dish soap, raw eggs, or mustard powder. They are not effective.
- use syrup of ipecac and activated charcoal at the same time. Charcoal will bind the ipecac and may prevent vomiting. Many toxicologists now recommend the use of activated charcoal over that of ipecac.

Although activated charcoal is an inexpensive, safe, and effective means for decreasing poison absorption, pharmacies do not routinely stock it.

8. Save poison containers, plants, and the victim's vomit to help medical personnel identify the poison.

⚠️ **CAUTION: DO NOT**

- follow the first aid procedures or recommendations on a container label without first getting confirmation from a medical source. Many labels are incorrect or out of date.
- try to neutralize a poison. Giving weak acids, such as lemon juice or vinegar, is not safe, contrary to the advice given on many drain cleaner and lye-product labels. Chemical neutralization releases large quantities of heat that can burn sensitive tissues.
- think that a specific antidote exists for most poisons. An *antidote* is a substance that counteracts a poison's effects. Few poisons have specific antidotes that will effectively block their toxic effects.
- think that there is a "universal antidote." *No* product is effective in treating most or all poisons.

Alcohol and Drug Emergencies
Alcohol Intoxication

Alcohol is a depressant, not a stimulant. It affects a person's judgment, vision, reaction time, and coordination. In very large amounts, it can cause death by paralyzing the respiratory center of the brain.

Alcohol is the most commonly used *and* abused drug in the United States, possibly even the world. It is also one of the most lethal, being implicated as a cofactor in 40 percent of drownings, about 50 percent of traffic deaths, 67 percent of homicides, and 25 percent of successful suicides. It directly affects more than 12 million people annually (10 percent of all males and 3 percent of all females) and causes more than 200,000 deaths. Alcohol abuse is the third greatest national health problem, after heart disease and cancer.

Lack of data makes it difficult to assess the actual number of alcohol-related injuries. It is estimated, however, that 20 to 25 percent of patients treated in many urban hospital emergency departments are intoxicated.

Helping an intoxicated person is often difficult since the individual may be belligerent and combative. Also, personal hygiene is sometimes less than optimal. However, it is important that alcohol abusers be helped and not just labeled as "drunks." Their condition may be quite serious, even life threatening.

Occasionally, a person will have consumed so much alcohol that there are signs that the central nervous system is depressed. In such cases, complete respiratory support may be necessary. Death can result from the excessive consumption of alcohol.

What to Look For

The following signs are indicators of alcohol intoxication. (Some of these symptoms can also mean illness or injury other than alcohol abuse, such as diabetes or heat injury.)

- the odor of alcohol on a person's breath or clothing
- unsteady, staggering walking
- slurred speech and the inability to carry on a conversation
- nausea and vomiting
- flushed face

What to Do

First aid for an intoxicated person includes these steps:

1. Look for any injuries. Alcohol can mask pain.
2. Check the ABCs and treat accordingly.
3. If the intoxicated person is lying down, place him or her in the recovery (left-side) position, to reduce the likelihood of vomiting and aspiration of vomit and to delay absorption. Be sure to check that the victim is breathing and does not have a spine injury before you move him or her. The recovery position can be used for both responsive and unresponsive persons.
4. Call the poison control center for advice or the local emergency number for help. It may be best to let EMS personnel decide if the police should be alerted.

5. If the victim becomes violent, leave the scene and find a safe place until police arrive.
6. Provide emotional support.
7. Assume that an injured or unconscious victim has a spine injury and needs to be stabilized against movement. Because of decreased pain perception, an intoxicated victim cannot be assessed reliably. If you suspect a spine injury, wait for the EMS to arrive. They have the proper equipment and training to stabilize and move a victim.
8. Since many intoxicated individuals have been exposed to the cold, suspect hypothermia and move the person to a warm environment. Remove wet clothing and cover the individual with warm blankets. Handle a hypothermic victim gently, since rough handling could induce a heart attack.

CAUTION: DO NOT

- **let an intoxicated person sleep on his or her back.**
- **leave an intoxicated person alone.**
- **try to handle a hostile drunk by yourself. Find a safe place, then call the police for help.**

Alcohol-induced seizures, from either alcohol ingestion or alcohol withdrawal, are usually brief and self-limiting.

The consumption of alcohol is deeply imbedded in our society. Because of alcohol's widespread use, those whose lives are affected directly or indirectly by alcohol abuse should be educated to recognize problems and what to do should an emergency arise.

Drugs

Drugs are classified according to their effects on the user:

- **Uppers** are stimulants of the central nervous system. They include amphetamines, cocaine, and caffeine.
- **Downers** are depressants of the central nervous system. They include barbiturates, tranquilizers, marijuana, and narcotics.
- **Hallucinogens** alter and often enhance the sensory and emotional information in the brain

centers. They include LSD, mescaline, peyote, and PCP (angel dust). Marijuana also has some hallucinogenic properties.

- **Volatile chemicals** usually are inhaled and can cause serious damage to many body organs. They include plastic model glue and cements, paint solvents, gasoline, spray paint, and nail polish remover.

Amphetamines and Cocaine

Amphetamines and cocaine provide relief from fatigue and a feeling of well-being. Blood pressure, breathing, and general body activity are increased. Some users take a "speed run" of repeated high doses. Results are hyperactivity, restlessness, and belligerence. Such persons need to be protected from hurting themselves and others. Acute cases need medical attention.

Hallucinogens

Hallucinogens produce changes in mood and sensory awareness—a person may "hear" colors and "see" sounds. They can cause hallucinations and bizarre behavior that may make users dangerous to themselves or to others. Acute cases need medical attention. Users should be protected from hurting themselves.

Marijuana

Marijuana provides a feeling of relaxation and euphoria. Users report distortions of time and space. In some persons, marijuana can cause a reaction similar to a bad LSD trip.

Barbiturates

Barbiturates induce relaxation, drowsiness, and sleep. Overdose can produce respiratory depression, coma, and death. Withdrawal can cause anxiety, tremors, nausea, fever, delirium, convulsions, and ultimately death.

Tranquilizers

Tranquilizers are used to calm anxiety. High doses and withdrawal produce the same effects as barbiturate overdose and withdrawal.

Inhaled Substances

Inhaling glue or other solvents (gasoline, lighter fluid, nail polish) produces effects similar to those from ingesting alcohol. Persons who "sniff" these substances can die from suffocation. In addition, some inhalants can cause death by changing the rhythm of the heartbeat.

Opiates

Opiates, or narcotics, are used medicinally to relieve pain and anxiety. Overdoses can result in deep sleep (coma), respiratory depression, and death. The pupils of opiate users are described as "pinpoint" in size. Withdrawal symptoms include intense agitation, abdominal discomfort, dilated pupils, increased breathing and body temperature, and a strong craving for a "fix."

What to Do

1. Check the ABCs.
2. Call the poison control center for advice or the EMS for help.
3. Check for injuries.
4. Keep the person on the *left* side to reduce the likelihood of vomiting and aspiration of vomit and to delay absorption.
5. Provide reassurance and emotional support.
6. If the person becomes violent, find a safe place until the police arrive. Let law enforcement officers handle dangerous situations.
7. Seek medical attention.

Carbon Monoxide Poisoning

Carbon monoxide (CO) is not the most dangerous poison around, but its common presence in our environment, along with its insidious nature, makes it the leading cause of poisoning death in the United States each year. According to a report from the Centers for Disease Control and Prevention, CO poisoning kills at least 1,500 people and sends 10,000 more to the hospital annually.

People who ride long distances in older, poorly maintained cars are at increased risk. Rust is a major factor in damaging an automobile's exhaust system and creating holes in the car's body through which CO can enter. Many deaths involve people sleeping inside a running car, often because of drinking. Many deaths also involve parking in remote areas for romantic purposes.

Persons in a closed room where there is cigarette smoking experience mild increases in the level of CO in their blood. Less familiar, and therefore more dangerous, sources of CO are faulty furnaces, water heaters, and kerosene heaters. Recreational fires, whether open-flame, charcoal, sterno, or hibachi grills, also give off CO.

CO victims often are unaware of its presence. The gas is invisible, tasteless, odorless, and nonirri-

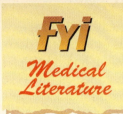

Carbon Monoxide Poisoning Riding in the back of an open pickup truck is extremely dangerous. Every year, people are maimed or killed when they are thrown out of the vehicle in which they are riding or when the truck rolls over. A recent report now maintains that riding in the enclosed back of a pickup exposes children to another danger: carbon monoxide poisoning.

Investigators at Seattle's Virginia Mason Medical School found that 20 out of 68 pediatric patients treated for carbon monoxide poisoning had been passengers in the back of pickup trucks. In 17 cases, the rear was enclosed by a rigid cap, and in three incidents, the children had been riding beneath tarpaulins. In all cases, exhaust fumes had built up in the enclosed space. One child died from cerebral edema, and one had permanent neurologic damage. The remaining patients apparently recovered well. Several states specifically outlaw riding in the back of pickup trucks.

Source: N. B. Hampson and D. M. Norkool, "Carbon Monoxide Poisoning in Children Riding in the Back of Pickup Trucks," *Journal of American Medical Association* 267:538–540 (January 22, 1992).

tating. It is produced by the incomplete burning of organic material such as gasoline, wood, paper, charcoal, coal, and natural gas.

CO poisons its victims by causing **hypoxia,** or lack of oxygen, in two ways. First, red blood cells (hemoglobin) are about 200 times more likely to bind to CO than to oxygen if both are present in the blood; thus, even a small amount of CO can greatly reduce the amount of oxygen carried in the bloodstream. Second, CO does not allow the cells to use what little oxygen is delivered. In short, CO deprives the body parts that need oxygen the most—the heart and the brain.

What to Look For

It is difficult to tell if a person is a CO victim. Sometimes, a complaint of having the "flu" is really a symptom of CO poisoning. Although many symptoms of CO poisoning resemble those of the flu, there are differences. For example, CO poisoning does not cause low-grade fever or generalized aching or involve the lymph nodes.

The traditionally cited sign of CO poisoning is a cherry-red color of the skin and the lips. This sign

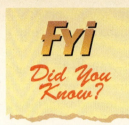

Carbon Monoxide Detectors Can Save Lives The U.S. Consumer Product Safety Commission recommends that consumers purchase and install carbon monoxide (CO) detectors with labels showing they meet the requirements of the Underwriters Laboratories, Inc. (UL) voluntary standard (UL 2034). The standard requires detectors to sound an alarm when exposure to CO reaches potentially hazardous levels over a period of time.

Properly working CO detectors can provide an early warning before the deadly gas builds up to a dangerous level. Exposure to a low concentration over several hours can be as dangerous as exposure to high carbon monoxide levels for a few minutes. The new detectors will detect both conditions. Each home should have at least one CO detector in the area outside individual bedrooms. CO detectors are as important to home safety as smoke detectors are.

Source: U.S. Consumer Product Safety Commission.

is uncommon, however, and occurs only at death; therefore, it is a poor initial indicator of CO poisoning. The following conditions are earmarks of possible CO poisoning:

- The symptoms come and go.
- The symptoms worsen or improve in certain places or at certain times of the day.
- People around you have similar symptoms.
- Pets seem ill.

The signs and symptoms of CO poisoning are as follows:

- headache
- ringing in the ears (tinnitus)
- angina (chest pain)
- muscle weakness
- nausea and vomiting
- dizziness and visual changes (blurred or double vision)
- unconsciousness
- respiratory and cardiac arrest

What to Do

1. Remove the victim from the toxic environment and into fresh air *immediately.*

2. Call the EMS, which will be able to give the victim 100 percent oxygen, improving oxygenation and disassociating the linkage between the CO and the hemoglobin. For a responsive victim, it takes four to five hours with ordinary air (21 percent oxygen) or 30–40 minutes with 100 percent oxygen to reverse the effects of CO poisoning.

3. Monitor the ABCs.

4. Place an unresponsive victim on one side.

5. Seek medical attention. All suspected CO victims should obtain a blood test to determine the level of CO.

Poison Ivy, Poison Oak, and Poison Sumac

Fifty percent of the United States population is sensitive to poison ivy, and with more people venturing into the outdoors, episodes of dermatitis caused by exposure to poison ivy, poison oak, and poison sumac are increasing. (Actually, more than 60 plants can cause allergic reactions, but these three are by far the most common offenders.) Of those who do react, 15–25 percent will have incapacitating swelling and blistering eruptions that require medical treatment with systemic corticosteroids. There is no routine test to determine an individual's degree of sensitivity—a history of past dermatitis is the most reliable indicator.

The resin (urushiol) of these plants is a colorless or slightly yellow, light oil. It runs in resin canals just under the surface, from the roots through the stems, into the leaves and flowers, and just under the surface of the fruit. It is not present in the nectar. The leaves of the plants are fragile and easily ruptured by high winds or by humans or animals brushing against them. The oil immediately oozes onto the surface.

The light oil generally is not visible on human skin. On the sole of a shoe, the palm of a hand or glove, or on the surface of an animal's fur, it can be spread by direct contact. On some objects, the oil

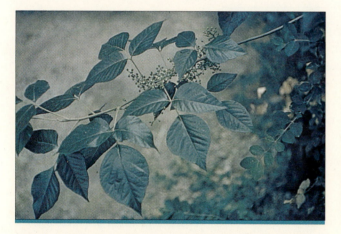

Poison ivy, found in all 48 contiguous U.S. states

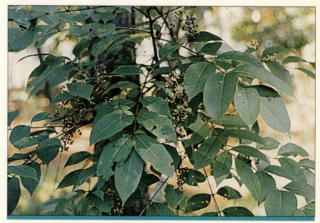

Poison sumac

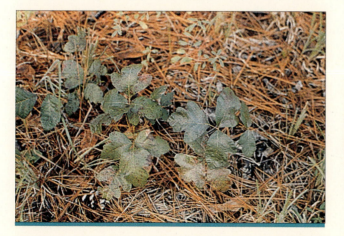

Poison oak

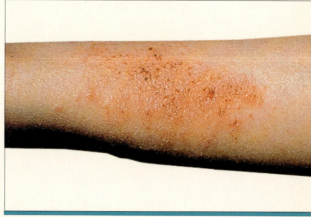

Poison ivy dermatitis

POISON IVY

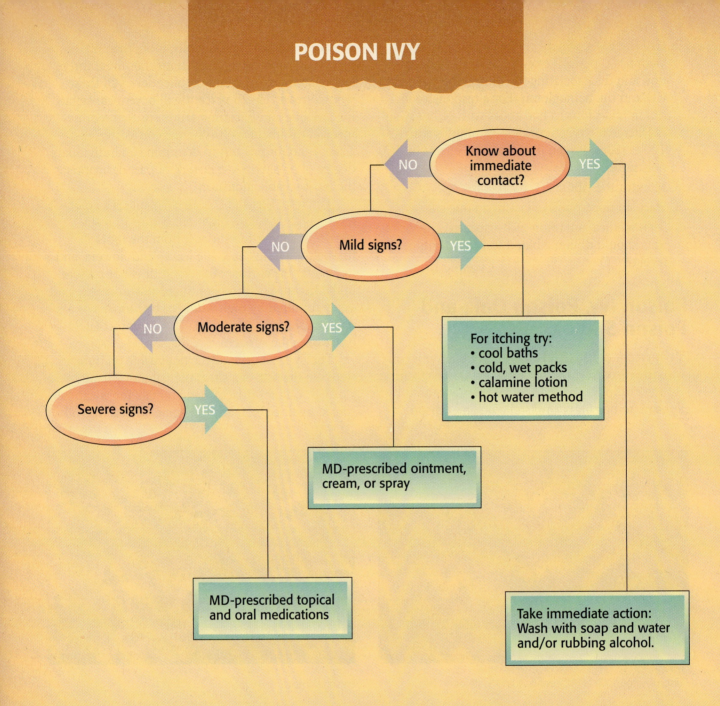

Know about immediate contact?

NO

YES

Mild signs?

NO

YES

Moderate signs?

NO

YES

Severe signs?

YES

For itching try:
• cool baths
• cold, wet packs
• calamine lotion
• hot water method

MD-prescribed ointment, cream, or spray

MD-prescribed topical and oral medications

Take immediate action: Wash with soap and water and/or rubbing alcohol.

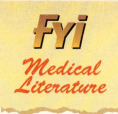

Black-Spot Test Most poison ivy dermatitis victims fail to recognize the plant. Poison ivy and poison oak leaves have three leaflets; poison sumac has 7 to 13 leaflets per leaf. The mature fruit is an off-white berry. These botanical characteristics explain the axioms "Leaflets three, let it be" and "Berries white, poisonous sight!"

The "black-spot test" is another means of identifying these plants. To check a suspicious plant, grasp a leaf with a piece of white paper (do not touch the leaf) and crush it with a rock. The clear sap of poison ivy, poison oak, and poison sumac on the paper will turn dark brown in 10 minutes and turn black in a day.

Source: J. D. Guin, "The Black Spot Test for Recognizing Poison Ivy and Related Species," *Journal of the American Academy of Dermatology* 2:332–333 (February 1980).

---

can stay in an active form for months or years. Smoke from burning plants can produce severe dermatitis. Firefighters and picnickers downwind from a campfire often are affected by airborne oil.

Most people cannot identify these irritating plants. Poison ivy and poison oak are low bushes or climbing vines with waxy, broad, green leaves in the summer that change to a brown-to-red color in the fall. The leaflets of poison ivy and poison oak grow in groups of three (three leaves radiating from a single attachment point), giving rise to the warning "Leaves of three, let them be." Poison ivy flourishes throughout most of the United States, except in Alaska and Hawaii, while poison oak is found in the West in low wooded areas, on mountain slopes, and along trails. Poison sumac is found chiefly in damp, swampy areas in the eastern United States. These plants tend not to grow at elevations above 5,000 feet or in hot, dry deserts. A helpful method of identifying these plants is the "black-spot test." When the sap is exposed to the air, it turns brown in a matter of minutes and by the next day is black.

Allergic people can come in contact with the urushiol of these plants from their clothes or shoes, pet fur, or the smoke from burning plants. Contrary to popular belief, no one can develop a rash by touching the fluid from the blisters (their own or others'), since the fluid does not contain the oily resin. Any apparent spreading is actually a delayed reaction to contact with the resin.

What to Look For

Most people do not realize they have come in contact with a poisonous plant until the rash erupts. Reactions can range from mild to severe:

- mild itching
- mild to moderate itching and redness
- moderate itching, redness, and swelling
- severe itching, redness, swelling, and blisters

Severity is important, but so is the amount of skin affected. The greater the amount of skin affected, the greater the need for medical attention. A day or two is the usual time between contact and the onset of signs and symptoms.

What to Do

1. For those who know they have contacted a poisonous plant, decontaminate the skin as soon as possible (within five minutes for sensitive people, up to one hour for moderately sensitive individuals). (Most victims do not know about their contact until several hours or days later, when the itching and rash begin.) Use soap and water to clean the skin of the oily resin or apply rubbing (isopropyl) alcohol liberally (not in swab-type dabs). If too little isopropyl alcohol is used, the oil will actually be spread to another site and enlarge the injury. Other solvents (e.g., paint thinner, gasoline) can be used, but they are hard on the skin. Rinse with water to remove the solubilized material. Water removes urushiol from the skin, oxidizes and inactivates it, and does not penetrate the skin as do solvents.

2. For the mild stage, have the victim soak in a lukewarm bath sprinkled with one to two cups of colloidal oatmeal (e.g., Aveeno™) (colloidal oatmeal makes a tub slick, so take appropriate precautions) or apply any of the following:
   - wet compresses soaked with Burow's solution (aluminum acetate) for 20–30 minutes three or four times a day
   - calamine lotion (calamine ointment if the skin becomes dry and cracked) or zinc oxide
   - baking soda paste, which is one teaspoon of water mixed with three teaspoons of baking soda

3. For the mild to moderate stage, care for the skin as you would for the mild stage and use a physician-prescribed corticosteroid ointment.

To reduce the likelihood of developing poisonous-plant dermatitis, follow these steps:

- Avoid the plants.
- Wear protective clothing and use appropriate commercial barrier preparations.
- Replenish the barrier protection every four to six hours, if practical.
- Decontaminate after known exposure with liberal amounts of soap and water and then reapply the barrier preparation.
- Decontaminate at the end of the day with isopropyl alcohol and a water rinse.
- Dispose of all contaminated clothing and equipment.

For itching, immerse or run hot water over the area. The water should be hot enough to redden the skin but not burn it. Do not use soap. Heat releases histamine, the substance in the skin's cells that causes severe itching. A hot shower or bath causes intense itching as the histamine is released. That depletes the cells of histamine, and the victim will then get up to eight hours of relief from itching.

CAUTION: DO NOT

- use nonprescription hydrocortisone creams, ointments, and sprays in strengths of 1 percent or less. They offer little benefit.
- use over-the-counter anti-itch lotions like Caladryl™ because they may cause further skin irritation. Oral antihistamines (such as Benadryl™) often are used in conjunction with prescription creams to help decrease itchiness.
- let the victim to rub or scratch the rash or itching skin.

4. For the severe stage, care for the skin as you would for the mild and moderate stages and use a physician-prescribed oral corticosteroid (e.g., prednisone). Apply a topical corticosteroid

ointment or cream, cover it with a transparent plastic wrap, and lightly bind the area with an elastic or self-adhering bandage.

Stinging Nettle

The stinging nettle plant has stinging hairs on its stem and leaves. The stinging hair is a fine, hollow tube with a bladder at its base that contains a chemical irritant. When the stinging hair is touched, a fine needlepoint is formed that penetrates the skin and injects an irritating chemical.

What to Look For

Stinging nettle affects almost all people. Its effects are not an allergic response, as with poison ivy, but rather are due to a direct irritant effect of the plant's sap. The effects are limited to the exposed area, and the response is usually immediate.

Stinging nettle produces some degree of redness, burning, and itching for an hour or more, depending on the area of the body exposed to the plant. For example, the thicker skin on the soles and the palms retards the stinging hairs better than areas of thinner skin, such as the backs of the hands and the arms. Humans vary in sensitivity when the plant actually contacts exposed skin.

The typical response to contact with stinging nettle is a rapid, intense burning sensation at the site of the injection. The area then may itch for an hour or more. Usually, no systemic (whole-body) effects are noted.

What to Do

1. Wash the exposed area with soap and water to remove irritant chemicals.
2. Apply a cold, wet pack to help soothe the painful itching. Other treatments might include a paste of colloidal oatmeal, an over-the-counter hydrocortisone cream (1 percent), or calamine lotion.
3. Take Benadryl, an over-the-counter antihistamine, if desired. Be sure to follow package directions and be aware that it causes drowsiness.

The duration of the stinging nettle reaction is measured in hours rather than days, so little therapy is needed.

BITES AND STINGS

Animal Bites

It is estimated that one of every two Americans will be bitten at some time by an animal* or by another person. Dogs are responsible for about 80 percent of all animal-bite injuries. Of the one million to two million dog bites that occur yearly, 80 percent are trivial or minor, and medical attention is not required or sought, which demonstrates the importance of knowing first aid. The remainder account for about 1 percent of all emergency department and physician office visits. Ten to 20 dog bite–related fatalities occur each year in the United States. Animal bites represent a major, largely unrecognized public health problem.

Two concerns result from an animal bite: immediate tissue damage and later infection from microorganisms. A dog's mouth may carry more than 60 different species of bacteria, some of which are dangerous to humans. Two examples of infection—tetanus and rabies—have been almost eradicated by medical advances, but they still pose a potential problem.

Though less mutilating, cat bites are common, about 400,000 bites annually in the United States. Cat bites have a much higher rate of infection than dog bites. Cats have very sharp teeth, which can create deep puncture wounds and involve muscle, tendon, and bone.

Other pets that are especially likely to bite children include ferrets, which are often unpredictable and can cause severe facial injury to infants. Ferrets sometimes unleash frenzied, rapid-fire bite-and-slash attacks on infants, usually on their heads and throats, and can inflict hundreds of bites.

Besides children, elderly persons and invalids are especially prone to animal bites since they are sometimes unable to detect or prevent a dangerous situation. Many of the animal-related deaths occurred when the victim was left alone with the offending dog, which was a pet. Contrary to popular belief, wild or stray dogs seldom are involved in fatal attacks.

Damage mostly occurs on the hands (48–59 percent of all bites), 16 to 26 percent on the arms, 15 percent on the legs, and 8 to 30 percent on the face. A damaged face presents several problems since it is susceptible to copious bleeding because of the closeness of blood vessels to the skin's surface. Facial disfigurement and scarring can result in emotional trauma. Complete or partial loss of an eye can also happen.

*As it is commonly interpreted, the term *animal bite* in this section refers to a bite by a mammal, not by an insect or reptile.

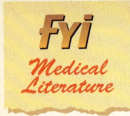

Dog Bites   During the past few years, there has been a rash of news stories about vicious attacks by pit bull terriers. The public hysteria has spurred some communities to such action as outlawing pit bulls.

The Centers for Disease Control undertook a study of fatalities related to dog bites. The researchers found 157 fatalities that occurred in a 10-year period. Pet dogs were responsible for almost 70 percent of fatalities, strays were involved in 27 percent of cases, and police or guard dogs in only 2.8 percent of the deaths. No significant "obvious" seasonal trends were noted, except that strays seemed to be involved more often in the fall, while pets were involved more often in the winter. Seventy percent of the victims were children under 10 years of age, with a "particularly high" death rate noted for infants less than one month old.

Pit bulls were implicated in more than 40 percent of the fatalities, "almost three times more than German shepherds, the next most commonly reported breed." Deaths attributed to pit bulls increased from 20 percent to 62 percent during the period. The researchers concluded that dog bite fatalities had been underestimated and suggest "strong animal control laws, public education regarding dog bites, and more responsible dog ownership."

Source: J. J. Sacks et al., "Dog Bite–Related Fatalities from 1979 through 1988," *Journal of the American Medical Association* 262:1489–1492 (September 15, 1989).

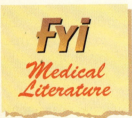

Dog Bites: Which Breeds Are Most Dangerous? Researchers who checked Denver records during a recent year found 178 reports of dog bites to people outside the dog owners' households (this is more common than bites to family members). They also identified 178 nonbiting dogs from the same neighborhoods. Results showed that male dogs (especially unneutered males), German shepherds, and Chow Chows were the most likely to bite outsiders, especially children. Children under age 12 were the victims in 51 percent of cases. Too few pit bulls, Akitas, and collies were involved in this study to rate their risks.

Source: K. A. Gershman et al., *Pediatrics* 93:913 (June 1994).

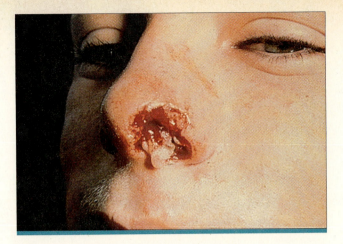

Dog bite

Rabies

Rabies is one of the most ancient and feared of diseases. Although human rabies rarely occurs in the United States or in other industrialized nations, it remains a scourge in developing countries. For example, reliable estimates place the annual number of deaths from rabies in India at 25,000–50,000, in Bangladesh at 2,000, in China at 4,500, and in Pakistan at 6,500.

A virus found in warm-blooded animals causes rabies and spreads from one animal to another in the saliva, usually through a bite or by licking. Bites from animals that are not warm-blooded (e.g., reptiles) do not carry the danger of rabies. (Such bites can become infected, however, and should be washed well and watched for signs of infection.)

Although there have been 12 human rabies infections since 1966 in the United States caused by rabid dogs, the exposures themselves were outside the continental United States.

Table 17-1: Human Deaths Caused by Animals in the United States, 1992	
Species Causing Deaths	**Number of Deaths**
Humans (homicide)	25,488
Farm animals	49
Hornets, wasps, bees	48
Dog bites	13
Venomous snakes, spiders	7
Unspecified venomous animal	13
Unspecified animal	99

Source: National Safety Council, *Accident Facts,* 1995.

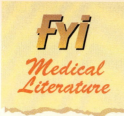

FYI Medical Literature

Rabies Seventeen cases of rabies in the United States were reported to the CDC between 1980 and 1992. Of these, 10 were acquired outside the United States. Worldwide, there are an estimated 25,000 to 50,000 deaths from rabies each year.

The dog is the most common animal carrier of rabies in Asia, Africa, the Indian subcontinent, and Latin America. In the United States, nearly 97 percent of identified rabid animals were raccoons, skunks, bats, and foxes. In Europe, the red fox is the principal host, with rabies also found in deer, cattle, dogs, and cats. England and Hawaii are free of rabies.

Source: R. A. Harrigan and F. Kauffman, *Emergency Medicine Reports* 14(5):37–44 (May 1993).

healthy after 10 days of observation. If an attacking dog or cat is rabid or suspected to be rabid, treatment should be started at once.

Report animal bites to the police or animal control officers; they should be the ones to capture the animal for observation. If the dog or cat escapes and is not suspected to be rabid, consult local public health officials.

If the victim was bitten in the United States by a skunk, raccoon, bat, fox, or other mammal, it should be considered a rabies exposure and treatment started *immediately*. The only exception is when the bite occurred in a part of the continental United States known to be free of rabies. If the wild animal is captured, it should be killed and its head shipped to a qualified laboratory immediately. In developing countries, except for those few areas where rabies does not occur, all attacking animals that elude capture should be considered rabid.

2. Thoroughly cleanse the bite wound with soapy water under pressure *immediately*. For best results, clean the wound with a soap solution, rinse it completely, then irrigate the area with a 1-percent solution of Zephiran™. (Soap neutralizes Zephiran and must be totally rinsed from the wound before irrigation with Zephiran.) For deep wounds, only Zephiran has been found to be effective against the rabies virus. If it is not available, instill 70-percent alcohol (ethanol) (produces extreme pain) or Betadine™ (diluted to 1%) in the wound.

3. Stop the bleeding and give wound care.

CAUTION: DO NOT

- try to capture the animal yourself.
- get near the animal.
- kill the animal unless absolutely necessary. If it must be killed, protect the head and brain from damage so they can be examined for rabies. Transport a dead animal intact to limit exposure to potentially infected tissues or saliva. The animal's remains should be refrigerated to prevent decomposition.
- handle the animal without taking appropriate precautions. Infected saliva may be on the animal's fur, so wear heavy gloves or use a shovel if you have to move a dead animal.

4. Seek medical attention for further wound cleaning and a possible tetanus shot. The physician will determine if sutures are needed to close the wound. If needed, a vaccination against rabies will be started. The old series of 20 painful abdominal injections has been replaced by a five-shot vaccine, which is given in the deltoid muscle of the arm.

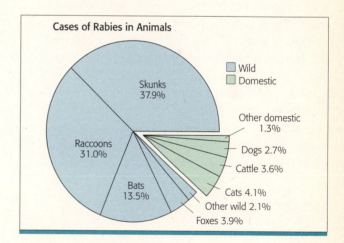

Cases of rabies in animals

Human Bites

After dogs and cats, the animal most likely to bite humans is another human. Human bites can cause severe injury, often more so than other animal bites. The human mouth contains a wide range of bacteria, so the chance of infection is greater from a human bite than from bites of other warm-blooded animals.

Most human bites are inflicted by young persons in a fight, by children at play, by persons in mental institutions, or during sexual assaults. Embarrassment sometimes causes a victim not to seek medical attention immediately, which greatly increases the risk of infection.

Although most human bites occur during acts of violence, about one-fourth are (1) accidental or sports related, (2) sustained by hospital workers trying to restrain children or seizure patients, or (3) self-inflicted during nail chewing or thumb sucking.

Men are more often victims than women, mostly during aggressive altercations, with the peak age being 25. The most common injury location is the hand, sustained on a closed fist as the result of a punch.

Types of Human Bites

There are two types of human bites. **True bites** occur when any part of the body's flesh is caught between teeth, usually deliberately. True bites happen during fights and in cases of abuse. *Note:* Mandatory-reporting laws apply if spousal or child abuse is involved. A "schoolyard bite," with one child biting another, generally is not reportable. Transmission of HIV by a bite has not been documented and is unlikely.

Much worse than a true bite is the **clenched-fist injury,** which results from cutting a fist on teeth. It is associated with a high likelihood of infection. The injury is usually a laceration over the fourth and fifth metacarpal joints. Although clenched-fist injuries usually result from a fight, unintentional injury can happen during sports and play.

What to Do

1. If the wound is not bleeding heavily, wash it with soap and water (under the pressure from a faucet) for 5 to 10 minutes. Avoid scrubbing, which can traumatize tissues.
2. Rinse the wound thoroughly with running water under pressure. Then use an antiseptic solution (diluted Betadine™) to rinse the wound. This helps kill any bacteria.
3. Control bleeding with direct pressure. See page 112 for details.
4. Cover the wound with a sterile dressing. Do *not* close the wound with tape or butterfly bandages.

That traps bacteria in the wound, increasing the chance of infection.

5. Seek medical attention for possible further wound cleaning, a tetanus shot, and sutures applied to close the wound.

Snakebites

Throughout the world, about 50,000 people die each year from snakebites. Each year in the United States, 40,000 to 50,000 people are bitten by snakes, 7,000 to 8,000 of them by venomous snakes. Amazingly, fewer than a dozen Americans die each year from snakebites. Victims who die from snakebites in the United States usually do so in the first 48 hours.

Only four snake species in the United States are poisonous: rattlesnakes (which account for about 65 percent of all venomous snakebites and nearly all the snakebite deaths in the United States), copperheads, water moccasins (also known as cottonmouths), and coral snakes. The first three are pit vipers, which have three characteristics in common:

- triangular, flat heads wider than their necks
- elliptical pupils (i.e., "cat's eyes")
- a heat-sensitive "pit" between the eye and the nostril on each side of the head

The coral snake is small and colorful, with a series of bright red, yellow, and black bands around its body (every other band is yellow). It also has a black snout.

Exotic snakes, whether imported legally or smuggled into the United States and found in zoos, schools, snake farms, and amateur and professional collections, account for at least 15 bites a year.

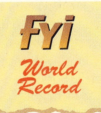

Most Venomous Snake in the U.S. The most venomous snake in the United States is the coral snake. In a standard LD99-100 test, which kills 99–100 percent of all mice injected with the venom, it takes 0.55 grain of venom per 2.2 lbs. of mouse weight injected intravenously. In this test, the smaller the dosage, the more toxic the venom. However, the teeth of the coral snake point back into its mouth; therefore, it cannot inject the venom until it has a firm hold on the victim.

Source: The Guinness Book of Records, New York: Bantam Books, 1995, p. 72.

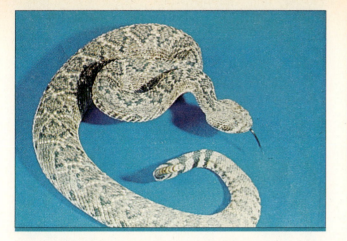

Rattlesnake

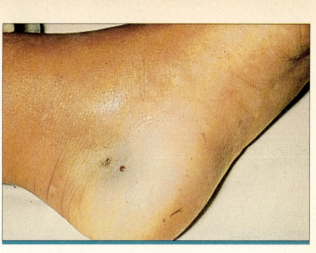

Rattlesnake bite (Note two fang marks)

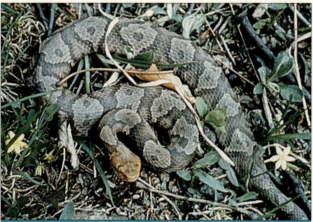

Copperhead snake

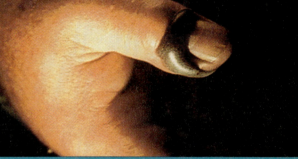

Copperhead bite two hours after bite

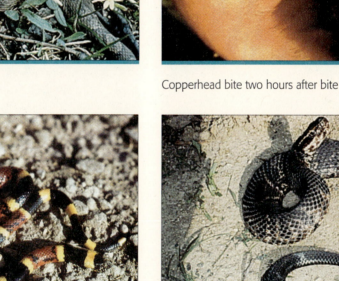

Coral snake, America's most venomous snake

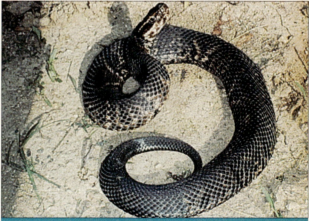

Water moccasin (cottonmouth)

Little information can be found describing the circumstances surrounding snakebites (such as what the victim was doing to get bitten by a rattlesnake). A "legitimate" snakebite is one in which the victim was bitten before the encounter with a snake was recognized or while trying to move away from the snake. They most often involve the lower extremities and are "accidental."

An "illegitimate" snakebite means that, before being bitten, the victim recognized the encounter with a snake but did not attempt to move away from the snake. Most illegitimate bites occur on the

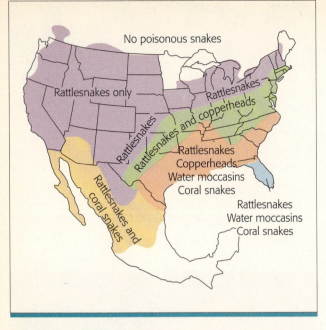

Location of venomous snakes

upper extremities. Most bites of this type happen when the victim tries to kill, capture, play with, or move a snake.

Adult snakes deliver more serious bites because they inject more venom than do young snakes, even though a young snake's venom is two to three times more toxic than an adult's.

Pit Viper Bites

What to Look For

- severe burning pain at the bite site
- two small puncture wounds about one-half inch apart (some cases may have only one fang mark)
- swelling (happens within 5 minutes and can involve an entire extremity)
- discoloration and blood-filled blisters possibly developing in 6 to 10 hours
- in severe cases, nausea, vomiting, sweating, and weakness

In about 25 percent of poisonous snakebites, there is no venom injection, only fang and tooth wounds (known as a "dry" bite).

What to Do

Most snakebites occur within a few hours of a medical facility, where antivenin is available. Bites showing no sign of venom injection require only a possible tetanus shot and care of the bite wounds.

Preventing Snakebites

A 16-percent reduction in bites from rattlesnakes would occur if they were not kept as pets. Researchers suggest that more than one-half of all rattlesnake bites would be eliminated if people simply would attempt to move away from the snake.

Follow these guidelines to prevent snakebites:

- Do not handle venomous snakes.
- Avoid hiking and camping in snake-infested areas and exploring caves, rock crevices, dens, lairs, stone walls, and wood piles.
- Know the outdoor terrain and be alert for snakes in thick foliage.
- Watch where you sit, step, and stretch; do not reach into holes or hidden ledges.
- Wear protective gear such as boots, trousers, long pants, long-sleeved shirts, and gloves when you are in possible snake habitats.
- Take a friend with you; it may save your life.
- Do not alarm a sleeping snake (even a newborn snake) or tease or molest an awake snake.
- Do not keep poisonous snakes as pets; zoos are better qualified to care for them.
- When you are in snake country, carry a Sawyer Extractor device.
- Don't sit on or step over logs until you closely scrutinize the area.
- Don't handle a dead venomous snake. The reflex action of the jaws can still inflict a wound 20 minutes or more after the snake has died.
- Don't surprise or corner a snake. Use a walking stick to prod uncleared ground and make noise so a snake can sense you coming.

Identifying the type of pit viper is of minimal importance, since the same antivenin is used to counteract all North American pit viper venom.

The Wilderness Medical Society lists the following guidelines for dealing with bites by pit vipers.

1. Get the victim and bystanders away from the snake. Snakes have been known to bite more than once. Pit vipers can strike about one-half their body length. Be careful around a decapitated snake head—head reactions can persist for 20 minutes or more.

2. Keep the victim quiet. If possible, carry the victim or have the victim walk very slowly to help.

3. Gently wash the bitten area with soap and water.

4. If you are more than one hour from a medical facility with antivenin or if the snake was large and the victim's skin is swelling rapidly, immediately apply suction with the Extractor™ (from Sawyer Products). It does not require an incision (cutting). If the Extractor is applied within 3 minutes of the bite and left on for 30 minutes, up to 30 percent of the venom can be removed. This procedure is seldom necessary, because most bites happen a relatively short distance from a medical facility.

5. Seek medical attention *immediately*. This is the most important thing to do for the victim. Antivenin must be given *within four hours* of the bite (not every venomous snakebite requires antivenin). Antivenin is found only in hospitals for several reasons: (1) it has a short shelf life; (2) the victim needs to be tested for sensitivity to horse serum (an allergic person will develop anaphylaxis); (3) the minimum dose is 5 to 10 vials for each incident; and (4) it is very expensive, over $100 per vial.

CAUTION: DO NOT

- **apply cold or ice to a snakebite. It does not inactivate the venom and poses a danger of frostbite.**
- **use the "cut-and-suck" procedure— you could damage underlying structures (e.g., blood vessels, nerves)**
- **apply mouth suction. Your mouth is filled with bacteria, increasing the likelihood of wound infection.**
- **apply electric shock. No medical studies support this method.**

Coral Snake Bites

The coral snake is America's most venomous snake, but it rarely bites people. The coral snake has short fangs and tends to hang on and "chew" its venom into the victim rather than to strike and release, like a pit viper. Coral-snake venom is neurotoxic, and symptoms may begin one to five hours after the bite.

What to Do

1. Keep the victim calm.
2. Gently clean the bite site with soap and water.

3. Apply mild pressure by wrapping several elastic bandages (e.g., Ace™ bandage) over the bite site and the entire arm or leg. Applying such pressure is recommended only for bites from elapid (e.g., coral) snakes, not pit vipers. The technique originated in Australia, where it has been very successful. Do *not* cut the victim's skin or use an Extractor.

4. Seek medical attention for antivenin. No deaths have occurred since 1961 with the development of an antivenin.

Nonpoisonous Snakebites

A nonpoisonous snake leaves a horseshoe shape of toothmarks on the victim's skin. If you are not positive about a snake, assume it was venomous. Some so-called nonpoisonous North American snakes (e.g., hognose and garter snakes) have venom that can cause painful local reactions but no systemic (whole-body) symptoms.

What to Do

1. Gently clean the bite site with soap and water.
2. Care for the bite as you would a minor wound.
3. Seek medical advice.

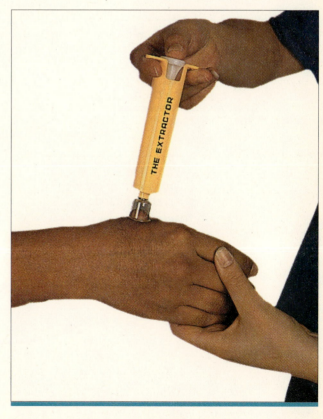

Extractor™ use does not require cutting the skin.

SNAKEBITES

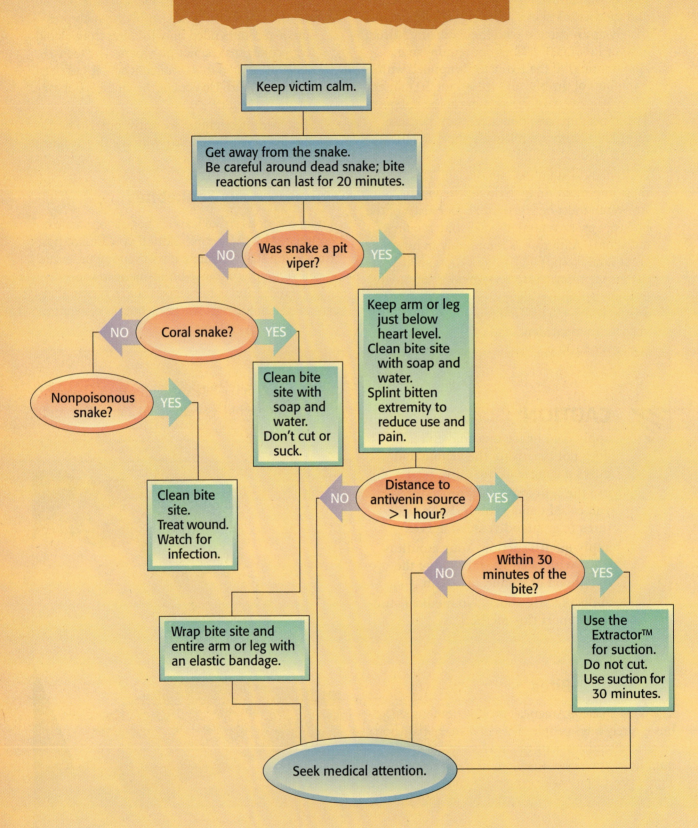

Keep victim calm.

Get away from the snake.
Be careful around dead snake; bite reactions can last for 20 minutes.

Was snake a pit viper? — NO / YES

YES: Keep arm or leg just below heart level. Clean bite site with soap and water. Splint bitten extremity to reduce use and pain.

NO: Coral snake? — NO / YES

Coral snake? YES: Clean bite site with soap and water. Don't cut or suck.

Coral snake? NO: Nonpoisonous snake? — YES

Nonpoisonous snake? YES: Clean bite site. Treat wound. Watch for infection.

Distance to antivenin source > 1 hour? — NO / YES

YES: Within 30 minutes of the bite? — NO / YES

Within 30 minutes YES: Use the Extractor™ for suction. Do not cut. Use suction for 30 minutes.

Wrap bite site and entire arm or leg with an elastic bandage.

Seek medical attention.

Insect Stings

The order of Hymenoptera includes honeybees, bumblebees, yellow jackets, white-faced hornets, yellow-faced hornets, wasps, and fire ants.

Hymenopterans kill between 50 and 100 people in the United States each year. The actual number is probably higher because an unknown number of deaths due to hymenopteran-caused anaphylaxis are mistakenly attributed to cardiac arrest. These insects account for more deaths and illnesses each year than all other venomous animals combined. Severe allergic reactions to insect stings are reported by about 0.5 percent of the population in the United States. Fortunately, localized pain, itching, and swelling—the most common consequences of an insect bite—can be treated with first aid.

Generally, venomous flying insects are aggressive only when threatened or when their hives or nests are disrupted. Under such conditions, they sting, sometimes in swarms. Honeybees and bumblebees have barbed stingers that become embedded in the victim's skin during the sting. After injecting its venom, the bee flies away, but the embedded stinger is torn from the bee's body, causing it to die. Honeybees and bumblebees do not release all their venom during the initial injection; some remains in the stinger left embedded in the victim's skin. If the stinger is not removed properly, additional venom may be released and worsen the victim's reaction.

In contrast, the stingers of wasps and hornets are not barbed and do not become embedded in the victim. Thus, these insects can sting multiple times, and most species (with a few exceptions, such as some yellow jacket species) do not die as a result of the stinging.

Most stings cause only self-limited, local inflammatory reactions consisting of pain, itching, redness, and swelling. These reactions are usually more

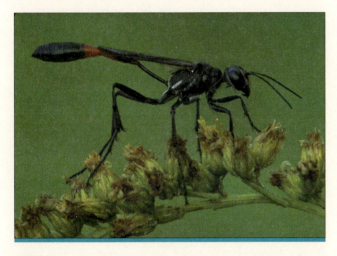

Wasp

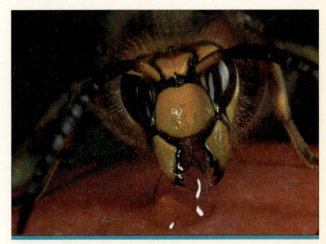

Hornet

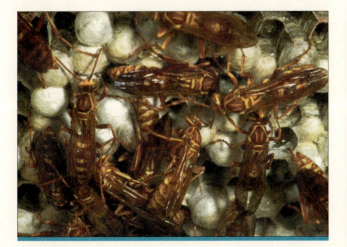

Yellow jacket

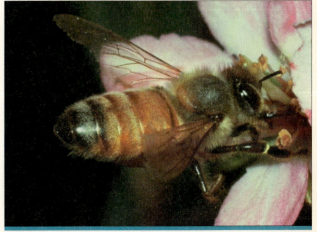

Honeybee

a nuisance than a medical emergency. However, local reactions can be extensive, involving the victim's entire arm. When that occurs, the swelling and redness may peak two to three days after the sting and last a week or longer. Signs and symptoms of life-threatening reactions include nausea, vomiting, bronchospasm, wheezing, fever, or drippy nose. A victim may go into anaphylaxis almost immediately or first progress through a variety of symptoms. Most people who have anaphylactic reactions have no history of them. In a study of 400 fatal bee stings, only 15 percent of the victims had a known sensitivity.

Reactions generally happen within a few minutes to one hour after the sting. Bee-sting victims who have anaphylactic reactions develop throat swelling and bronchospasm, which are manifested by difficulty in speaking, tightness in the throat or chest, wheezing, shortness of breath, and chest pain. Respiratory-tract obstruction accounts for the majority of deaths among victims of flying-insect stings (hymenoptera).

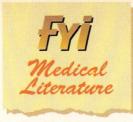

Honeybee Venom Delivery Envenomation by a honeybee is initiated by the insertion of the stinging apparatus or stinger into the victim's skin. Researchers found that at least 90 percent of the venom sac contents were delivered within 20 seconds of the initiation of the sting and that venom delivery was completed within one minute. This suggests that a bee stinger must be removed within a few seconds to prevent anaphylaxis in an allergic person.

Source: M. J. Schumacher et al., "Rate and Quantity of Delivery of Venom from Honeybee Stings," *Journal of Allergy and Clinical Immunology* 92:831–835 (April 1994).

For the severely allergic person, a single sting may be fatal within minutes. And although accounts exist of individuals who have survived some 2,000 stings at one time, 500 stings will usually kill even those people who are not allergic to stinging insects.

Massive multiple stings are rare. Such a case might happen if a person stumbled into a hive, or if a truck carrying a load of hives crashed. With the slow migration of Africanized bees (so-called "killer bees") from South and Central America into the United States, the number of multiple-sting cases is likely to increase. The venom of the Africanized bee is no more potent than that of the European type; it is just that the African type is extremely aggressive and thus more likely to be involved in multiple stings. A number of child deaths have resulted from the multiple stings of fire ants, which are common in the southeastern United States.

What to Look For

A rule of thumb is that the sooner symptoms develop after a sting, the more serious the reaction will be.

- Usual reactions are momentary pain, redness around the sting site, itching, and heat.
- Worrisome reactions include skin flush, hives, localized swelling of lips or tongue, a "tickle" in the throat, wheezing, abdominal cramps, and diarrhea.

Preventing Insect Stings

People who know they are allergic to insect stings need to exercise extra care to avoid being stung. They should carry a bee-sting kit and follow these guidelines:

- Wear long pants and long-sleeved shirts.
- Insects are attracted to bright colors and floral patterns. Wear white, green, tan, and khaki—the least attractive colors to insects.
- Wear shoes outdoors.
- Avoid yardwork and other activities where insect contact is frequent.
- Keep garbage cans away from the house.
- Remove insect-attracting plants from inside and the immediate proximity of the house.
- Do not use scented soaps, lotions, or perfumes.
- Keep car windows closed.
- If you are confronted by an insect, avoid quick movements and do not provoke it. Turn away, lower your face, and walk away slowly. Do not run about wildly or move erratically when bees are nearby.
- Do not eat when bees are nearby.
- Have insect nests around the house removed by professional exterminators.

- Life-threatening reactions are bluish or grayish skin color, seizures, unconsciousness, and an inability to breathe due to swelling of the vocal cords.

About 60–80 percent of anaphylactic deaths are caused by the victim's not being able to breathe because swollen airway passages obstruct airflow to the lungs. The second most common cause of death is shock, caused by insufficient blood circulating through the body.

One of the difficulties in dealing with stings is the lack of uniformity in victims' responses. One sting is not necessarily equivalent to another, even within the same species, because the amount of venom injected varies from sting to sting.

A person who goes into anaphylactic shock after being stung by a hornet may respond to a bee sting with only a small amount of swelling. One person may have a local reaction involving an entire limb, while the more typical response is a small circle of redness and swelling that disappears without incident in a few days. In beekeepers, for whom stings are an accepted occupational hazard, the response is likely to be even less than in most other people, because they have become tolerant to the toxins in the venom from having been stung many times on different occasions. There seems to be no easy way to predict how a person may react. Most people who get stung, however, do have local reactions: redness, swelling, and pain.

Stings to the mouth or eye tend to be more dangerous than stings to other body areas. Also, victims tend to react more severely to multiple stings, especially 10 or more.

The most dangerous single stings in nonallergic individuals are those inside the throat, which can result from swallowing an insect that has dropped into a soft drink can or from inhaling one that flies into the victim's open mouth. A sting in the mouth or throat can cause swelling that obstructs the airway even in a person who is not allergic to insect stings. If the sting is not life threatening, have the victim suck on ice or flush his or her mouth with cold water. For a bee sting, dissolve a teaspoon of baking soda in a glass of water. Have the victim rinse his or her mouth and then hold the water in the mouth for several minutes.

What to Do

Most people who have been stung can be treated on site, but everyone should know what to do if a life-threatening allergic reaction (anaphylaxis) occurs. In particular, those who have had a severe reaction to an insect sting should be instructed on what they can do to protect themselves. They also should be advised to wear a medical-alert identification tag identifying them as insect allergic.

1. Look at the sting site for a stinger embedded in the skin. Bees are the only stinging insects that leave their stingers behind. If the stinger is still embedded, remove it or it will continue to inject poison for two or three minutes. Scrape the

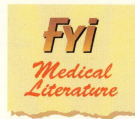

Doctors Not Giving Aftercare Instructions to Sting Anaphylaxis Victims A survey of 124 emergency department or urgent care center physicians found that 58 percent of them never provided written avoidance instructions to those suffering anaphylaxis from an insect sting. Twenty-four percent provided or prescribed medical-alert identification bracelets, 44 percent referred all their patients to an allergist for further evaluation, and 73 percent reported prescribing an Epi-pen or Ana-kit to all hymenoptera sting anaphylaxis victims. Twenty-four percent of physicians did not know where to obtain anaphylaxis identification bracelets. This survey demonstrated that a substantial number of physicians practicing emergency medicine are not providing appropriate aftercare instructions to patients.

Source: L. McDougle et al., "Management of Hymenoptera Sting Anaphylaxis," *Journal of Emergency Medicine* 13(1):9–13 (January 1995).

CAUTION: DO NOT

- pull the stinger with tweezers or your fingers because you may squeeze more venom into the victim from the venom sac. Bee stingers can continue to secrete poison for up to 20 minutes, and squeezing the wound may inject more venom.

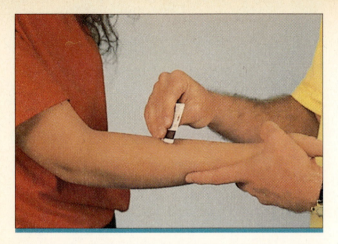

Scraping stinger away with credit card

stinger and venom sac away with a hard object such as a long fingernail, credit card, scissor edge, or knife blade. If applied in the first three minutes, a Sawyer Extractor can remove a portion of the venom.

2. Wash the sting site with soap and water to prevent infection.

3. Apply an ice pack over the sting site to slow absorption of the venom and relieve pain. Use a commercial "sting stick" containing a topical anesthetic like xylocaine (unless the victim is known to be allergic to the drug). Because bee venom is acidic, a paste made of baking soda and water can help. Sodium bicarbonate is an alkalinizing agent that draws out fluid and reduces itching and swelling. Wasp venom, on the other hand, is alkaline, so apply vinegar or lemon juice.

   A paste made of unseasoned meat tenderizer can help a bee sting victim if it comes in direct contact with the venom. That generally is not possible, however, because the bee will have injected the venom through too small a hole and too deeply into the victim's skin.

4. To further relieve pain and itching, some type of analgesic (e.g., aspirin, acetaminophen) usually is adequate. A topical steroid cream, such as hydrocortisone, can help combat local swelling and itching. An antihistamine may prevent some local symptoms if given early, but it works too slowly to counteract a life-threatening allergic reaction.

5. Observe the victim for at least 30 minutes for signs of an allergic reaction. For a person having a severe allergic reaction, a dose of epineph-rine is the only effective treatment. A person with a known allergy to insect stings should have a physician-prescribed emergency kit that includes prefilled syringes of epinephrine or a spring-loaded device that automatically injects epinephrine. (The spring-loaded device is useful for those reluctant to use a syringe with a visible needle.) The allergic person should take along the kit whenever he or she is going someplace where stinging insects are known to exist. (Appendix B describes these kits in more detail.) Because epinephrine is short-acting, watch the victim closely for signs of returning anaphylaxis. Inject another dose of epinephrine as often as every 15 minutes if needed.

Do *not* use epinephrine to treat a sting unless the victim has a severe allergic reaction. Epinephrine has a shelf life of one to three years, or until it has turned brown.

Watch for signs and symptoms of a delayed allergic reaction, especially in the first 6 to 24 hours. If the victim develops difficulty in breathing, facial swelling, fever, chills, or dizziness, call the local emergency telephone number.

Spider Bites

Most spiders are venomous, which is how they paralyze and kill their prey, but lack an effective delivery system—long fangs and strong jaws to bite a human. About 60 species of spiders in North America have been implicated in human bites of medical importance, although only 15 species or so have produced significant poisonings. Most bites are by female spiders. Male spiders almost always are smaller than females and have fangs that are too short and fragile to bite humans. Death occurs rarely and only from bites by brown recluse and black widow spiders.

The number of deaths from spider bites is not accurately known. A spider bite is difficult to diagnose, especially when the spider was not seen or recovered, because the bites typically cause little immediate pain. In a study of 600 suspected spider bites, 80 percent were caused by other arthropods (e.g., kissing bugs, ticks, fleas, mites, bedbugs) and 10 percent by other disease states (e.g., poison ivy, diabetic ulcer, bedsore, Lyme disease, gonococcus). Spiders rarely bite more than once, and they do not always release venom.

INSECT STINGS
(Flying Insects)

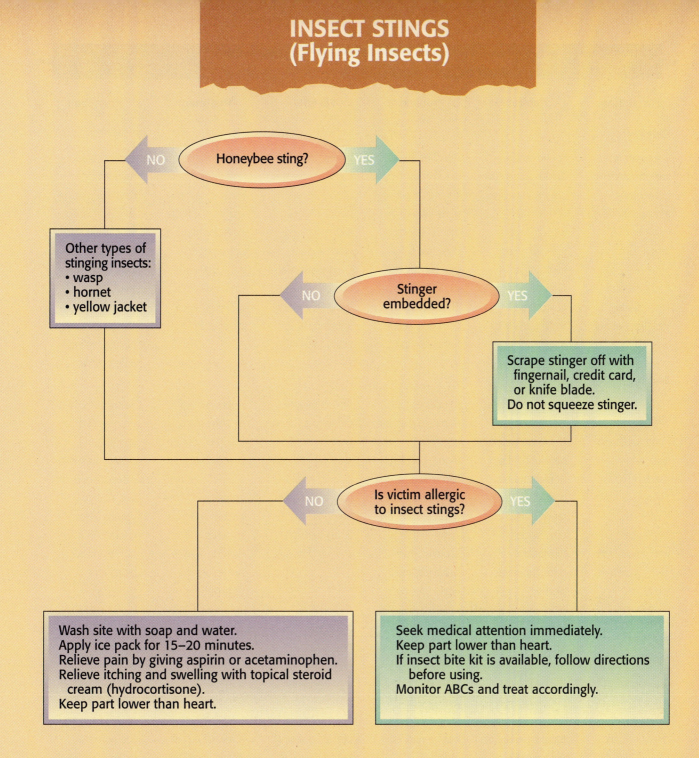

Honeybee sting?

NO → Other types of stinging insects:
• wasp
• hornet
• yellow jacket

YES →

Stinger embedded?

YES → Scrape stinger off with fingernail, credit card, or knife blade.
Do not squeeze stinger.

NO →

Is victim allergic to insect stings?

NO → Wash site with soap and water.
Apply ice pack for 15–20 minutes.
Relieve pain by giving aspirin or acetaminophen.
Relieve itching and swelling with topical steroid cream (hydrocortisone).
Keep part lower than heart.

YES → Seek medical attention immediately.
Keep part lower than heart.
If insect bite kit is available, follow directions before using.
Monitor ABCs and treat accordingly.

Table 17-2: Facts About Troublesome Insects

Description	Habitat	Problem	Severity	Treatment	Protection
Chigger Oval with red velvety covering. Sometimes almost colorless. Larva has six legs. Harmless adult has eight and resembles a small spider. Very tiny—about $\frac{1}{20}$-inch long.	Found in low damp places covered with vegetation: shaded woods, high grass or weeds, fruit orchards. Also lawns and golf courses. From Canada to Argentina.	Attaches itself to the skin by inserting mouthparts into a hair follicle. Injects a digestive fluid that causes cells to disintegrate. Then feeds on cell parts. It does not suck blood.	Itching from secreted enzymes results several hours after contact. Small red welts appear. Secondary infection often follows. Degree of irritation varies with individuals.	Lather with soap and rinse several times to remove chiggers. If welts have formed, dab antiseptic on area. Severe lesions may require antihistamine ointment.	Apply proper repellent to clothing, particularly near uncovered areas such as wrists and ankles. Apply to skin. Spray or dust infested areas (lawns, plants) with suitable chemicals.
Bedbug Flat oval body with short broad head and six legs. Adult is reddish brown. Young are yellowish white. Unpleasant pungent odor. From $\frac{1}{8}$- to $\frac{1}{4}$-inch in length.	Hides in crevices, mattresses, under loose wallpaper during day. At night travels considerable distance to find victims. Widely distributed throughout the world.	Punctures the skin with piercing organs and sucks blood. Local inflammation and welts result from anticoagulant enzyme that bug secretes from salivary glands while feeding.	Affects people differently. Some have marked swelling and considerable irritation; others aren't bothered. Sometimes transmits serious diseases.	Apply antiseptic to prevent possible infection. Bug usually bites sleeping victim, gorges itself completely in 3 to 5 minutes and departs. It's rarely necessary to remove one.	Spray beds, mattresses, bed springs, and baseboards with insecticide. Bugs live in large groups. They migrate to new homes on water pipes and clothing.
Brown Recluse Spider Oval body with eight legs. Light yellow to medium dark brown. Has distinctive mark shaped like a fiddle on its back. Body from $\frac{3}{8}$- to $\frac{1}{2}$-inch long, $\frac{1}{4}$-inch wide, $\frac{3}{4}$-inch from toe-to-toe.	Prefers dark places where it's seldom disturbed. Outdoors: old trash piles, debris, and rough ground. Indoors: attics, storerooms, closets. Found in southern and midwestern United States.	Bites produce an almost painless sting that may not be noticed, at first. Shy, it bites only when annoyed or surprised. Left alone, it won't bite. Victim rarely sees the spider.	In 2 to 8 hours pain may be noticed, followed by blisters, swelling, hemorrhage, or ulceration. Some people experience rash, nausea, jaundice, chills, fever, cramps, or joint pain.	Summon doctor. Bite may require hospitalization for a few days. Full healing may take from 6 to 8 weeks. Weak adults and children have been known to die.	Use caution when cleaning secluded areas in the home or using machinery usually left idle. Check firewood, inside shoes, packed clothing and bedrolls—frequent hideaways.

Table 17-2: Facts About Troublesome Insects (continued)

Description	Habitat	Problem	Severity	Treatment	Protection
Black Widow Spider Color varies from dark brown to glossy black. Densely covered with short microscopic hairs. Red or yellow hourglass marking on the underside of the female's abdomen. Male does not have this mark and is not poisonous. Overall length with legs extended is 1½ inch. Body is ¼-inch wide.	Found with eggs and web. Outside: in vacant rodent holes, under stones, logs, in long grass, hollow stumps, and brush piles. Inside: in dark corners of barns, garages, piles of stone, wood. Most bites occur in outhouses. Found in southern Canada, throughout United States, except Alaska.	Bites cause local redness. Two tiny red spots may appear. Pain follows almost immediately. Larger muscles become rigid. Body temperature rises slightly. Profuse perspiration and tendency toward nausea follow. It's usually difficult to breathe or talk. May cause constipation, urine retention.	Venom is more dangerous than a rattlesnake's but is given in much smaller amounts. About 5% of bite cases result in death. Death is from asphyxiation due to respiratory paralysis. More dangerous for children; to adults its worst feature is pain. Convulsions result in some cases.	Use an antiseptic such as alcohol on the bitten area to prevent secondary infection. Keep victim quiet and call a doctor. Do not treat as you would a snakebite since this will only increase the pain and chance of infection; bleeding will not remove the venom.	Wear gloves when working in areas where there might be spiders. Destroy any egg sacs you find. Spray insecticide in any area where spiders are usually found, especially under privy seats. Check them out regularly. General cleanliness, paint, and light discourage spiders.
Tick Oval with small head; the body is not divided into definite segments. Gray or brown. Measures from ¼ to ¾ inch when mature.	Found in all United States areas and in parts of southern Canada, on low shrubs, grass, and trees. Carried around by both wild and domestic animals.	Attaches itself to the skin and sucks blood. After removal there is danger of infection, especially if the mouthparts are left in the wound.	Sometimes carries and spreads Rocky Mountain spotted fever. Lyme disease, Colorado tick fever. In a few rare cases, causes paralysis until removed.	Gently remove with tweezers so none of the mouthparts are left in skin. Wash with soap and water; apply antiseptic.	Cover exposed parts of body when in tick-infested areas. Use proper repellent. Remove ticks attached to clothes, body. Check neck and hair. Bathe.
Mosquito Small dark fragile body with transparent wings and elongated mouthparts. From ⅛- to ¼-inch long.	Found in temperate climates throughout the world where the water necessary for breeding is available.	Bites and sucks blood. Itching and localized swelling result. Bite may turn red. Only the female is equipped to bite.	Sometimes transmits yellow fever, malaria, encephalitis, and other diseases. Scratching can cause secondary infections.	Don't scratch. Lather with soap and rinse to avoid infection. Apply antiseptic to relieve itching.	Destroy available breeding water to check multiplication. Place nets on windows and beds. Use proper repellent.

Table 17-2: Facts About Troublesome Insects (continued)

Description	Habitat	Problem	Severity	Treatment	Protection
Scorpion					
Crablike appearance with clawlike pincers. Fleshy post-abdomen or "tail" has five segments, ending in a bulbous sac and stinger. Two poisonous types: solid straw yellow or yellow with irregular black stripes on back. From 2½ to 4 inches long.	Spends days under loose stones, bark, boards, floors of outhouses. Burrows in the sand. Roams freely at night. Crawls under doors into homes. Lethal types are found only in the warm desert-like climate of Arizona and adjacent areas.	Stings by thrusting its tail forward over its head. Swelling or discoloration of the area indicates a nondangerous, though painful, sting. A dangerously toxic sting doesn't change the appearance of the area, which does become hypersensitive.	Excessive salivation and facial contortions may follow. Temperature rises to over 104°F. Tongue becomes sluggish. Convulsions, in waves of increasing intensity, may lead to death from nervous exhaustion. First 3 hours most critical.	Apply ice pack. Keep victim quiet and call a doctor immediately. Do not cut the skin or give painkillers. They increase the killing power of the venom. Antitoxin, readily available to doctors, has proved to be very effective.	Apply a petroleum distillate to any dwelling places that cannot be destroyed. Cats are considered effective predators, as are ducks and chickens, though the latter are more likely to be stung and killed. Don't go barefoot at night.
Bee					
Winged body with yellow and black stripes. Covered with branched or feathery hairs. Makes a buzzing sound. Different species vary from ½ to 1 inch in length.	Lives in aerial or underground nests or hives. Widely distributed throughout the world wherever there are flowering plants—from the polar regions to the equator.	Stings with tail when annoyed. Burning and itching with localized swelling occur. Usually leaves venom sac in victim. It takes between 2 and 3 minutes to inject all the venom.	If a person is allergic, more serious reactions occur—nausea, shock, unconsciousness. Swelling may occur in another part of the body. Death may result.	Gently scrape (don't pluck) the stinger so venom sac won't be squeezed. Wash with soap and antiseptic. If swelling occurs, contact doctor. Apply ice pack.	Have exterminator destroy nests and hives. Avoid wearing sweet fragrances and bright clothing. Keep food covered. Move slowly or stand still in the vicinity of bees.
Tarantula					
Large dark "spider" with a furry covering. From 6 to 7 inches in toe-to-toe diameter.	Found in southwestern United States. The tropical varieties are poisonous.	Bites produce pinprick sensation with negligible effect. It will not bite unless teased.	Usually no more dangerous than a pinprick. Has only local effects.	Wash and apply antiseptic to prevent the possibility of secondary infection.	Harmless to man, the tarantula is beneficial since it destroys harmful insects.

Source: National Safety Council, *Family Safety,* Spring 1980, pp. 20–21.

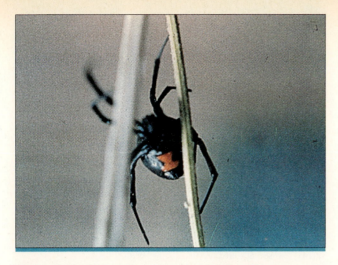

Black widow spider. Note red hourglass configuration on abdomen.

Black Widow Spiders

Black widow spiders are also commonly known as brown widow spiders and red-legged spiders, depending on the species. The term *black widow* is actually inaccurate, because only three of the five species of widow spider are actually black, the others being brown and gray. Newly hatched spiders are almost entirely red. Males have white stripes along the outside of the abdomen.

The female black widow spider is one of the largest spiders, with a body that ranges up to one-half inch in length and a leg span of up to two inches. It is precisely her large size that allows the female black widow's fangs to be large and strong enough to penetrate human skin. The female black widow may live as long as three years. Black widow spiders have round abdomens that vary in color from gray to brown to black, depending on the species. In the female black widow, the abdomen is shiny black with a red or yellow spot (often in the shape of an hourglass) or white spots or bands.

The male is only one-third the size of the female. Contrary to popular myth, the male usually mates safely with the female. Because of his small size, the male's fangs are incapable of penetrating human skin, so bites are from the female. Black widow spiders produce one of the most potent venoms known in terms of volume. The venom is chiefly a neurotoxin in humans, with symptoms most often manifested as severe muscle pain and cramping.

Black widow spiders are found throughout the world. In the western hemisphere, these spiders are found from southern Canada, throughout every state in the continental United States, to the tip of South America, and in Hawaii.

The web of the black widow spider is an extensive, irregular, shaggy trap for the insects she normally eats. The black widow rarely leaves the web and stays close to her egg mass. She aggressively defends the egg mass and bites if it is disturbed. When she is not guarding eggs, the spider often attempts to escape rather than bite.

Frequent cleaning to remove spiders and their webs from buildings, outbuildings, and outdoor living areas decreases the chance of accidental contact with black widow spiders. Insecticides may decrease the population of the food for the black widows but do not usually affect the spiders themselves.

What to Look For

If the spider is trapped against the skin or crushed, it will bite. It is difficult to determine if a person has been bitten by a black widow spider or, for that matter, by any spider.

- The victim may feel a sharp pinprick when the spider bites, but some victims are not even aware of the bite. Within 15 minutes, a dull, numbing pain develops in the bite area.
- Two small fang marks might be seen as tiny red spots.
- Within 15 minutes to 4 hours, muscle stiffness and cramps occur, usually affecting the abdomen when the bite is on a lower part of the body and the shoulders, back, or chest when the bite is on an upper part. Victims often describe the pain as the most severe they have ever experienced.
- Headache, chills, fever, heavy sweating, dizziness, nausea, and vomiting appear next. Severe pain around the bite site peaks in 2 to 3 hours and can last 12 to 48 hours.

Brown Recluse Spiders

Brown recluse spiders are also known in North America as fiddle-back, violin, and brown spiders. They have a violin-shaped figure on their backs (several other spider species have a similar configuration on their backs). Color varies from fawn to dark brown, with darker legs. Both male and female spiders are venomous.

Brown recluse spiders are found primarily in the southern and midwestern states, with other less toxic related spiders throughout the rest of the country. They are absent from the Pacific Northwest.

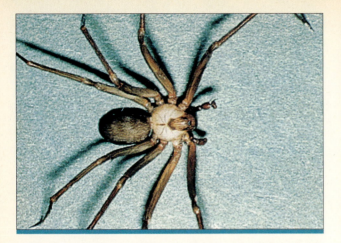

Brown recluse spider. Note violin or fiddle configuration on back.

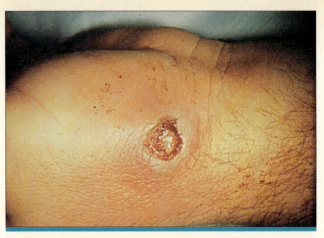

Brown recluse spider bite. Note bull's-eye approach.

What to Look For

The brown recluse spider bites only when it is trapped against the skin.

- A local reaction is usually manifested within two to eight hours by mild to severe pain at the bite site and the development of redness, swelling, and local itching.
- In 48 to 72 hours, a blister develops at the bite site, becomes red, and bursts. During the early stages, the affected area often takes on a bull's-eye appearance, with a central white area surrounded by a reddened area, ringed by a whitish or blue border. A small, red crater remains, over which a scab forms. When that scab falls away in a few days, a still larger crater remains. That too scabs over and falls off, leaving a yet larger crater. The craters are known as *volcano lesions*. This process of slow tissue destruction can continue for weeks or even months. The ulcer sometimes requires skin grafting.
- Fever, weakness, vomiting, joint pain, and a rash may occur.
- Stomach cramps, nausea, and vomiting may occur. Death is rare.

Tarantulas

Tarantulas bite only when vigorously provoked or roughly handled. The bite varies from almost painless to a deep throbbing pain lasting up to one hour. The tarantula, when upset, will roughly scratch the lower surface of its abdomen with its legs and flick hairs onto the invader's skin. The hairs cause itching and hives that can last several weeks. Treatment is cortisone cream and antihistamines.

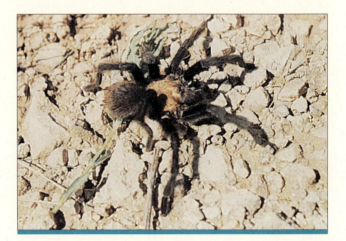

Tarantula

Common Aggressive House Spider

Another biter is the common aggressive house spider, or hobo spider. It arrived in the Pacific Northwest in 1936 and slowly made its way across Washington state and into surrounding states. In those areas, the hobo spider is the most common large spider. The signs and symptoms of its bite are similar to those of the brown recluse.

What to Do (for All Spider Bites)

1. If possible, catch the spider to confirm its identity. Even if the body has been crushed, save it for identification (although most spider-bite victims never see the spider). The species helps determine the treatment, so the dead spider (if it can be found) should be taken with the victim to the hospital.
2. Clean the bite area with soap and water or rubbing alcohol.

3. Place an ice pack over the bite to relieve pain and delay the effects of the venom.

4. Monitor the ABCs.

5. Seek medical attention immediately. For black widow spider bites, an antivenin exists. It is usually reserved for children (under 6 years), the elderly (over 60 and with high blood pressure), pregnant women, and victims with severe reactions. The antivenin will give relief within one to three hours. Antivenin for brown recluse and other spider bites is not currently available.

Scorpion Stings

Scorpions look like miniature lobsters, with lobster-like pincers and a long upcurved "tail" with a poisonous stinger. Several species of scorpions inhabit the southwestern United States, but only the bark scorpion poses a threat to humans. Severe cases, which usually appear only in children, may include paralysis, spasms, or breathing difficulties. Death from scorpion stings in the United States is rare.

The bark scorpion is found in the desert Southwest. There are rare colonies on the north side of the Colorado River in Nevada and Utah and occasional colonies in New Mexico. Rare stings have been reported in other parts of the United States, after the scorpions traveled from Arizona as "hitchhikers" in luggage or in car trunks. The bark scorpion is pale tan in color and is ¾ to 1¼ inches long, not including the so-called tail.

Stings to adult victims usually are not life threatening. Stings to small children, however, often are dangerous. When a child is stung, every effort should be made to get the victim to a medical facility as quickly as possible. Pay close attention to making sure the victim's airway is open and that he or she is breathing.

What to Look For

The most frequent symptom of a scorpion sting, especially to an adult victim, is local, immediate pain and burning around the sting site. Later, numbness or tingling occurs. There is no swelling or blanching. Tapping a finger over the sting site may cause pain (the "tap test") and may serve to indicate a scorpion sting. More severely affected individuals will experience pain along the stung arm or leg, even paralysis. In even more serious stings, uncontrolled jerking movements of the legs or arms and facial twitching may occur.

Victims with a severe reaction will have a fast heart rate, will salivate, and will experience breathing distress. Symptoms begin from within minutes to half an hour and reach their height within the first few hours. Symptoms usually last from 6 to 24 hours.

What to Do

1. Monitor the ABCs.

2. Gently clean the sting site with soap and water or rubbing alcohol.

3. Apply an ice pack over the sting site.

4. Seek medical attention. Small children are prime candidates for receiving antivenin. An antivenin, supplied by the Antibody Production Laboratory at Arizona State University, is available at most hospitals in Arizona. This product has been approved by the Arizona Board of Pharmacy but has never been tested by the U.S. Food and Drug Administration. Therefore, transportation of the antivenin across state lines is illegal, and it is not available outside Arizona. Antivenin should be given only in a hospital emergency department or intensive care unit, because anaphylaxis is a potential complication.

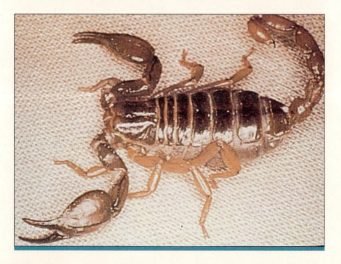

Scorpion

Centipede Bites

Centipedes come in various sizes and colors and are found all over the United States and throughout the world. The giant desert centipede, which can be up to eight inches in length, is the only U.S. centipede that is dangerous to humans.

SPIDER BITES AND SCORPION STINGS

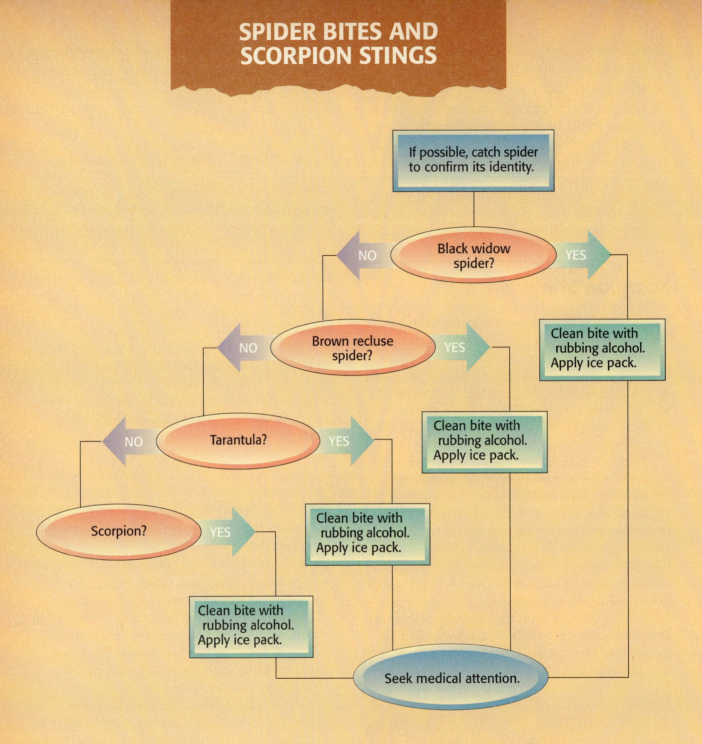

Like spiders, any centipede whose fangs can penetrate human skin can inject venom. These arthropods inject toxic substances into the skin from a pair of hollow jaws that act like fangs. Contrary to popular belief, centipedes do not inject venom with their feet. Exaggerated stories about the deadly effects of their bites and reports that the tip of each leg carries a poisonous spur have caused many people to have an unreasonable fear of centipedes. Their venom is relatively weak.

What to Look For

Generally, bite indications are burning pain and local inflammation of the wound site, with mild swelling of the lymph nodes. The bite of the giant desert centipede causes inflammation, swelling, and redness that last 4 to 12 hours. Swelling and tenderness may last as long as three weeks or may disappear and recur.

What to Do

1. Clean the wound with soap and water.
2. Apply an ice pack at the bite site.
3. Give an analgesic for pain: aspirin, acetaminophen, or ibuprofen.
4. Seek medical attention for inflamed lymph glands.

Centipedes, which have one pair of legs per body segment, are sometimes confused with millipedes, which have two pairs of legs per body segment. Millipedes cannot inject venom, but their secretions can irritate the skin. Treat by washing the area of contact with soap and water and applying a cortisone cream or ointment.

Mosquitoes

Millions of people are bitten by mosquitoes. Mosquitoes not only are a nuisance, they also are the carriers of many diseases. In developing countries, mosquitoes transmit malaria, yellow fever, and dengue fever; in the United States, they carry encephalitis. There is no evidence that mosquitoes transmit HIV, the virus that causes AIDS.

Female mosquitoes need blood to lay their eggs. Because they breed in water, mosquitoes are most often found in marshes, wetlands, and wooded areas. Mosquitoes usually can be separated into daytime and nighttime biters, but most will bite at twilight.

Preventing Mosquito Bites

To minimize being bitten by mosquitoes, follow these guidelines:

- Wear protective clothing: pants, long-sleeved shirt, full-brimmed hat. Mosquito netting draped over a hat will protect the face and neck.
- Use insect repellents on exposed skin. DEET-containing repellents are most effective against mosquitoes and to a lesser extent helpful in repelling ticks and black flies.

DEET is considered to have low toxicity. However, it is absorbed through the skin, and hives, skin rashes, and blisters can result when it is used for prolonged periods or in excessive amounts. The new long-acting 35-percent solution has a polymer that prevents evaporation as well as skin absorption.

Products that contain 100 percent DEET are available but unnecessary, especially in children. Long-acting formulations of 35-percent DEET appear equally effective in protecting against mosquitoes and have far less potential for toxicity.

DEET products can be applied over other creams such as sunscreens and moisturizers. Use DEET only on exposed skin and avoid the hands of young children since children often put their hands in their mouths. Keep DEET out of the reach of small children since ingestion may be fatal. Children under the age of 5 should not be exposed to concentrations greater than 10 percent, according to the American Academy of Pediatrics. For others, the amount should not exceed 30 percent.

Other, nontoxic insect repellents appear to be less effective than DEET. They may be only 25 percent as effective as DEET and are likely to require reapplication every half hour. Mixed opinions exist about taking 100 mg of vitamin B1 (thiamine) daily for one week prior to being exposed as an effective preventative agent. Some experts believe that a diet high in garlic will render a person undesirable to a mosquito.

Permethrin is a pesticide, not a repellent. It should be applied to clothing and not the skin.

What to Do

1. Wash the bitten area with soap and water.
2. Apply an ice pack.
3. Apply calamine lotion to decrease redness and itching.

4. For a victim suffering a number of bites or a delayed allergic reaction, an antihistamine (Benadryl) every six hours or a physician-prescribed cortisone may prove useful.

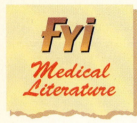

Mosquito Bites   In tropical climates, mosquitoes are important carriers of infectious diseases such as malaria and yellow fever. Mosquito bites can also, by themselves, provoke unpleasant skin lesions. In many areas of the world, massive and disturbing mosquito infestations may occur. For example, in Alaska it is possible to be bitten by mosquitoes as many as 1,000 times in one hour. Under such conditions, complete avoidance of bites is impossible without use of effective repellents and protective clothing. Topical treatment with over-the-counter sticks, creams, and lotions containing antihistamines, hydrocortisone, or other antipruritic agents is common. However, only a few studies have been made on the effects of these products.

Source: T. Reunala et al., "Treatment of Mosquito Bites with Cetirizine," *Clinical and Experimental Allergy* 23:72–75 (January 1993).

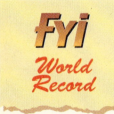

Most Dangerous Animal
The malarial parasites of the genus *Plasmodium* carried by mosquitoes of the genus *Anopheles,* if we exclude wars and accidents, have probably been responsible for half of all human deaths since the Stone Age.

Source: The Guinness Book of Records. New York: Bantam Books, 1995, p. 42.

Tick Bites

Ticks are not insects but are close relatives of mites and spiders. They have eight legs and are classified as hard ticks and soft ticks. Hard ticks are more familiar because of their wide distribution and common occurrence on domestic animals. Soft ticks are found mainly in western states. In the United States, seven kinds of hard ticks and five kinds of soft ticks carry diseases (e.g., Lyme disease), are a nuisance (e.g., itching, swelling), or cause paralysis (toxin injected).

Preventing Tick Bites

- Wear light-colored clothing so you can see any ticks on your clothes.
- Wear a long-sleeved shirt that fits tightly at the wrists and neck and tuck the shirt into your pants.
- Wear long pants and tuck the pant legs into your boots or socks. Or use masking tape to tape the pant legs tightly to your socks, shoes, or boots.
- Check your clothes while you are outdoors and before entering a house. If possible, wash your clothes as soon as possible.
- Inspect your pets for ticks before they come inside.
- After coming indoors, shower or bathe and check your body for ticks, especially in areas that have hair or where clothing was tight. Another person could do the checking.
- Treat your body and clothing with a repellent. The most common, EPA-approved, and effective tick repellent is DEET (N,N-diethyl-metatoluamide).

You can buy DEET under the trade names Off! and Cutters and apply it directly to your skin. Ticks crawling on the treated area are irritated by the repellent and drop off. DEET is most effective against ticks when applied to clothing from a spray can.

There have been a few reports of adverse toxic reactions to DEET, such as seizures, allergic responses, and skin irritation. To minimize reactions,

- Apply DEET sparingly to your skin.
- Avoid applying high-concentration products (no greater than 30 percent DEET) to the skin.
- Do not inhale or ingest DEET-containing products or get them in your eyes.
- Do not treat wounds or irritated skin.
- Wash your skin after coming indoors.
- Do not put these products with concentrations greater than 10 percent on infants and small children.

You can also use 0.5-percent preparations of permethrin (a pesticide). Permethrin should be applied *only* to clothing (especially shirt sleeves, pants legs, and collars), never directly on the skin.

Ticks hatch from eggs and grow through three distinct stages: nymph (too small to see), larva (just visible), and adult (ready to lay eggs). The adult is most likely to be seen. Ticks at any stage of develop-

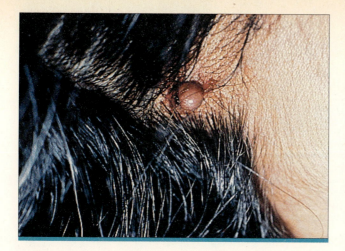

Tick embedded and engorged with victim's blood.

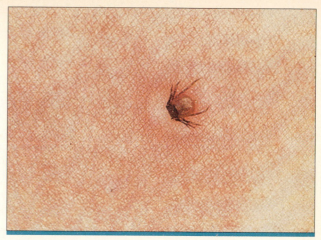

Tick embedded

ment can use humans for food; at each stage, they need what those who study them casually call a "blood meal" before they can grow to the next stage.

Ticks are limited in their ability to find their meals. They cannot fly, they crawl very slowly, and they cannot travel without some help more than a few yards from where they were hatched. When they are ready for their next meal, they may wait months, years, or even decades for the right host to come along. Bites are nearly painless, so the tick attachment is not noticed until later.

The front part of a tick consists of the head area and the mouthparts. The mouthparts have a central structure, the **hypostome,** which is shaped like a blunt harpoon. A tick pushes its hypostome into a hole in the victim's skin that has been made by sharp teeth on the front of the hypostome. The barbs anchor the tick to the skin and make it difficult to pull the tick out. Some ticks produce a substance that helps cement them to the host. As they feed, some ticks increase in size 20 to 50 times.

Removing Ticks

Remove ticks as soon as possible. If a tick is carrying a disease, the longer it stays embedded, the greater the chance of the disease being transmitted.

Because its bite is painless, a tick can remain embedded for days without the victim realizing it. Most tick bites are harmless, although ticks can carry Lyme disease, Rocky Mountain spotted fever, and other serious diseases.

1. To pull a tick off,
   • Use tweezers if possible. If you have to use your fingers, protect your skin by using a paper towel or disposable tissue or gloves.

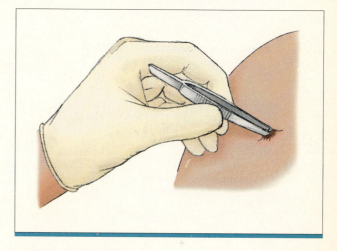

Removing a tick with tweezers

CAUTION: DO NOT

• use the following popular methods of tick removal, which have been proved useless:

  • petroleum jelly
  • fingernail polish
  • rubbing alcohol
  • a hot match
  • a petroleum product, such as gasoline
  • grab a tick at the rear of its body. The internal gut may rupture and the contents squeezed out, causing infection.
  • twist or jerk the tick, which may result in incomplete removal.

TICK REMOVAL

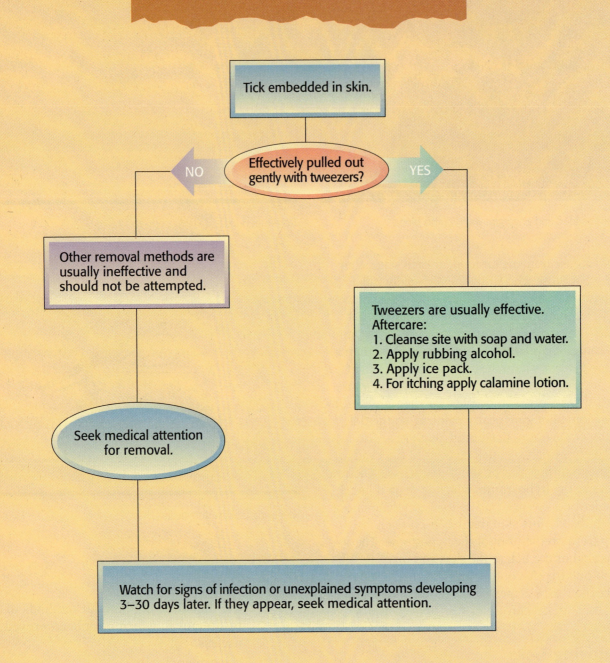

Tick embedded in skin.

Effectively pulled out gently with tweezers?

NO

YES

Other removal methods are usually ineffective and should not be attempted.

Tweezers are usually effective.
Aftercare:
1. Cleanse site with soap and water.
2. Apply rubbing alcohol.
3. Apply ice pack.
4. For itching apply calamine lotion.

Seek medical attention for removal.

Watch for signs of infection or unexplained symptoms developing 3–30 days later. If they appear, seek medical attention.

- Grasp the tick as close to the skin surface as possible and pull away from the skin with a steady pressure. Or lift the tick slightly upward and pull parallel to the skin until the tick detaches.

2. Wash the bite site with soap and water. Apply rubbing alcohol to further disinfect the area.

3. Apply an ice pack to reduce pain.

4. Apply calamine lotion to relieve any itching. Keep the area clean.

5. Continue to watch the bite site for one month for a rash. If a rash appears, see a physician. Watch for other signs such as fever, muscle aches, sensitivity to bright light, and paralysis that begins with leg weakness.

Lyme Disease

In 1975, many children living near Lyme, Connecticut, developed painful swelling of the body joints. The swelling looked like arthritis but was not. Researchers finally determined that people got the sickness after being bitten by deer ticks. Infected people got rashes, and about the same time flu-like symptoms. Eventually, they developed swollen joints. The sickness was named **Lyme disease**, after the town where it was first reported. (Actually, what we now call Lyme disease has been around, under other names, since the early 1900s.)

Lyme disease is caused by a bacterium that is carried by the deer tick. A deer tick is about the size of a poppy seed, except when it is swollen with blood. The ticks are carried into new areas by two animals, the white-tailed deer and the white-footed mouse. The ticks feed and mate on the deer, drop off, and later, as larvae, attach themselves to the mice, from which they obtain the bacteria.

While in the eastern United States, it is the deer tick that carries the bacteria, in the western states, the western black-legged tick is the carrier. Other tick species, including the dog tick and the Lone Star tick, have been known to carry the disease. Migrating birds may carry the ticks into new areas.

Not all ticks are infected, nor do all tick bites cause Lyme disease. Other types of ticks carry other diseases, for example, Rocky Mountain spotted fever and Colorado tick fever.

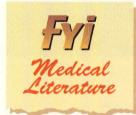

The Right Way to Remove a Tick In one study, researchers allowed adult ticks to attach to sheep. After three to four days, they covered some ticks with petroleum jelly, some with clear nail polish, and others with rubbing alcohol. They also lit wooden kitchen matches, blew them out, and touched some ticks with the hot, smoking ends of the matches. None of these folklore methods made the ticks detach. The researchers removed other ticks by grasping them with medium-tipped, angled tweezers as closely as possible to where the mouthparts entered the skin, then steadily pulling the ticks from the skin. They found no crushed ticks or broken mouthparts. A small piece of skin may come off painlessly with the tick, which usually means that the tick was completely removed. If the tick's head or mouthparts remain in the skin, remove them as you would a splinter, with a sterilized needle. The researchers obtained the same results with ticks that had been attached for only 12 to 15 hours.

Source: G. R. Needham, "Evaluation of Five Popular Methods for Tick Removal," *Pediatrics* 75(6): 997–1002 (June 1985).

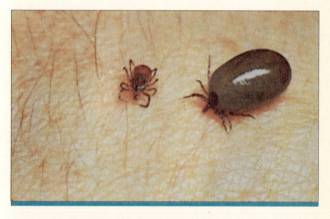

Deer ticks: not engorged and blood engorged

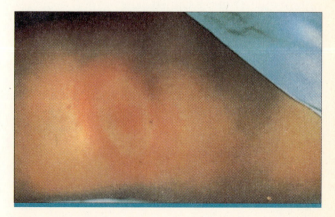

Lyme disease rash

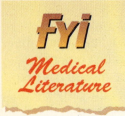

Imported Fire Ant Stings

The fire ant bites its victim by securing itself to the skin with its mandibles, causing pain. Then, using its head as a pivot, the ant swings its abdomen in an arc, repeatedly stinging the victim with an abdominal stinger.

The imported fire ant (IFA) made its first appearance in the United States around 1918, when it was introduced from Uruguay and Argentina via sea shipments to Mobile, Alabama. A second species arrived about two decades later from Brazil and Paraguay. Since then, these two species have spread rapidly throughout the southeastern United States, displacing many of the native species of insects. The ants are believed to inhabit about 13 southern states, Puerto Rico, and the Virgin Islands, with isolated colonies reported in a few western states. The spread of the IFA appears to be limited by its sensitivity to cold. Unfortunately, hybrids of the IFA have been discovered that show increased resistance to cold climates. This resistance may permit the ants to increase their territory beyond the current areas of infestation. Since the IFA was introduced to the United States, its spread has become a hazard to animals, agriculture, and humans. Inhabitants of infested areas report stings occurring in 30–60 percent of the population annually. The ant is capable of delivering a painful sting that produces a characteristic localized pustule. The true hazard to humans, however, does not occur with this localized reaction but with the less frequent systemic (whole-body) reactions. A survey of physicians showed that of 20,755 IFA stings reported, 16 percent of the people stung had a systemic reaction, and 2 percent had a life-threatening reaction (anaphylaxis). The IFA has become the most common cause of insect venom hypersensitivity in the southeastern quarter of the United States.

The South American fire ants range in color from red to dark brown. They are about ⅛ – ¼ inch long and usually live in foot-high, dome-shaped mounds.

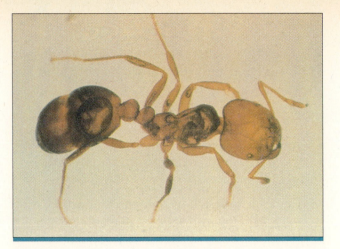

Fire ant

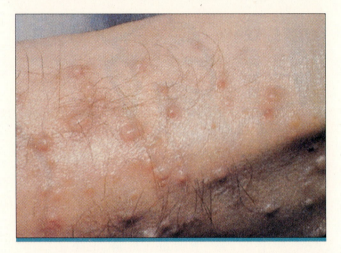

Fire ant stings

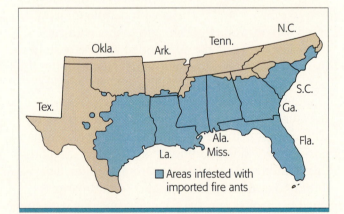

Areas infested with imported fire ants

Source: K. A. Candiotti and A. M. Lamas, "Adverse Neurologic Reactions to the Sting of the Imported Fire Ant," *International Archives of Allergy and Immunology* 102:417–420 (1993).

What to Look For

Signs and symptoms of Lyme disease occur any time from 3 to 30 days following a bite from an infected deer tick. The disease begins with flu-like symptoms: fever, chills, headaches, and joint stiffness.

The only visible sign of Lyme disease is the appearance of a slowly expanding, red bull's-eye rash that develops at the bite site. The rash is common to about 70 percent of all Lyme disease victims. The rash may grow over a period of a few days or weeks, eventually fading in time, even without treatment. It varies in shape, but its size usually is two inches or more. The rash appears as a circle of white surrounded by an area of redness, thus the term "bull's eye." It is painless, but hot to the touch.

The rash alone is a good indication that a person has been exposed to Lyme disease and may be infected. Other signs and symptoms include extreme fatigue, fever as high as 104°F, mild to severe headache, meningitis, and Bell's palsy.

Weeks after the initial tick bite, the victim may experience nerve and joint problems. In the later stages of Lyme disease, the most common symptom is arthritis-like swelling but little pain in a weight-bearing joint, such as the knee. In many cases, however, the diagnosis of Lyme disease comes down to a physician's judgment. The physician should always ask, "Was there ever a rash?" and "Do you live in or did you visit a tick-infested area up to a month before the symptoms appeared?"

Without proper antibiotic treatment, the disease can invade the central nervous system, resulting in meningitis, encephalitis, and Bell's palsy. Without treatment, the disease can cause stiffness in the large joints (knees and shoulders). The diagnosis of arthritis is often made by mistake. The stiffness comes and goes for periods lasting from several weeks to several years.

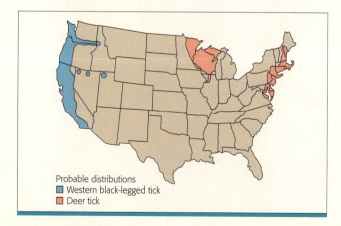

Probable distributions
- Western black-legged tick
- Deer tick

Carriers of Lyme disease

Medical diagnosis is difficult, because Lyme disease is often mistaken for the flu, especially if the rash is absent. Another problem is that over half the victims do not remember having been bitten by a tick. That is due to the extremely small size of the deer tick while it is in its infectious nymph stage of development. (The ticks do not look like the common wood or dog ticks familiar to most people.) Also, when the tick bites, it secretes a substance that acts like an anesthetic, so the human does not feel the bite.

Marine-Animal Injuries

Most marine animals bite or sting in defense, rather than attack per se. Marine venoms are similar in nature to many venoms found in reptiles and arthropods and may cause anaphylaxis or other types of reactions. The general first aid guidelines are similar to those for any disorder involving trauma, allergy, or cardiopulmonary failure. Serious allergic reactions require primary attention to keeping the airway open.

Animals That Bite, Rip, or Puncture

Sharks

Sharks are the most feared of all marine animals, but the chance of being attacked by a shark along the North American coastline is less than 1 in 5,000,000. Although exact figures are unavailable, it is estimated that, worldwide, no more than 50 attacks and no more than a dozen fatalities occur each year.

Most attacks occur within 100 feet of shore, and most victims are attacked by a single shark without warning. In the majority of attacks, the victim does not see the shark before the attack. The leg is the most frequently bitten part. Sharks are clearly more attracted to persons on the surface than to underwater scuba divers. The greatest attraction for sharks appears to be chemicals found in fish blood—sharks can detect them in quantities as small as one part per million parts water. Shark bite wounds, among the most devastating of all animal bites, are similar to injuries caused by boat propellers or chainsaws. Immediate control of bleeding and treatment for shock are essential.

What to Do

1. Control bleeding.
2. Treat for shock.
3. Seek medical attention.

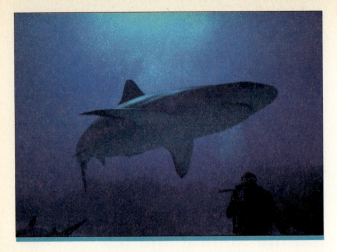
Shark

Barracudas and Eels

Barracudas are fearsome in appearance, but they have an undeserved reputation as attackers of humans. The risk of a barracuda bite is exceedingly small. First aid for a barracuda bite is identical to that for a shark bite.

Moray eels are also fierce in appearance. They are not infrequent biters of divers who handle or tease them, usually in competition for food or in pursuit of lobsters. The multiple puncture wounds created by moray eel bites have a high infection risk. Treat as you would shark bites.

Animals That Sting

Stings from marine animals lead the list of adverse marine-animal encounters. It is important to identify the offending animal, because in many cases first aid is quite specific.

Each year, jellyfish, Portuguese man-of-wars, corals, and anemones that lie along the shallow ocean waters of the United States sting more than

Preventing Shark Attacks

No shark repellents are universally effective. Explosive and electronic devices may threaten diver safety instead of sharks. Prevention of shark attacks includes the following guidelines:

- Avoid swimming in areas frequented by sharks or where shark attacks have previously occurred. (In the United States, the greatest concentration of great white shark attacks is off the northern California coast.)
- Do not swim or dive alone.
- Do not swim far offshore, in murky water, or incautiously along deep dropoffs.
- People with open wounds and menstruating women should avoid swimming in areas where there is risk of shark attack.
- Avoid swimming in the vicinity of seal or sea lion colonies or turtle haulouts.
- Do not spearfish for an extended period in the same area and do not attach fish to your body.
- Avoid swimming at dawn, dusk, or night in potentially dangerous waters.

one million people. Reactions to being stung by Portuguese man-of-wars and jellyfish vary from mild dermatitis to severe reactions. Most victims recover without medical attention.

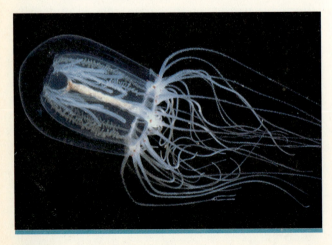
Jellyfish

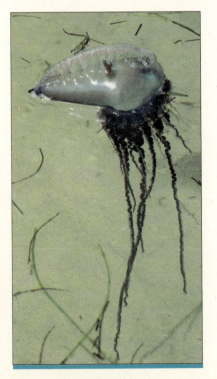
Portuguese man-of-war

MARINE-ANIMAL INJURIES

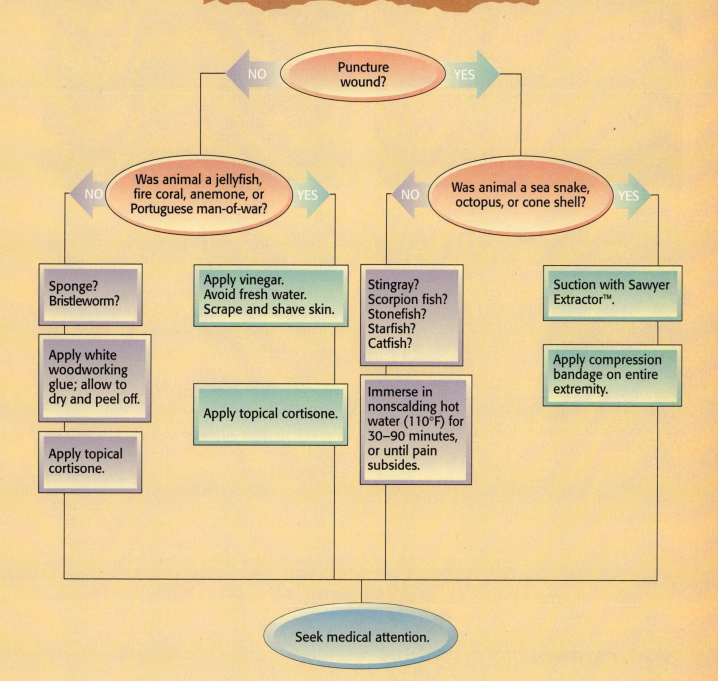

Puncture wound?

NO → Was animal a jellyfish, fire coral, anemone, or Portuguese man-of-war?

YES → Was animal a sea snake, octopus, or cone shell?

Was animal a jellyfish, fire coral, anemone, or Portuguese man-of-war?

NO:
- Sponge? Bristleworm?
- Apply white woodworking glue; allow to dry and peel off.
- Apply topical cortisone.

YES:
- Apply vinegar. Avoid fresh water. Scrape and shave skin.
- Apply topical cortisone.

Was animal a sea snake, octopus, or cone shell?

NO:
- Stingray? Scorpion fish? Stonefish? Starfish? Catfish?
- Immerse in nonscalding hot water (110°F) for 30–90 minutes, or until pain subsides.

YES:
- Suction with Sawyer Extractor™.
- Apply compression bandage on entire extremity.

Seek medical attention.

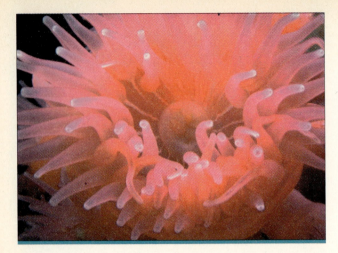

Anemones

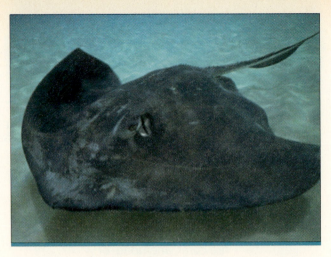

Stingray

Jellyfish and Portuguese man-of-wars have long tentacles equipped with stinging devices called *nematocysts*. When cast ashore or onto rocks, detached nematocysts retain their ability to sting for a long period of time, usually until they are completely dried out.

The Portuguese man-of-war sting is usually in the form of well-defined linear welts or scattered patches of welts with redness, which usually disappear within 24 hours. The jellyfish sting produces severe muscle cramping with multiple thin lines of welts crossing the skin in a zigzag pattern. Pain usually is a burning type that lasts 10 to 30 minutes. The welts on the skin usually disappear within an hour.

Anemones are beautiful but potentially dangerous. Many anemone stings result from the improper handling of aquarium animals.

What to Do

1. Apply vinegar to the sting area. Combine the vinegar with unseasoned meat tenderizer to prevent the nematocysts from further discharging.

 CAUTION: DO NOT

- try to rub the tentacles off of the victim's skin—that will activate the stinging cells.
- use fresh water for rinsing because it will cause the nematocysts to fire.
- apply cold packs—they also will cause the nematocysts to fire.
- touch the tentacles with your bare hands.

2. Immediately scrape off any tentacles remaining on the skin by using a credit card, stick, comb, knife blade, or similar object. Or apply shaving cream or a baking soda paste and shave the area. For large tentacles use tweezers or pliers.
3. Reapply vinegar or alcohol and soak the area for 15 minutes.

Animals That Puncture (by Spine)

Stingrays, commonly found in tropical and subtropical waters, are peaceful, reclusive bottom feeders that generally lie buried in the sand or mud. Most wounds inflicted by sting rays are produced on the ankle or foot when the victim steps on a ray. The ray reacts by thrusting its barbed tail upward and forward into the victim's leg or foot. At least 2,000 stingray injuries occur each year in coastal U.S. waters. The stingray's venomous tail barb easily penetrates human skin. The sting usually is more like a laceration, since the large tail barb can do significant damage. The venom causes intense burning pain at the site.

What to Do

1. Relieve pain by immersing the injured body part in hot water (110°F) for 30–90 minutes. Make sure the water is not hot enough to cause a burn.
2. Wash the wound with soap and water.
3. Irrigate the area with water under pressure to wash out as much of the toxin and foreign material as possible.
4. Treat the wound like any puncture wound.

STUDY QUESTIONS 17

Name _____ Course _____ Date _____

Activities

Activity 1
Mark each statement as true (T) or false (F).

T   F   1. An antivenin exists for black widow spider bites.

T   F   2. Honeybees and wasps leave a stinger embedded in the victim's skin.

T   F   3. Long and strong fangs enable black widow and brown recluse spiders to bite humans.

T   F   4. No venom injection occurs in about one-fourth of all venomous snakebites.

T   F   5. The same antivenin is used for all pit viper snakebites in the United States.

T   F   6. Covering an embedded tick with petroleum jelly causes the tick to back out.

T   F   7. Ticks can transmit disease.

T   F   8. Apply ice on all animal and insect bites and stings.

Activity 2
Mark each statement true as (T) or false (F).

T   F   1. Reactions to being stung by an ocean animal can be severe.

T   F   2. Examples of marine animals that sting include jellyfish and Portuguese man-of-wars.

T   F   3. The intense burning pain from a jelly-fish sting is produced by nematocysts on the tentacles.

T   F   4. Remove jellyfish tentacles on the skin by scraping them off with a credit card.

T   F   5. Use rubbing alcohol or vinegar to inactivate the tentacles.

T   F   6. Water can be used to inactivate the nematocysts.

Case Situations

Case 1
A 16-year-old male is stung by a swarm of bees. According to his friends, he was outside mowing the lawn when he was suddenly and repeatedly stung. He is responsive, but his face is swollen (especially around the eyes) and cyanotic about the lips. You can hear a wheezing sound when he breathes. Several large red welts appear on his back and neck. His friends report that he has asthma.

_____ 1. This victim is most likely experiencing
   a. a minor allergic reaction
   b. anaphylaxis
   c. an acute asthma attack
   d. neurogenic shock

T   F   2. The sooner symptoms develop after a sting, the more serious the reaction will be.

T   F   3. The majority of anaphylactic deaths are caused by inability of the victim to breathe because of swollen airway passages.

_____ 4. Treatment for this victim would include
   a. giving the victim prescribed epine-phrine, if available
   b. giving syrup of ipecac
   c. giving activated charcoal
   d. giving CPR
   e. giving rescue breaths

Case 2
While showering after an overnight camping trip, you discover a tick embedded in your skin.

_____ What should you do?
   a. Hold a heated needle or a blown-out, glowing match head to the tick.
   b. Squeeze the protruding end of the tick with your fingers and allow the blood to drain out. The body will fall out within 24 hours.
   c. Do nothing. The tick will die in 24 to 48 hours and then fall out.
   d. Use tweezers to remove as much of the tick as possible, then clean the wound with soap and water.

Case 3

While you are camping, a friend is bitten on the hand by a rattlesnake.

_____ 1. How do you know it is a rattlesnake bite?
   a. The snake was brightly colored—red, yellow, and black.
   b. The snake had a triangular-shaped head.
   c. The victim's skin had two puncture marks.
   d. Both a and c.
   e. Both b and c.

_____ 2. What should you do for a pit viper snakebite?
   a. Cool the bite site with an ice pack.
   b. Avoid using cold on the bite site.

_____ 3. a. Do not cut through any snake bite wound.
   b. Cut through the fang marks if you are more than one hour from a medical facility.

_____ 4. a. First aiders can give antivenin.
   b. Only a qualified physician should give antivenin.

_____ 5. a. Apply a tourniquet.
   b. Apply suction with the Extractor device.

_____ 6. a. If possible, identify the snake and its size.
   b. Information about the snake usually is not necessary.

Case 4

A small girl is bitten by a neighbor's dog. You see an avulsed flap of skin on the girl's back.

1. How many people are bitten by dogs each year in the United States?

2. Animal bites raise what two concerns?
   a. _____
   b. _____

3. Which animal accounts for the most bites?
   a. dogs
   b. cats
   c. humans
   d. skunks

4. Which animal accounts for the most rabies cases?
   a. dogs
   b. skunks
   c. raccoons
   d. cats

Case 5

Your three-year-old daughter runs into the house crying and holding her arms. She complains about having a black bug on her. You look at her arm and notice a slight redness and swelling around what may be a bite.

1. A coal-black body with a red spot on its abdomen can be the identification of which poisonous spider?
   _____
   _____

2. The other poisonous spider that causes severe medical problems is the
   _____
   _____

3. Which of the following first aid procedures are appropriate for spider bites and scorpion stings? (Check _all_ that apply.)
   _____ a. Apply a cold pack.
   _____ b. Seek medical attention immediately.
   _____ c. Capture the spider or have a definite identification.
   _____ d. Maintain open airway and restore breathing, if necessary.
   _____ e. Wash area with soap and water or rubbing alcohol.
   _____ f. Apply a constriction band 2 to 4 inches above the bite.
   _____ g. Apply calamine lotion to relieve discomfort.

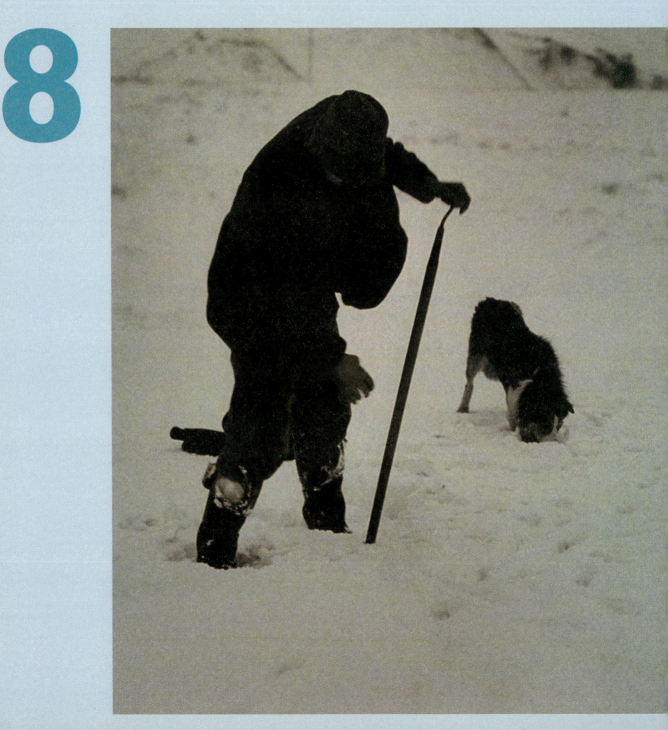

COLD-RELATED EMERGENCIES

Heat flows from an area with a higher temperature to an area with a lower temperature. When a person is surrounded by air or water cooler than body temperature, the body will lose heat. If heat escapes faster than the body produces heat, body temperature will fall. Normal body temperature is 98.6°F, and if body temperature falls much below that, cold injuries can result.

How Cold Affects the Body

Humans protect themselves from cold primarily by avoiding or reducing cold exposure through the use of clothing and shelter. When that protection proves inadequate, the body has biological defense mechanisms to help maintain correct body temperature. The body's internal mechanisms to defend its temperature during cold exposure include vasoconstriction and shivering. When those responses are triggered, it is a signal that clothing and shelter are inadequate.

Vasoconstriction is the tightening of blood vessels in skin that is exposed to cold. The reduced skin blood flow conserves body heat but can lead to discomfort, numbness, loss of dexterity in the hands and fingers, and eventually cold injuries.

Cold triggers shivering, which increases internal heat production, which helps to offset the heat being lost. Shivering is the body's main involuntary defense against the cold. Shivering produces body heat by forcing muscles to contract and relax rapidly. About 80 percent of the muscle energy used in shivering is turned into body heat. When the core temperature rises, shivering is no longer needed and is shut down by the hypothalamus (in the brain). When the core temperature falls to about 86°F, the shivering reflex stops. Likewise, when there is no further fuel (glycogen) for the body, shivering stops. Several drugs suppress the shivering response, including barbiturates, beta-blocking agents, and alcohol.

Internal heat production is also increased by physical activity; the more vigorous the activity, the greater the heat production. In fact, heat production during intense exercise or strenuous work usually is sufficient to completely compensate for heat loss, even when it is extremely cold. However, high-intensity exercise and hard physical work are fatiguing, can cause sweating, and cannot be sustained indefinitely.

Susceptibility to cold injuries can be minimized by maintaining proper hydration and nutrition, avoiding alcohol, caffeine, and nicotine, and limiting periods of inactivity in cold conditions. Humans do not acclimatize to cold weather nearly as well as they acclimatize to hot weather.

The colder the surrounding temperature is, the greater the potential for body heat to escape. When the skin is exposed to cold, the brain signals the blood vessels in the skin to tighten, and blood flow to the skin decreases. This is the body's attempt to prevent heat inside the body from being carried to the skin, where it will be lost. However, due to reduced blood flow to the skin, the skin temperature falls.

When cold exposure lasts more than an hour, cooling of the skin and reduced blood to the hands leads to blunted sensation, touch, and pain and loss of dexterity and agility. That can impair a person's ability to perform manual tasks and, since symptoms may go unnoticed, lead to more severe cold injuries.

Heat Loss from the Body

Normal body temperature is maintained by a balance of heat production and heat loss. Heat is produced by food metabolism and muscle activity, and production can be increased up to 500 percent with shivering. Shivering causes a large increase in heat production, but it consumes calories stored in the liver and muscles as glycogen rapidly. Lack of food limits the body's ability to produce heat; when glycogen stores become depleted, heat output decreases.

Heat loss occurs primarily through the skin. Blood flow to the skin varies in different parts of the body, and some areas lose more heat than others. Thermograms demonstrate high losses from the head and neck (up to 50 percent), axillary area (armpits), and groin area. Blood vessel constriction caused by cold conserves heat.

Body heat can be lost by four mechanisms:

- **Conduction**, or direct contact with a colder object (e.g., lying on the snow), normally accounts for only a small fraction of heat loss. The exception is immersion in cold water, where heat loss can be 25 to 30 times greater than in air, even more with water movement.
- **Convection** is the loss of heat from the body by air blowing over the skin or through porous clothing. **Windchill** is the combined effect of the ambient temperature and wind speed.
- **Evaporation**, or conversion of liquid on the skin to a vapor, normally accounts for about 20 percent of heat loss (two-thirds through sweating and one-third through respiration).

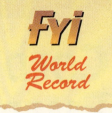

- **Radiation** is the primary method of heat loss, accounting for about 65 percent of the body's heat loss. A warm object gives off (radiates) heat to cooler air. It has been demonstrated that up to 50 percent of the body's total heat production can be lost by radiation through a person's unprotected head.

Susceptibility to Cold Injury

An individual's susceptibility to cold injury (nonfreezing and freezing injuries, and hypothermia) is affected by many factors. The physically unfit are more susceptible to cold injury. They tire more quickly and are unable to stay active to keep warm as long as those who are physically fit.

Dehydration reduces skin blood flow, which increases susceptibility to cold injury. Fat functions as an insulator against heat loss because it has less blood flow than muscle and loses less heat. Therefore, a very lean person may be susceptible to the effects of cold, if clothing is inadequate or wet, or the individual is relatively inactive. Persons 50 years old and older may be less tolerant of the cold than younger persons, due to the decline in physical fitness that often occurs with aging.

Alcohol and, to a lesser extent, caffeine cause the blood vessels in the skin to open, which can accelerate body heat loss. Also, alcohol and caffeine both increase urine formation, leading to dehydration, which can further degrade the body's defenses against cold. Most important, alcohol blunts the senses and impairs judgment, so an individual may not feel the signs and symptoms of developing cold injury.

Because nicotine decreases blood flow to the skin, smoking and chewing tobacco can increase susceptibility to frostbite. Inadequate nutrition, illness, and injury compromise the body's responses to cold and an individual's ability to recognize and react appropriately to the symptoms of developing cold injury.

Persons who have experienced a cold injury in the past are at greater risk of experiencing a cold injury.

Effects of Altitude

Assessment of weather conditions in mountainous regions needs to take into account altitude if that assessment is based on weather measurements obtained at lower elevations. Temperatures, windchill, and the risk of cold injury at high altitudes can differ considerably from those at lower elevations.

In general, it can be assumed that air temperature is 3.6°F lower for every 1,000 feet above where the temperature was measured. Winds usually are more severe at high altitudes, and there is less cover above the tree line. People are more susceptible to frostbite and other cold injuries at altitudes above 8,000 feet than at sea level, because of lower temperatures, higher winds, and lack of oxygen.

Effects of Water

Water can conduct heat away from the body much faster than air of the same temperature. When clothing becomes wet due to snow, rain, splashing

---

Table 18.1: How Cold Is It?

In addition to coldness, two other factors account for body heat loss: moisture and wind. Moisture—whether from rain, snow, or perspiration—speeds the conduction of heat away from the body.

Wind causes sizable amounts of body-heat loss. If the thermometer reads 20°F and the wind speed is 20 mph, the exposure is comparable to −10°F. This is called the windchill factor. Use the following rough measures of wind speed: If you feel the wind on your face, the speed is about 10 mph; if small branches move or dust or snow is raised,

20 mph; if large branches are moving, 30 mph; and if a whole tree bends, about 40 mph.

To determine the windchill factor:

1. Estimate the wind speed by checking for the signs described above.

2. Look at a thermometer reading (in Fahrenheit degrees) outdoors.

3. Match the estimated wind speed with the actual thermometer reading in the table below.

Windchill Factor

Estimated Wind Speed (mph)	Actual Thermometer Reading (°F) Equivalent Temperature (°F)											
	50	40	30	20	10	0	−10	−20	−30	−40	−50	−60
Calm	50	40	30	20	10	0	−10	−20	−30	−40	−50	−60
5	48	37	27	16	6	−5	−15	−26	−36	−47	−57	−68
10	40	28	16	3	−9	−21	−33	−46	−58	−70	−83	−95
15	36	22	9	−5	−18	−32	−45	−58	−72	−85	−99	−112
20	32	18	4	−10	−25	−39	−53	−67	−82	−96	−110	−124
25	30	15	0	−15	−29	−44	−59	−74	−89	−104	−118	−133
30	25	13	−2	−18	−33	−48	−63	−79	−94	−109	−125	−140
35	27	11	−4	−20	−35	−51	−67	−82	−98	−113	−129	−145
40	26	10	−6	−21	−37	−53	−69	−85	−101	−117	−132	−148

(Wind speeds greater than 40 mph have little additional effect.)

Little danger. (In less than 5 hours with dry skin. Greatest hazard from false sense of security.)

Increasing danger. (Exposed flesh may freeze within 1 minute.)

Great danger. (Flesh may freeze within 30 seconds.)

water, or accumulated sweat, the body's loss of heat is accelerated, up to 25 times faster.

Swimmers and persons working or wading in water can lose a great deal of body heat even when the water temperature is only mildly cool. Individuals working in cold water should be closely watched as they enter the water, since sudden plunging into cold water can produce irregular heartbeats, gasping, and hyperventilation, which can cause inhalation of water, heart failure, and drowning.

Effects of Wind

For any given air temperature, the potential for body heat loss, skin cooling, and decreased internal temperature is increased by wind. Wind increases heat loss from skin exposed to cold air, in effect lowering the temperature. The windchill index integrates wind speed and air temperature to provide an estimate of the cooling power of the environment and the associated risk of cold injury.

Windchill temperatures obtained from weather reports do not take into account artificial wind, which worsens the windchill effect of natural wind. For example, riding in an open vehicle can subject the passengers to dangerous windchill, even when natural winds are low.

Effects of Metals and Liquid Fuels

Metal objects and liquid fuels that have been left outdoors in the cold pose a serious hazard. Both can conduct heat away from the skin rapidly. Fuels and solvents remain liquid at very low temperatures. Skin contact with fuel or metal at below-freezing temperatures can result in nearly instantaneous freezing. Fuel handlers must use great care and not allow exposed skin to come into contact with spilled fuel or metals.

Minimizing Effects of Cold on the Body

When adequately protected, humans can tolerate temperatures as low as −72°F. Adequate clothing maintains the "microclimate" surrounding the body. Air is an excellent insulator, and the basis for most clothing is to trap a layer of air around the body. Layering, which has been used for centuries, allows the removal or opening of a garment to vent excess heat during times of greater activity or changes in environment and accommodates an individual's own needs and preferences. Wearing layered clothing is especially important for people who fre-

quently change environments (e.g., go in and out of buildings) or who periodically undertake vigorous physical activity.

Three important layers are recommended for most outdoor activities. The first layer (undergarments) removes perspiration from the skin, the middle layers insulate, and the outer layer or outer shell protects against wind. By understanding this principle, individuals can vary their clothing to regulate protection and stay comfortable.

For the first layer, use underwear that wicks away perspiration, that is, it stays dry by drawing moisture away from the skin to the next layer of clothing. Wet clothing transfers heat away from the body. Cotton holds moisture next to the skin so you feel cold and clammy. Silk feels warm and soft, but it also retains moisture. Fabrics such as polypropy-

If a Blizzard Traps You While You Are Driving

- Don't panic.
- Stay in your vehicle. Do not attempt to walk out of a blizzard. Disorientation comes quickly in blowing and drifting snow. Being lost in open country during a blizzard is almost certain death. You are more likely to be found and certainly more likely to be sheltered in your car.
- Avoid overexertion and exposure. Exertion from attempting to push your car, shovel heavy drifts, and perform other difficult chores during the strong winds, blinding snow, and bitter cold of a blizzard may cause a heart attack—even in a person in apparently good physical condition.
- Keep fresh air in your car. Freezing, wet snow and wind-driven snow can completely seal the passenger compartment, causing suffocation.
- Beware the "gentle" killers: carbon monoxide and oxygen starvation. Run the motor and heater sparingly and only with the downwind window open for ventilation.
- Keep watch. Do not permit all occupants of the car to sleep at one time.
- Exercise by clasping hands and moving arms and legs vigorously from time to time. Do not stay in one position for long.
- Turn on your car's dome light at night, to make the vehicle visible to work crews.

Source: National Oceanic and Atmospheric Administration.

Winter Wardrobe

	Advantages	Disadvantages	Layer
Wool	Stretches without damage; insulates well even when wet	Heavy weight; absorbs moisture; may irritate skin	1, 2, or 3
Cotton	Comfortable and lightweight	Absorbs moisture	1 (for inactive people) or 2
Silk	Extremely lightweight and durable; very good insulator; washes well	More expensive; does not transfer moisture quickly	1
Polypropylene	Lightweight; transfers moisture quickly and dries quickly	Does not insulate well; low melting point; surface may pill	1 or 2 (for active people)
Down	Durable, lightweight; most effective insulator by weight	Expensive; loses insulative quality when wet; difficult to dry	2 or 3 (especially in dry, extreme cold)
Nylon	Lightweight; wind- and water-resistant; durable	May not allow perspiration to evaporate; low melting point; flammable	3
Synthetic Polyester Insulation	Does not absorb moisture, therefore insulates even when wet	Heavier than down; does not compress as well	2 or 3 (especially in wet weather)

Source: National Safety Council, *Family Safety & Health.*

lene or one of the new types of polyesters such as Capilene™ or Thermax™ should be considered.

The middle layer can be a synthetic pile or fleece jacket that is warm and dries quickly or a wool or synthetic sweater. Synthetic insulative materials such as Thinsulate™, unlike down or wool, provide warmth without bulk or heavy weight. Insulation should be effective even when wet. In that respect, synthetics are clearly superior to natural fibers and products. Duck or goose down, for example, is virtually useless when wet, and it dries out slowly. One exception, however, is the insulating ability of wool, even when wet.

Physically active people may sweat even in extremely cold weather. Therefore, the best choice for an outside layer is a jacket that is waterproof, wind resistant, and "breathable." Materials like Gore-Tex™ allow perspiration to evaporate. A zipper is preferable, so the clothing can be opened easily to increase ventilation. Nylon and vinyl are poor choices because they produce a sauna effect by holding in perspiration.

Because the head loses more body heat than any other part (50 percent), heed the admonition, "If the feet are cold, cover the head." A wool or synthetic cap serves well.

Nonfreezing Cold Injuries

Nonfreezing cold injuries can occur when conditions are cold and wet (air temperatures between 32° and 55°F) and the hands and feet cannot be kept warm and dry. The most prominent nonfreezing cold injuries are chilblain and trenchfoot.

Chilblain is a nonfreezing cold injury that, while painful, causes little or no permanent damage. It appears as red, swollen skin that is tender, hot to the touch, and possibly itchy. This can worsen to an aching, prickly ("pins and needles") sensation and then numbness. Chilblain can develop in only a few hours in skin exposed to cold.

Trenchfoot is a serious nonfreezing cold injury that develops when the skin on the feet is exposed to moisture and cold for prolonged periods (12 hours or longer). The combination of cold and moisture softens the skin, causing tissue loss and, often, infection. Untreated, trenchfoot can eventually require amputation. Often, the first sign of trenchfoot is itching, numbness, or tingling pain. Later the feet may appear swollen and the skin mildly red, blue, or black. Commonly, trenchfoot shows a distinct waterline that coincides with the water level in the boot. Red or bluish blotches appear on the skin, sometimes with open weeping or bleeding. The risk of this potentially crippling injury is high during wet weather. Persons who wear rubberized or tight-fitting boots are at risk for trenchfoot regardless of weather conditions, because sweat accumulates inside the boots and keeps the feet wet.

Freezing Cold Injuries

Freezing cold injuries can occur whenever the air temperature is below freezing (32°F). Freezing limited to the skin surface is **frostnip.** Freezing that extends deeper through the skin and into the flesh is **frostbite.**

Frostbite is prevalent during military campaigns and is a known hazard for mountain climbers and explorers. As more and more recreationalists pursue cross-country skiing and snowmobiling, the number of frostbite cases probably will increase. However, it is still thought to be rare in nonmilitary situations.

Frostnip involves the freezing of water on the skin surface. The skin becomes reddened and possibly swollen. Although painful, there usually is no further damage after rewarming. Repeated frostnip in the same spot can dry the skin, causing it to crack and become sensitive. It is difficult to tell the difference between frostnip and frostbite. Frostnip should be taken seriously since it may be the first sign of impending frostbite. First aid for frostnip consists of gently warming the affected area by placing it against a warm body part (e.g., bare hands, armpit, stomach) or by blowing warm air on the area. Do not rub the area. After rewarming, the affected area may be red and tingling.

Frostbite occurs when temperatures drop below freezing. Tissue is not composed of water alone, so it will not freeze until it has been cooled to about 28°F. Tissue is damaged in two ways: (1) actual tissue freezing, which results in the formation of ice crystals between the tissue cells (the ice crystals enlarge by extracting water from the cells), and (2) the

obstruction of the blood supply to the tissue, which causes "sludged" blood clots, which further prevent blood from flowing to the tissues. The second type of tissue damage is more extensive than the first. In severe cold temperatures, flesh can freeze in under a minute.

Frostbite affects mainly the feet, hands, ears, and nose. Those areas do not contain large heat-producing muscles and are some distance from the body's heat-generation sources. The most severe consequences of frostbite are gangrene and amputation.

What to Look For

The severity and extent of frostbite are difficult to judge until hours after thawing, although before thawing it can be classified as *superficial* or *deep*. Even physicians have to wait until thawing has occurred before they can judge the extent of the injury.

The signs and symptoms of superficial frostbite are as follows:

- Skin color is white, waxy, or grayish-yellow.
- The affected part feels very cold and numb. There may be tingling, stinging, or an aching sensation.

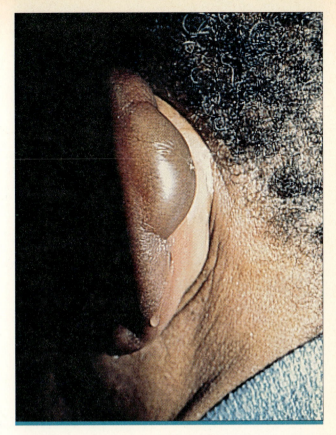

Frostbitten ear 8 hours old

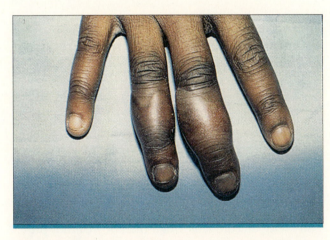

Frostbitten fingers, 6 hours after rewarming in 108°F water

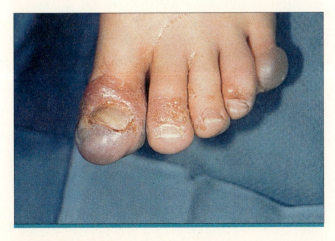

Second-degree frostbite

- The skin surface feels stiff or crusty and the underlying tissue soft when depressed gently and firmly.

Deep frostbite is indicated by the following signs and symptoms:

- The affected part feels cold, hard, and solid and cannot be depressed.
- Blisters may appear after rewarming.
- The affected part is cold, with pale, waxy skin.
- A painfully cold part suddenly stops hurting.

After a part has thawed, frostbite can be categorized by degrees, similar to the classification of burns. First-degree frostbite is superficial, while the other three are degrees of deep frostbite.

- **First-degree frostbite:** The affected part is warm, swollen, and tender.
- **Second-degree frostbite:** Blisters form minutes to hours after thawing and enlarge over several days.
- **Third-degree frostbite:** Blisters are small and contain reddish-blue or purplish fluid. The surrounding skin may have a red or blue color and may not blanch when pressure is applied.

- **Fourth-degree frostbite:** No blisters or swelling occurs. The part remains numb, cold, and white to dark purple in color.

What to Do

All frostbite injuries require the same first aid treatment. *Seek medical attention immediately.* Rewarming of frostbite seldom needs to take place outside a medical facility, because such facilities usually are nearby.

1. Get the victim out of the cold and to a warm place.

⚠ CAUTION: DO NOT

- use water hotter than 108°F—burns can result.
- use water cooler than 100°F—it will not thaw frostbite rapidly enough.
- break any blisters.
- rub or massage the part—ice crystals can be pushed into body cells, rupturing them.
- rub the affected part with ice or snow.
- rewarm the part with a heating pad, hot-water bottle, stove, sunlamp, radiator, or exhaust pipe or over a fire. Excessive temperatures cannot be controlled, resulting in burns.
- allow the victim to drink alcoholic beverages. Alcohol dilates blood vessels and causes a loss of body heat.
- allow the victim to smoke. Smoking constricts blood vessels, thus impairing circulation.
- rewarm if there is any possibility of refreezing.
- allow the thawed part to refreeze since ice crystals formed will be larger and more damaging. If refreezing is likely or even possible, it is better to leave the part frozen.
- use the "dry" rewarming technique (putting the victim's hands in your armpits) since that takes three to four times longer than the wet, rapid method to thaw frozen tissue. Slow rewarming results in greater tissue damage than rapid rewarming.

2. Remove any clothing or constricting items that could impair blood circulation (e.g., rings).

3. Seek immediate medical attention.

4. If the affected part is partially thawed or the victim is in a remote or wilderness situation (more than 1 hour from a medical facility), use the following wet, rapid rewarming method.

   Place the frostbitten part in warm (102°–105°F) water. If you do not have a thermometer, pour some of the water over the inside of your arm or put your elbow into it to test that it is warm, not hot. Maintain water temperature by adding warm water. Rewarming usually takes 20 to 40 minutes or until the tissues are soft. To help control the severe pain during rewarming, give the victim aspirin or ibuprofen. For ear or facial injuries, apply warm moist cloths, changing them frequently.

5. After thawing,
   - Treat victim as a "stretcher" case—the feet will be impossible to use after they are rewarmed.
   - Protect the affected area from contact by clothing and bedding.
   - Place dry, sterile gauze between the toes and the fingers to absorb moisture and to keep them from sticking together.
   - Slightly elevate the affected part to reduce pain and swelling.
   - Apply aloe vera gel to promote skin healing.
   - Give the victim aspirin or ibuprofen to limit pain and inflammation.

Hypothermia

Body temperature falls when the body cannot produce heat as fast as it is being lost. **Hypothermia** is a life-threatening condition in which the body's core temperature falls below 95°F.

Generally, the core temperature will not fall until after many hours of continuous exposure to cold air, if the individual is healthy, physically active, and reasonably dressed. However, because wet skin and wind accelerate body heat loss and the body produces less heat during inactive periods, the core body temperature can fall even when the air temperature is above freezing if conditions are windy, clothing is wet, or the individual is inactive.

Hypothermia can occur year round. Most people think of hypothermia as related only to cold outdoor exposure. It can happen indoors, in the southern states, and even on a summer day. It does not require subfreezing temperatures.

FROSTBITE

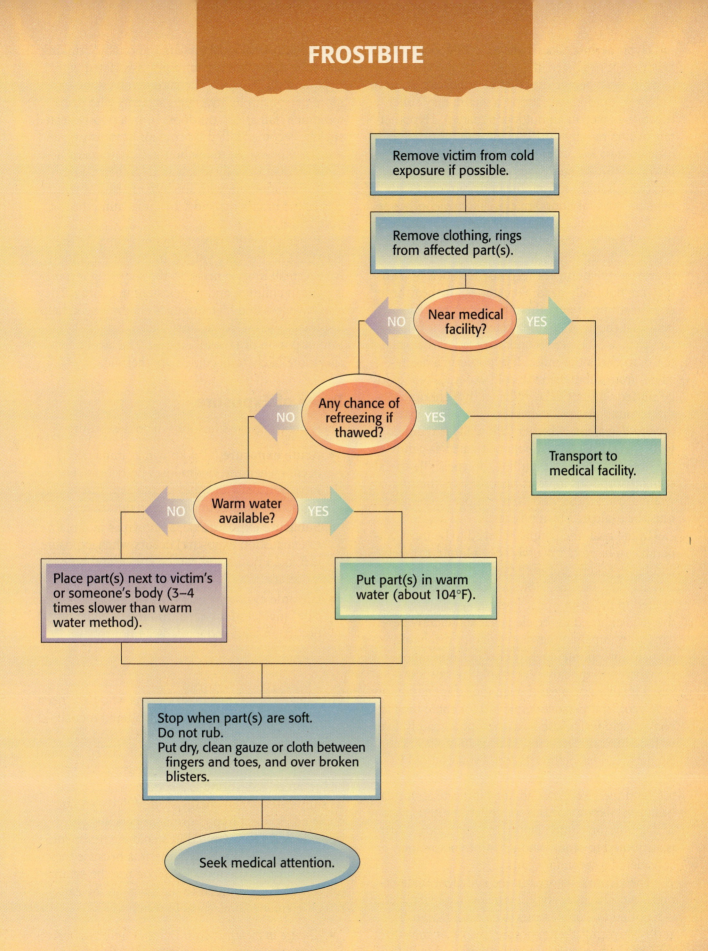

Remove victim from cold exposure if possible.

Remove clothing, rings from affected part(s).

Near medical facility?

NO

YES → Transport to medical facility.

Any chance of refreezing if thawed?

NO

YES

Warm water available?

NO → Place part(s) next to victim's or someone's body (3–4 times slower than warm water method).

YES → Put part(s) in warm water (about 104°F).

Stop when part(s) are soft.
Do not rub.
Put dry, clean gauze or cloth between fingers and toes, and over broken blisters.

Seek medical attention.

Hypothermia occurs when the body loses more heat than it produces. If the body temperature falls to 80°F, most people die. Hypothermia can occur in indoor or outdoor situations; a victim may suffer frostbite as well in an outdoor situation. Hypothermia occurs rapidly during cold-water immersion (one hour or less when the water temperature is below 45°F). Because water has a tremendous capacity to drain heat from the body, prolonged immersion (several hours) in even slightly cool water (< 70°F) can cause hypothermia. Hypothermia is a medical emergency. Untreated, it results in death.

Even though hypothermic victims may show no heartbeat, breathing, or response to touch or pain, they are not really dead. Sometimes, the heartbeat and breathing of hypothermic victims will be so faint that they can go undetected. Thus, it is important to take 30 to 45 seconds, instead of the usual 5 to 10, to check the pulse. If hypothermia has resulted from submersion in cold water, CPR should be started without delay. When a hypothermic victim is found on land, however, take a little extra time to determine whether CPR really is required. Hypothermic victims should be treated as gently as possible, since rough handling can cause life-threatening disruptions in heart rate. All hypothermic victims, even those who do not appear to be alive, must be evaluated by a physician.

In the past, the people believed to be most vulnerable to hypothermia have been hunters, hikers, and backpackers, not to mention careless drinkers and accident victims. However, the condition is not limited to those groups. Disadvantaged urban dwellers exposed to the elements and elderly persons with impaired thermoregulatory mechanisms also are susceptible. Lightly clad persons almost anywhere can quickly become chilled outdoors when it is raining even though the temperatures are only cool, and persons immersed for some time in cool or cold water lose heat even more readily. Even well-conditioned athletes, such as long-distance runners, can be victims. Hypothermia should be considered whenever the victim's behavior and history and the weather conditions indicate abnormal heat loss. Hypothermia is an underreported cause of death in the United States. In most cases, death is attributed to other factors, with hypothermia considered a secondary cause.

The victim's history may be sufficient to determine hypothermia. Hypothermia is likely if a victim is reported by companions to be acting strangely and is shivering after exposure to cold or moisture if he or she has been suddenly immersed in cold water. Predisposing factors are important: drinking alcoholic beverages is commonly associated with hypothermia. A typical scenario involves one or more persons in lightweight garments who drink too much, fall asleep outdoors or in a poorly heated shelter, become chilled by cold air or moisture, and remain exposed for many hours. Certain medications predispose individuals to hypothermia because they interfere with the hypothalamus, which acts as the brain's thermostat in regulating the body's heat.

Especially vulnerable to hypothermia are the very old and the very young. Infants and children have a small muscle mass, so the shivering response is poor in children and nonexistent in infants. They also have less body fat. Younger children need help to protect themselves against the cold since they cannot put on or take off clothes. The less fit are also more likely to become hypothermic.

Types of Exposure

There are three classifications of cold exposure:

- **Acute exposure** (also known as immersion) occurs when the victim loses body heat very rapidly, usually in water. Acute exposure is considered to be 6 hours or less in duration.
- **Subacute exposure** (also known as mountain or exhaustion exposure) occurs when exposure is 6 to 24 hours and can be either land based or in water.
- **Chronic exposure** (also known as urban exposure) involves long-term cooling. It generally occurs on land and exceeds 24 hours.

What to Look For

Consider hypothermia in all victims who have been exposed to cold and who have an altered mental status. Suspect hypothermia in any person who has a temperature reading less than 95°F. (Keep in mind that some thermometers do not measure below that temperature.) Shivering is a good clue, but it may be suppressed when energy stores (glycogen) are depleted. Suspect hypothermia in persons with frostbite and those injured in a cold environment.

Some people die of hypothermia because they or those around them do not recognize the symptoms, which are difficult to recognize in the early stages. Here are some signs to watch for:

- *Change in mental status.* Deteriorated responsiveness or mental status is one of the first symptoms of developing hypothermia. Examples are disorientation, apathy, and changes in personality, such as unusual aggressiveness.

- *Shivering.* Shivering is the first, and most important, body defense against a falling body temperature. *Shivering* starts when the body temperature drops 1°F and *can produce more heat than many rewarming methods.* As the core temperature continues to fall, shivering decreases and usually stops at about 90°F. Shivering also stops as body temperature rises. If shivering stops while responsiveness is decreasing, assume that the core temperature is falling. If, on the other hand, shivering stops while the victim is becoming more coordinated and feeling better, assume that the core temperature is rising.

- *Cool abdomen.* Place the back of your hand between the clothing and the victim's abdomen to assess the victim's temperature. When the victim's abdominal skin under clothing is cooler than your hand, consider the victim hypothermic until proved otherwise.

- *Low core body temperature.* The best indicator of hypothermia is a thermometer reading of the core body temperature. The ability to reliably measure core temperature depends on the availability of an appropriate thermometer and access to the victim's rectum. Normal thermometers do not register below 94°F and so do not indicate whether the hypothermia is mild or severe. Because first aid for mild hypothermia is different from that for severe hypothermia, it is helpful to have a thermometer that registers below 90°F. Oral and axillary (armpit) temperatures are influenced by too many external factors to make them reliable.

- Measuring rectal temperatures in wilderness or remote locations is seldom done, mainly because low-reading rectal thermometers usually are not readily available. Also, taking a rectal temperature can be difficult, inconvenient, and embarrassing to victim and rescuer. If done outdoors, such a procedure can expose the already cold victim.

Types of Hypothermia

The difference between mild and severe hypothermia is based on the core body temperature, but taking a rectal temperature often is not possible. The other most significant difference is that with severe hypothermia the victim becomes so cold that shiv-

ering stops. That means the victim's body cannot rewarm itself internally and will require external heat for recovery.

Victims of mild hypothermia have a core body temperature above 90°F. Symptoms are shivering, slurred speech, memory lapses, and fumbling hands. Victims frequently stumble and stagger, but they are usually conscious and can talk. While many people suffer cold hands and feet, victims of mild hypothermia experience cold abdomens and backs.

Victims of profound or severe hypothermia have a core body temperature below 90°F. Shivering has stopped. Muscles may be stiff and rigid, similar to rigor mortis. The victim's skin is ice cold and has a blue appearance. Pulse and breathing slow down, and the pupils dilate. The victim appears to be dead. Fifty to 80 percent of all profoundly hypothermic victims die.

The National Association of Emergency Medical Service Physicians recommends that CPR *not* be started on a profoundly hypothermic victim if one of the following applies:

- The victim's core body temperature is less than 60°F.
- The victim's chest is frozen (cannot be compressed).
- The victim was submerged in water for more than 60 minutes.
- The victim has a lethal injury.
- Transport for controlled rewarming will be delayed.
- Rescuers are endangered.

For CPR to be effective, heart activity must be restored within a short time, which requires defibrillation, oxygen, and medications. Rescue breathing can be continued for hours when there is a pulse, but chest compressions cannot support circulation very long. CPR is also difficult to continue during a remote setting evacuation.

Also, do *not* start CPR until you have checked the victim's pulse for 30–45 seconds. A hypothermic victim will have an extremely slow pulse rate. CPR can cause cardiac arrest in an already beating heart.

What to Do

1. For all hypothermic victims, stop further heat loss:
   - Get the victim out of the cold.
   - Add insulation (e.g., blankets, towels, pillows, newspapers) beneath and around the victim.

Cover the victim's head (50–80 percent of the body's heat loss is through the head).

- Replace wet clothing with dry clothing.
- Handle the victim gently. Rough handling can cause a cardiac arrest.
- Keep the victim in a horizontal (flat) position. Do *not* raise the legs. (Elevating the legs would cause cold blood from the legs to flow into the body core and adversely affect the heart.)
- Do not let the victim walk or exercise. Do not massage the victim's body. Either activity could drive cold blood from the extremities to the torso and produce what is known as **temperature afterdrop.**

2. Call the EMS for immediate medical transportation. Remember that hypothermia is more common in urban settings than in victims found in the wilderness.

3. For mild hypothermia in a remote or wilderness location, the goal is to prevent further heat loss. If protected from further heat loss, most mildly hypothermic victims are able to rewarm themselves by shivering, which generates heat.

4. For profound or severe hypothermia in a remote or wilderness situation:
   - Check the victim's ABCs (airway, breathing, circulation). Take 30 to 45 seconds to check the pulse before starting CPR.
   - Evacuate the victim by helicopter. Rewarming in a remote location is difficult and rarely effective.

   Remember: *The best care can be summarized simply as: Rescue, examine, insulate, and transport.*

Adding heat to a victim is extremely difficult. The longer the victim has been exposed to the cold, the longer it will take to raise the core temperature to normal. Trying to rewarm a hypothermic victim may cause a cardiac arrest.

Although surface rewarming suppresses shivering, it may be the only option when the victim is far from medical care. In that case, the victim must be warmed by any available external heat source.

There are problems with the commonly recommended rewarming methods*. *Warm water immersion* requires a lot of warm water (no hotter than 106°F) and a bathtub—both rarely found in remote locations. Hot baths can produce rapid changes in the blood that can produce cardiac arrest.

*Bruce C. Paton, MD, "Field Treatment of Hypothermia," Second World Congress on Wilderness Medicine, Wilderness Medical Society, 1995.

Recent studies show that *body-to-body* contact in an insulated sleeping bag is ineffective for rewarming. Reasons why include the following:

- All the heat produced by the rescuer's body is not enough to rewarm a victim. For example, heat loss of adults cooled to 91°F exceeds 300 kcal; heat production of a rescuer is only 100 kcal per hour.
- There usually is only a small amount (less than 50 percent) of direct skin contact, which is essential for effective heat transfer, between the victim and the rescuer.
- The victim's peripheral blood vessel constriction may impair heat transfer to the body's core.
- Skin warming may slow the victim's shivering response, which effectively rewarms the body.

Despite the problems, there are some reasons to use body-to-body contact:

- It may provide a psychological benefit to a victim.
- The victim, as a result of chronic cold exposure or physical exhaustion, may have depleted the body's energy stores (glycogen) and cannot shiver.
- The victim's thermoregulatory control may be impaired because of old age, alcohol ingestion, or brain or spine injury; thus, the victim cannot shiver.

Because skin rewarming suppresses shivering, which slows the rate of core rewarming, body-to-body rewarming should be used only when there will be a long delay in getting the victim to medical care and when more appropriate methods of adding heat are unavailable.

Several types of *chemical heating pads* are on the market. While they may be effective for warming hands and feet, there is no evidence that they are capable of rewarming a hypothermic victim. For example, one type of heating pad is 7 inches by 9 inches and provides 14.5 kcal total heat, with a maximum temperature of about 125°F. A minimum of 20 pads would be needed to provide enough heat to rewarm a 91°F victim, even if heat transfer were 100-percent efficient. This method may stop the desirable effects of shivering, still leaving the victim hypothermic.

Warm drinks have no warming effect and contain little energy. Warm drinks signal the brain to send more blood to the skin. Dilation of the skin's blood vessels produces a warm feeling but causes

HYPOTHERMIA

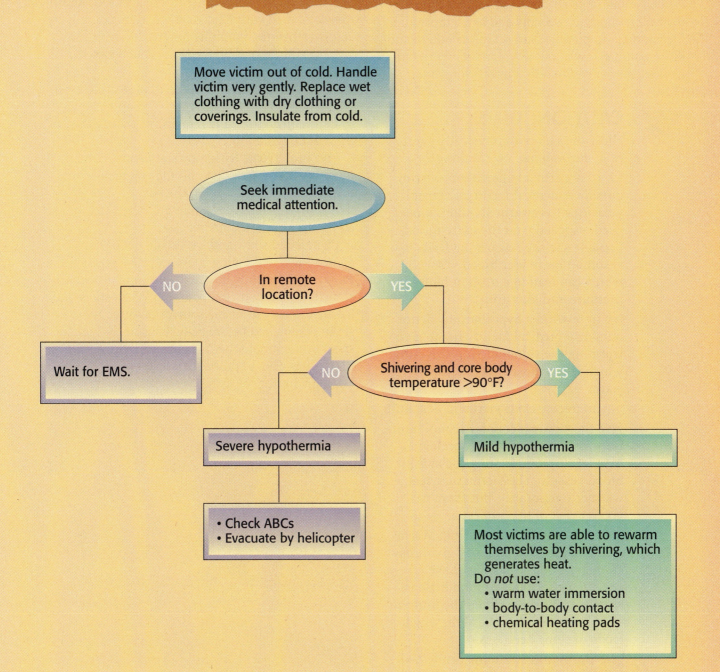

Move victim out of cold. Handle victim very gently. Replace wet clothing with dry clothing or coverings. Insulate from cold.

Seek immediate medical attention.

In remote location?

NO — Wait for EMS.

YES — Shivering and core body temperature >90°F?

NO — Severe hypothermia
- Check ABCs
- Evacuate by helicopter

YES — Mild hypothermia

Most victims are able to rewarm themselves by shivering, which generates heat.
Do *not* use:
- warm water immersion
- body-to-body contact
- chemical heating pads

some heat loss since the capillaries are dilated. Warm drinks taste good and provide a psychological boost, but to be effective it would take more than the stomach could hold and at a temperature high enough to produce burns. On the other hand, if the victim can swallow, fluids are highly recommended since dehydration is usually present.

CAUTION: DO NOT

- allow the victim to physically exert (e.g., no walking, no climbing).
- try to rewarm a hypothermic victim outside a medical facility. External measures to rewarm should not be used, especially on the extremities, because surface rewarming leads to vasodilation (wider blood vessels), which can lead to a drop in blood pressure and afterdrop.
- try to rewarm a hypothermic victim outside a medical facility because rewarming the skin will stop shivering, which is the most effective way to rewarm.
- put an unconscious victim in a bathtub.
- give the victim alcohol. Alcohol interferes with shivering and accelerates heat loss by vasodilating the skin's blood vessels. The victim may feel warmer temporarily, but there is a greater risk of hypothermia.
- give the victim a warm drink. Warm drinks taste good and may give a psychological boost, but they have no warming effect and contain little energy. Warm drinks signal the brain to send more blood to the skin, which leads to some heat loss.
- give the victim a caffeine drink. Caffeine has a diuretic effect, and the victim probably is already dehydrated.
- rub or massage the victim's arms or legs. Rubbing the skin suppresses shivering, dilates the skin's blood vessels (resulting in more heat loss), and produces temperature afterdrop.
- raise the victim's legs, which allows cold blood from the legs to flow into the body core and adversely affect the heart. Keep the victim in a flat position.

Dehydration

Dehydration occurs because of unperceived fluid loss combined with inadequate fluid intake. In very cold weather, the humidity approaches zero, and large quantities of fluid are lost through exhaled breath.

People in a cold environment must drink even when they are not thirsty. Inactive people in comfortable climates need two quarts of water a day to prevent dehydration.

An individual's hydration status can be monitored by noting the color and the volume of the urine. The lighter the color, the better hydrated; dark yellow urine is a definite indication that fluid consumption should be increased.

Unmelted snow and ice should *not* be consumed for water. Eating snow and ice irritates the mouth, wastes body heat, and, if enough is consumed, lowers body temperature. When snow and ice are the only available sources of water, they should be melted before being consumed. Melted snow or ice should not be considered drinkable until it has been appropriately disinfected (i.e., by boiling, filtering, or using chemicals).

HEAT-RELATED EMERGENCIES

When the temperature goes up, a multitude of problems can—and do—arise. Given the right (or wrong) conditions, anyone can get heat illness. Some victims are lucky enough to suffer only from heat cramps, while less fortunate ones may be laid low by heat exhaustion or devastated by heatstroke.

How the Body Stays Cool

The human body is constantly engaged in a life-and-death struggle to disperse the heat that it produces. If allowed to accumulate, the heat would quickly increase your body temperature beyond its comfortable 98.6°F. That does not normally happen, because your body is able to lose enough heat to maintain a steady temperature. Usually, you are aware of this struggle only during hard labor or exercise in a hot environment, when your body produces heat faster than it can lose heat. In certain circumstances, your body can build up too much heat, your temperature may rise to life-threatening levels, and you can become delirious or lose consciousness. This condition is called **heatstroke** and is a serious medical emergency. If you do not rid your body of excess heat fast enough, it "cooks" the brain and other vital organs. It is often fatal, and those who do survive may have permanent damage to their vital organs. Before your temperature reaches heatstroke level, however, you may suffer **heat exhaustion** with its flu-like symptoms. By treating the symptoms of heat exhaustion, you avoid heatstroke.

How does the body dispose of excess heat? Humans lose heat largely through their skin, much as a car loses heat through its radiator. Exercising muscles warm the blood, just like the car's hot engine warms its radiator fluid. Warm blood travels through the skin's dilated blood vessels, losing heat by evaporating sweat to the surrounding air, just like a car losing engine heat through the radiator.

When blood delivers heat to the skin, the body loses heat primarily in two ways: radiation and evaporation (vaporization of sweat). When the air temperature is 70°F or less, the body releases its heat into the surroundings by radiation. As the environmental temperature approaches the body's temperature, however, heat loss through radiation is greatly reduced. In fact, people working or exercising on a hot summer day actually gain heat through radiation from the sun. That leaves evaporation as the only way to effectively control body temperature.

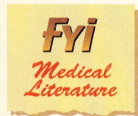
Water Loss

Water makes up about 50–60 percent of an adult's body weight. You lose about 2 quarts every day through breathing, urinating, bowel movements, and sweat. That lost fluid must be replaced. Although the amount of water used each day varies from person to person, an adult requires about 2 quarts a day from water, beverages, and food (about 70 percent of most food is water). Sweat produced by a working adult can reach 2 to 3 quarts an hour for short periods and up to 10 to 15 quarts a day. When the body's water absorption rate of 1.5 quarts per hour is pitted against a 2-quart sweat rate, **dehydration** results—drinking water cannot keep up with sweat losses.

If you drink only when you are thirsty, you are already dehydrated. Thirst is not a good guide for when to drink water. In fact, in hot and humid conditions, people may be so dehydrated by the time they become thirsty that they have trouble catching up with their fluid losses. One guideline regarding water intake is to monitor urine output. You are getting enough water if you are producing clear urine at least five times a day. Cloudy or dark urine or urinating fewer than five times a day means you probably should drink more.

If possible while working, especially in hot weather, drink one cup (8 ounces) of water every 20 minutes. Usually, one pint (16 ounces) is the most a person can comfortably drink at once. It takes time for water to pass from the stomach into the blood, so you cannot catch up by drinking extra water later; about one quart of water per hour can pass out of the stomach.

Cool water (50°F) is easier for the stomach to absorb than warm water, and a little flavoring may make the water more tasty. The best fluids are those that leave the stomach fast and contain little sodium and some sugar (less than 8 percent). Coffee and tea should be avoided because they contain caffeine, a diuretic that increases water loss through urination. Alcoholic beverages also dehydrate by increasing urination. Soda pop contains about 10 percent sugar and therefore is not absorbed as well as water or commercial sports drinks (which contain about 5 to 8 percent sugar). Fruit juices range from 11 to 18 percent sugar and have an even longer absorption time.

Electrolyte Loss

Sweat and urine contain potassium and sodium, essential electrolytes that control the movement of water in and out of the body's cells. These electrolytes can be found in many everyday foods. Bananas and nuts are rich in potassium, and most American diets have up to 10 times as much sodium as the body needs. Acclimatizing to heat can also reduce sodium loss tenfold. Getting enough salt (sodium chloride) rarely is a problem in the typical American diet. In fact, most Americans consume an excessive amount of sodium, averaging 5 to 10 grams of sodium per day, although we probably require only 1 to 3 grams. Sodium loss, therefore, is seldom a problem, unless a person is sweating profusely for long periods and drinking large amounts of water (more than 1 quart an hour).

Most people require only water most of the time. Commercial sports drinks can be useful if you are participating in vigorous physical activity longer than one hour. The human body needs water more

Water Intoxication in Grand Canyon Hikers Water intoxication (hyponatremia) has been reported in athletes participating in marathon and ultramarathon events. Water intoxication results from sweat loss replaced with plain water. Differentiating water intoxication from heat exhaustion is difficult. Recreational wilderness hikers performing sustained exercise in the heat may require electrolyte replacement similar to endurance athletes.

Source: H. Backer et al., "Hyponatremia in Recreational Hikers in Grand Canyon National Park," *Journal of Wilderness Medicine* 4:391–406 (November 1993).

than it needs salt. Whenever extra sodium is added to your diet, drink more water. Otherwise, excessive sodium can draw water out of the body cells, accelerating dehydration.

Drinking large amounts of water (more than 1 quart an hour) and profuse sweating for long periods can lead to a condition called **water intoxication,** in which electrolytes are flushed from the body. Symptoms of water intoxication include frequent urination and behavior changes (irrationality, combativeness, seizures, and coma).

Effects of Humidity

Sweat can cool the body only if it evaporates (vaporizes). In dry air, you will not notice sweat evaporating. In high humidity, no sweat can evaporate. It just drips off the skin, without cooling the body. At about 75-percent humidity, sweating is ineffective in cooling the body.

Because humidity can significantly reduce evaporative cooling, a very humid but mildly warm day can be more stressful than a very hot, dry day. The higher the humidity, the lower the temperature at which heat risk begins, especially for those individuals who are generating heat with vigorous work.

Who Is at Risk?

Everyone is susceptible to heat illness if environmental conditions overwhelm the body's temperature-regulating mechanisms. Heat waves can set the

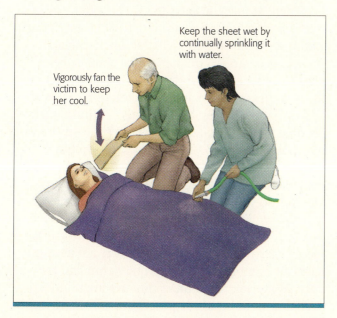

Vigorously fan the victim to keep her cool.

Keep the sheet wet by continually sprinkling it with water.

Spraying with water and fanning are effective in low humidity conditions.

Hot-Weather Precautions

These simple preventive measures can reduce heat stress:

1. Keep as cool as possible.
   - Avoid direct sunlight.
   - Stay in the coolest available location (usually indoors).
   - Use air-conditioning, if available.
   - Use electric fans to promote cooling.
   - Place wet towels or ice bags on the body or dampen clothing.
   - Take cool baths or showers.
2. Wear lightweight, loose-fitting clothing.
3. Avoid strenuous physical activity, particularly in the sun and during the hottest part of the day.
4. Increase intake of fluids, such as water and fruit or vegetable juices. Thirst is not always a good indicator of adequacy of fluid intake. Some studies indicate that fluid intake in hot weather should be 1½ times the amount that quenches thirst. Persons who are overweight or large in build or who engage in strenuous activities, such as sports, may require more than a gallon of fluid intake daily in very hot weather. Persons for whom salt or fluid is restricted should consult their physicians for instructions on appropriate fluid and salt intake.
5. Do not take salt tablets unless so instructed by a physician.
6. Avoid alcoholic beverages (beer, wine, and liquor).
7. Stay in daily contact with other people.

Source: Morbidity and Morality Weekly Report.

stage for a rash of heatstroke victims. For example, in the 1995 Chicago heat wave, the death toll reached 591 in five days. Several groups are at particular risk, including the obese, the chronically ill, and alcoholics.

The elderly are at higher risk because of their impaired cardiac output and decreased ability to sweat. Infants and young children also are susceptible to heatstroke. Children (and pets) are especially vulnerable when they are left in automobiles that overheat in shopping center parking lots. The temperature in a parked car can soar to 150°F, even when a window is slightly open. The fluid loss and dehydration resulting from physical activity put outdoor laborers and athletes at particular risk.

Certain medications predispose individuals to heatstroke. They include drugs that alter sweat production (e.g., antihistamines, antipsychotics, antidepressants) or interfere with thermoregulation.

Heat Illnesses

Several disorders exist along a spectrum of heat illnesses. Some of them are common, but only heatstroke is life threatening. Untreated heatstroke victims always die.

Heat Cramps

Heat cramps are painful muscular spasms that happen suddenly. They usually involve the back of the leg muscles (calf and hamstring muscles) or the abdominal muscles. They tend to happen immediately after exertion and some experts claim they are caused by salt depletion. Victims may be drinking water without adequate salt content. However, some experts disagree because the typical American diet is heavy with salt.

Heat Exhaustion

Heat exhaustion is characterized by heavy perspiration with normal or slightly above normal body temperatures. It is caused by water or salt depletion or both. Some experts believe that a better term would be severe dehydration. Heat exhaustion affects workers and athletes who do not drink enough fluids while working or exercising in hot environments. Symptoms include severe thirst, fatigue, headache, nausea, vomiting, and sometimes diarrhea. The affected person often mistakenly believes he or she has the flu. Uncontrolled heat exhaustion can evolve into heatstroke.

Heatstroke

Two types of heatstroke exist: classic and exertional. **Classic heatstroke,** also known as the "slow cooker," may take days to develop. It is often seen during summer heat waves and typically affects poor, elderly, chronically ill, alcoholic, or obese persons. Because the elderly, often with medical problems, are frequently afflicted, this type of heatstroke has a 50-percent death rate even with medical care. It results from a combination of a hot environment and dehydration. **Exertional heatstroke** is also more common in the summer. It is frequently seen

Table 19.1: Classic or Exertional Heatstroke?		
Characteristics	**Classic**	**Exertional**
Age group usually affected?	Elderly	Men aged 15–45 years
Claims many victims at the same time?	During heat waves	During athletic competition
Health status of victims?	Chronically ill	Healthy and physically fit
Activity at the time of incident?	Sedentary	Strenuous exercise
Medication use?	Common	Usually none
Sweating?	Absent	Often present (50% of victims)

in athletes, laborers, and military personnel, all of whom often sweat profusely. This type of heatstroke is known as the "fast cooker." It affects healthy, active individuals strenuously working or playing in a warm environment. Because its rapid onset does not allow enough time for severe dehydration to occur, 50 percent of exertional heatstroke victims usually are sweating. (Classic heatstroke victims are not sweating.)

There are several ways to tell the difference between heat exhaustion and heatstroke. First, if the victim's body feels extremely hot when touched, suspect heatstroke. Another major mark of heatstroke is altered mental status (behavior), ranging from slight confusion and disorientation to coma. Between those extreme conditions, victims usually become irrational, agitated, or even aggressive and may have seizures. In severe cases, the victim can go into a coma in less than an hour. The longer a coma lasts, the less the chance for survival.

A third way to distinguish heatstroke from heat exhaustion is by rectal temperature. That is not very practical, however, because a conscious heatstroke victim may not cooperate. Taking a rectal temperature can be embarrassing to both victim and rescuer. Moreover, rectal thermometers are seldom available, and the whole procedure of finding the right thermometer and then using it wastes time and distracts from important emergency care.

Other Heat Illnesses

Less serious heat illnesses include heat syncope, heat edema, and prickly heat:

- **Heat syncope,** in which a person becomes dizzy or faints after exposure to high temperatures, is a self-limiting condition. Victims should lie down in a cool place and, if not nauseated, drink water.
- **Heat edema,** which is also a self-limiting condition, causes the ankles and feet to swell from heat exposure. It is more common in women unacclimatized to a hot climate. It is related to salt and water retention and tends to disappear after acclimatization. Wearing support stockings and elevating the legs may help reduce the swelling.
- **Prickly heat,** also known as a heat rash, is an itchy rash that develops because of unevaporated moisture on skin wet from sweating. Treat by drying and cooling the skin.

What to Do

Heat Cramps

To relieve heat cramps (it may take several hours), follow these steps:

1. Rest in a cool place.
2. Drink lightly salted cool water (dissolve ¼ teaspoon salt in a quart of water) or a commercial sports drink. (A commercial sports drink is easier to absorb if diluted to half strength to reduce the sugar content.)
3. Stretch the cramped calf muscle. Also, try an acupressure method: pinch the upper lip just below the nose.

Heat Exhaustion

1. Move the victim immediately out of the heat to a cool place.
2. Give cool liquids, adding electrolytes (lightly salted water or a commercial sports drink) if plain water does not improve the victim's condition in 20 minutes. Do not give salt tablets; they can irritate the stomach and cause nausea and vomiting.
3. Raise the victims legs 8 to 12 inches (keep the legs straight).
4. Remove excess clothing.
5. Sponge with cool water and fan the victim.
6. If no improvement is seen within 30 minutes, seek medical attention.

Table 19.2: Heat Illnesses

Condition	Symptoms	What to Do
Heat cramps	Painful muscle spasms Sweaty skin Normal body temperature	1. Sit or lie down in the shade. 2. Drink cool, lightly salted water or sports drink. 3. Stretch affected muscles.
Heat exhaustion	Profuse sweating Flu-like symptoms Clammy or pale skin Dizziness Nausea, vomiting Rapid pulse Thirst Normal or slightly above normal body temperature	1. Treat mild cases the same as heat cramps (except do not stretch the muscles). 2. If persistent, gently apply wet towels and call EMS.
Heatstroke	Unresponsiveness (if responsive, victim will be confused, stagger, be agitated) Hot skin, which can be dry or wet	1. Move person to a half-sitting position in the shade. 2. Call EMS. 3. If humidity below 75%, spray victim with water and vigorously fan. If humidity above 75%, apply ice packs on neck, armpits, groin.

Heatstroke

Heatstroke is a medical emergency and must be treated rapidly! Every minute delayed increases the likelihood of serious complications or death.

1. Move the victim immediately out of the heat to a cool place.
2. Remove clothing down to the victim's underwear.
3. Keep the victim's head and shoulders slightly elevated.

4. Seek immediate medical attention, even if the victim seems to be recovering.

5. The only way to prevent damage is to cool the victim quickly and by any means possible. Cooling methods include the following:
   - An *ice bath* cools a victim quickly, but it requires a great deal of ice—at least 80 pounds—to be effective. The need for a big enough tub also limits this method.
   - A *cool water bath* (less than 60°F) can be successful if the water is stirred to prevent a warm layer from forming around the body. This is the most effective method in high-humidity (greater than 75 percent) conditions.
   - *Spraying* the victim with water and then *fanning* him or her is another method for cooling the body. The water droplets act as artificial sweat and cool through evaporation. This method is *not* effective in high-humidity (greater than 75 percent) conditions.
   - *Ice bags* wrapped in wet towels and placed against the large veins in the groin, armpits, and sides of the neck also cool the body, although not nearly as fast as immersion.

CAUTION: DO NOT

- delay initiating cooling while waiting for an ambulance. The longer the delay, the greater the risk of tissue damage and prolonged hospitalization.

- continue cooling after the victim's mental status has improved. Unnecessary cooling could lead to hypothermia.

- use rubbing alcohol to cool the skin. It can be absorbed into the blood and cause alcohol poisoning. Also, the vapors are a potential fire hazard.

- give the victim aspirin or acetaminophen. The brain's control center is not elevated, as it is with fever caused by diseases, so these products are not effective in lowering body temperature.

Preventing Heat Illness

Most heat illness occurs during the first days of working in the heat, so the main preventive measure is acclimatization (adjusting to heat). To better handle the heat, the body adjusts by decreasing the salt content in sweat and increasing the sweating rate.

Year-round exercise can help workers prepare for hot weather. Such activity raises the body's core temperature so it becomes accustomed to heat. Full acclimatization, however, requires exercise in hot weather. That can be accomplished by a minimum of 60 to 90 minutes of exercise in the heat each day for one to two weeks.

The acclimatized heart is able to pump more blood with each stroke than a heart not used to working in the heat. Sweating starts earlier, and the amount of sweat per hour doubles, from 1.5 quarts to 3 quarts or more.

Workers who live in a constantly hot climate have an advantage over those living in cooler temperatures.

Heat illnesses are avoidable. With knowledge, preparation, fluid replacement, and prompt emergency care, there is no need for heat illness to affect people working in warm weather. The following measures can help prevent heat illnesses:

- Avoid dehydration. A good rule of thumb for fluid replacement is to drink one cup (8 ounces) every 20 minutes while working.
- Dress in light-colored porous, loose-fitting clothing, which reflects heat, facilitates evaporative heat loss, and allows air to circulate around your body.
- Rest frequently, preferably in shade. This applies especially if you are not fully acclimatized, are older, are markedly overweight, or have heart disease.
- Wipe cool water on exposed areas of the skin.
- Dip clothing periodically in water.

HEAT-RELATED EMERGENCIES

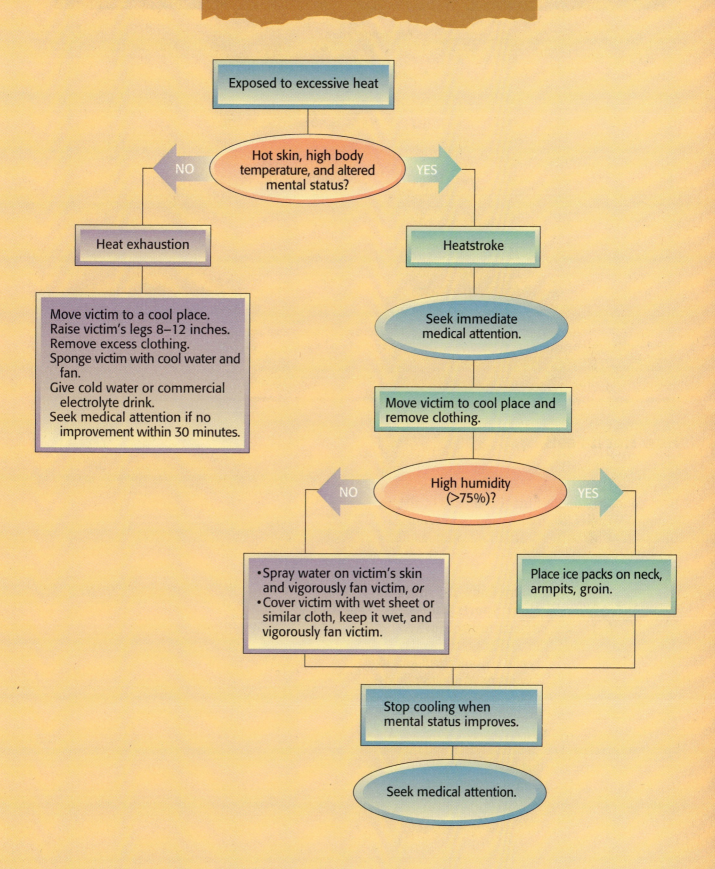

Exposed to excessive heat

Hot skin, high body temperature, and altered mental status?

NO → Heat exhaustion

Move victim to a cool place.
Raise victim's legs 8–12 inches.
Remove excess clothing.
Sponge victim with cool water and fan.
Give cold water or commercial electrolyte drink.
Seek medical attention if no improvement within 30 minutes.

YES → Heatstroke

Seek immediate medical attention.

Move victim to cool place and remove clothing.

High humidity (>75%)?

NO
• Spray water on victim's skin and vigorously fan victim, *or*
• Cover victim with wet sheet or similar cloth, keep it wet, and vigorously fan victim.

YES
Place ice packs on neck, armpits, groin.

Stop cooling when mental status improves.

Seek medical attention.

Table 19-3: Heat Index

Relative Humidity, %	Air Temperature, °F										
	70	75	80	85	90	95	100	105	110	115	120
	Apparent Temperature, °F										
0	64	69	73	78	83	87	91	95	99	103	107
10	65	70	75	80	85	90	95	100	105	111	116
20	66	72	77	82	87	93	99	105	112	120	130
30	67	73	78	84	90	96	104	113	123	135	148
40	68	74	79	86	93	101	110	123	137	151	
50	69	75	81	88	96	107	120	135	150		
60	70	76	82	90	100	114	132	149			
70	70	77	85	93	106	124	144				
80	71	78	86	97	113	136					
90	71	79	88	102	122						
100	72	80	91	108							

Above 130°F = heatstroke imminent
105°–130°F = heat exhaustion and heat cramps likely; heatstroke with long exposure and activity
90°–105°F = heat exhaustion and heat cramps with long exposure and activity
80°–90°F = fatigue during exposure and activity

Source: National Weather Service.

How Hot It Feels

Under normal conditions, temperature and humidity are the most important elements influencing body comfort. The Heat Index compiled by the National Weather Service lists **apparent temperatures**—how hot it feels—at various combinations of temperature and humidity.

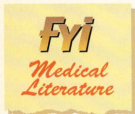

Water Loss: Do Athletes Need Sports Drinks?

An athlete who burns 4,000 to 5,000 calories per day needs to drink about four to five quarts of water or fluids. Water is best for people who work out for less than an hour. But for prolonged endurance exercise, sports drinks are better—they are absorbed slightly faster than water, and they replace carbohydrates that fuel the muscles.

Source: N. Clark, "Water: The Ultimate Nutrient," *Physician and Sportsmedicine* 23:21 (May 1995).

NOTES

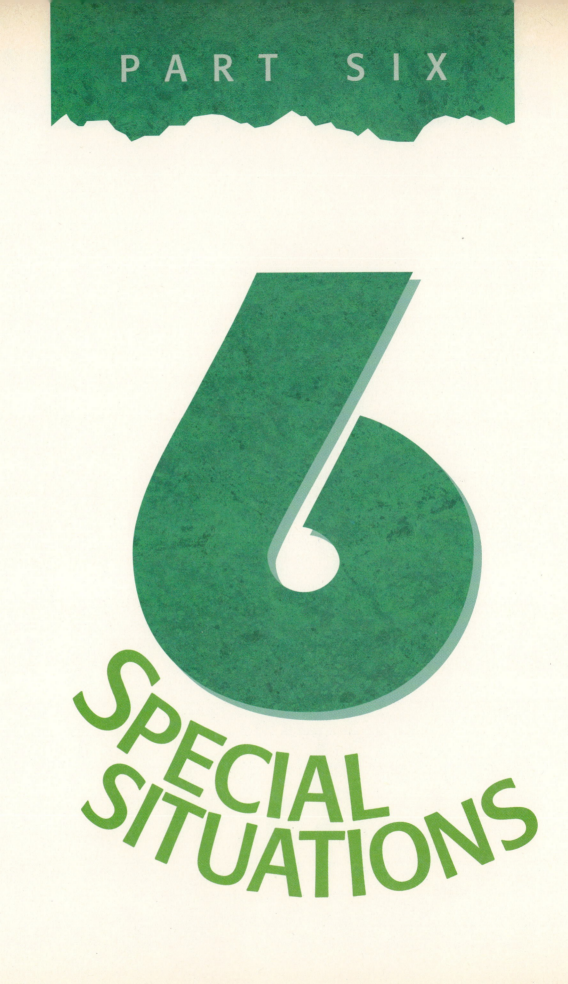

PART SIX

SPECIAL SITUATIONS

CHAPTER 20
Childbirth and Gynecologic Emergencies

CHAPTER 21
Behavioral Emergencies

CHAPTER 22
Wilderness Emergencies

CHAPTER 23
Rescuing and Moving Victims

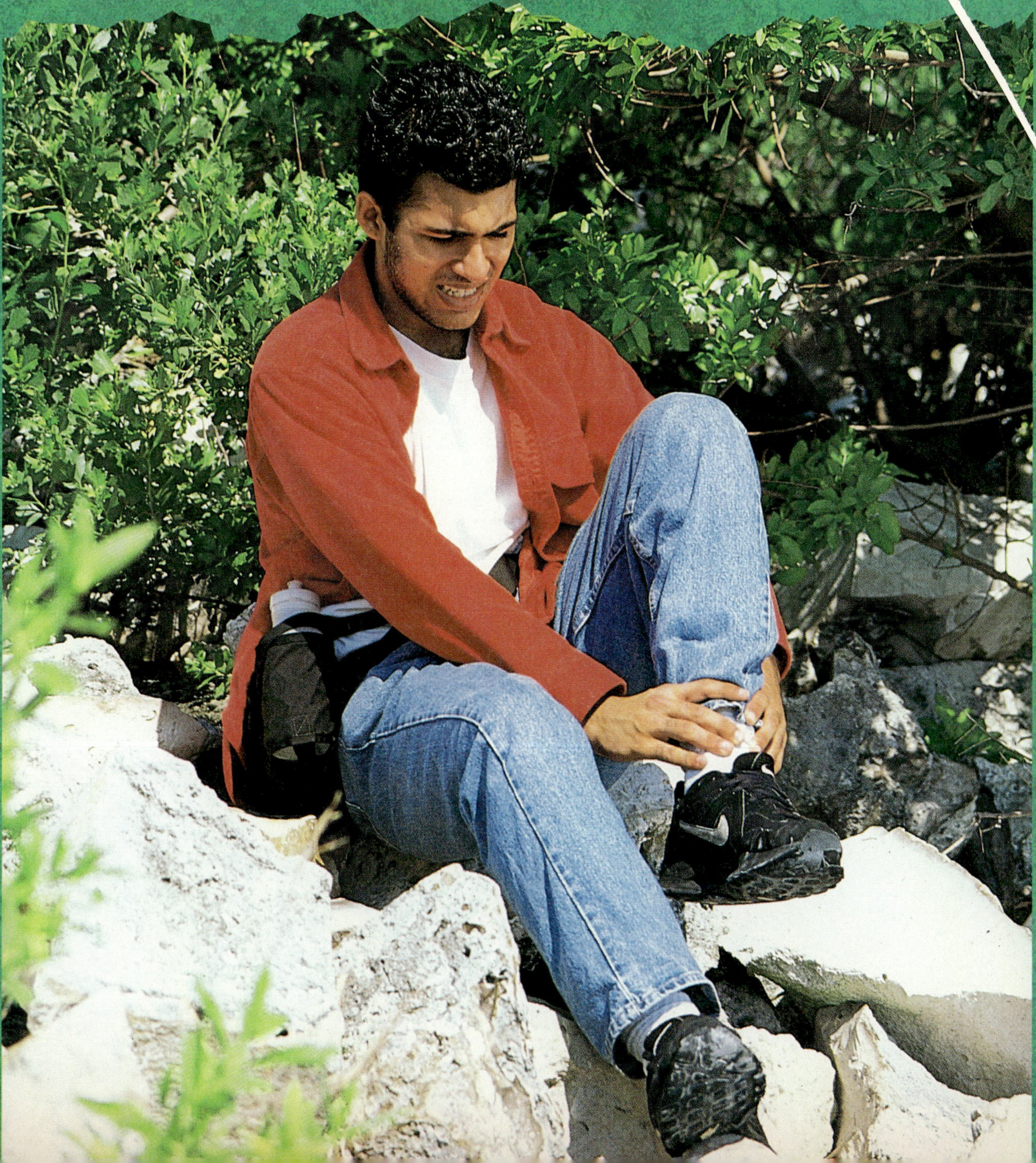

20

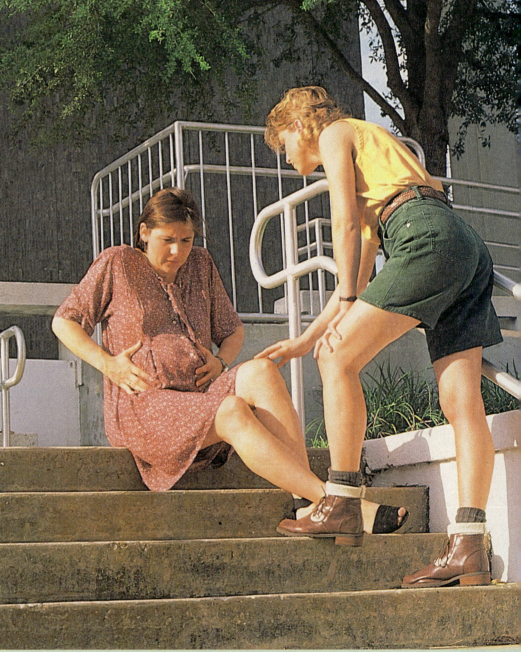

CHILDBIRTH AND GYNECOLOGIC EMERGENCIES

Handling emergency childbirth and gynecologic situations requires familiarity with the terminology used to describe female reproductive anatomy and physiology.

- The **birth canal** includes the vagina and lower part of the uterus.
- The **cervix** is the small opening at the lower end of the uterus through which the baby passes.
- The **placenta** (afterbirth) is the organ through which the mother and the fetus exchange nourishment and waste products during pregnancy. It is expelled after the baby's birth.
- The **umbilical cord** is the extension of the placenta through which the fetus receives nourishment while in the uterus.
- The **amniotic sac** ("bag of waters") surrounds the fetus inside the uterus. **Amniotic fluid** in the sac cushions the fetus and helps protect it from injury.
- **Crowning** is the bulging out of the vagina, which is opening as the fetus's head or presenting part presses against it.
- **Bloody show** is the mucus and blood that may be discharged from the vagina as labor begins.
- **Labor** is the time and the process of childbirth (defined in three stages), beginning with the first regular uterine-muscle contractions until delivery of the placenta.
- A **miscarriage** (medical term is **spontaneous abortion**) is the delivery of a fetus before it can live independently of the mother.

Predelivery Emergencies

Miscarriage

Miscarriages usually occur during the first three months (first trimester) of pregnancy. The signs and symptoms of a threatened miscarriage include vaginal bleeding and pain that resembles menstrual cramps. Signs of an inevitable miscarriage include heavy vaginal bleeding and uterine contractions. Gently remove anything (fetal tissue) protruding from the vagina. Apply sanitary pads over the outside of the vagina. Take fetal tissues to the hospital.

Vaginal Bleeding in Late Pregnancy

If a woman has vaginal bleeding late in her pregnancy (third trimester), save the pads so that medical personnel can estimate the amount of blood lost. What may seem like an alarming amount may be insignificant. The victim should be asked how long she has been bleeding and how many sanitary pads she has used. An increase in pulse rate of more than 20 beats per minute when the victim goes from a lying-down to a sitting position suggests blood loss greater than one pint. Should that be the case, treat the victim for shock by raising her legs 8 to 12 inches. Seek medical attention.

Vaginal Bleeding Caused by Trauma

External vaginal bleeding caused by trauma usually can be controlled by applying external pressure over the laceration. Internal vaginal bleeding, however, can be massive. It is both useless and dangerous to introduce packs blindly into the vagina in an attempt to control bleeding. A pack should be used *only* if bleeding is life threatening. Place the victim on her left side to help prevent vomiting, to prevent aspiration of vomitus, and to relieve pressure the fetus places on the mother's circulatory system (vena cava). Seek medical attention.

Delivery

Childbirth in an out-of-hospital setting rarely occurs. Because of the infrequency, taking care of an anxious mother and her newborn infant is a stressful event for a first aider. On the other hand, assisting in the birth of a baby is one of the few situations in which first aiders have the opportunity to participate in a happy event rather than an unpleasant one.

At the scene of a woman in labor, you will need to determine if delivery is imminent or whether there is time to transport the woman to the hospital. To make that decision, answer the following questions:

- *Has the woman had a baby before?* Labor during a first pregnancy is usually longer than in subse-

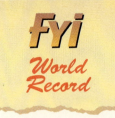

Heaviest Single Birth
Big babies (i.e., those over 10 lb.) are usually born to mothers who are large or overweight or have some medical problem such as diabetes. The heaviest baby born to a healthy mother was a boy weighing 22 lb. 8 oz. who was born to Carmelina Fedele of Aversa, Italy, in September 1955.

Source: The Guinness Book of Records. New York: Bantam Books, 1995, p. 10.

quent pregnancies. For a first pregnancy, there may be more time for transport to a hospital.

- *How frequent are the contractions?* Contractions more than five minutes apart are a good indication that there will be enough time to get the mother to a nearby hospital. Contractions less than two minutes apart and 45 to 60 seconds long, especially in a woman who has had more than one pregnancy, signal imminent delivery.

- *Has the amniotic sac ruptured? If so, when?* If the sac ruptures more than 18 hours before birth occurs, the likelihood of fetal infection is increased, and the hospital staff should be alerted. Delivery may be more difficult when the amniotic sac has ruptured prematurely, because amniotic fluid serves as a lubricant.

- *Does the mother feel as though she has to move her bowels?* That sensation is caused by the fetal head in the vagina pressing against the rectum and indicates that delivery is imminent.

Only if the answers to those questions seem to indicate an imminent birth should you examine the mother for crowning, that is, look to see if there is bulging at the vaginal opening or if part of the baby is visible. Crowning indicates that the baby is about

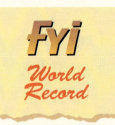

Lightest Single Birth   A premature baby girl weighing 9.9 oz. was reported to have been born on 27 June 1989 at the Loyola University Medical Center in Illinois.

Source: The Guinness Book of Records. New York: Bantam Books, 1995, p. 10.

to be born and that there is no time to get to a hospital before delivery. Because this step may be embarrassing to the mother, the father, bystanders, even you, it is important that you explain fully what you are doing and why. Make every effort to protect the woman from embarrassment during such an examination by removing only enough clothing to expose the vaginal area.

Consider transporting the woman to a hospital only if she is not straining or crowning and this is her first pregnancy. Making a hasty decision to transport the woman means that the delivery could take place under the worst possible circumstances. When there is enough time to transport the woman to a hospital, place her on her left side. That position prevents a possible drop in blood pressure caused by pressure on the inferior vena cava (large vein between the spine and the abdominal organs), which reduces venous blood returning to the heart.

CAUTION: DO NOT

- allow the mother to go to the toilet if delivery seems imminent.
- attempt to delay or restrain delivery in any way (e.g., holding the mother's legs together).

If the woman is straining or crowning, has had prior pregnancies, and there is not enough time to get to the hospital, you must prepare to assist in the delivery. First, call (or have a bystander call) the EMS. Then, if the woman is in a crowded or public place, try to find a private, clean area. The mother may find it reassuring to have a companion, such as her husband, a friend, or a relative present. Follow these guidelines:

- Wear disposable latex gloves. If available, wear mask, gown, and eye protection.
- Do not touch the vaginal area except during delivery and, if possible, with a witness present.
- Do not let the mother use the toilet.
- Do not hold the mother's legs together.

If the baby's head is not the presenting part, the delivery may be complicated. Tell the mother not to push and attempt to calm and reassure her.

Stages of Labor

Labor is a three-stage process that begins with the first regular uterine contractions, includes delivery of the baby, and ends with delivery of the placenta. The first stage usually lasts several hours (possibly 18 hours or more for a first baby), from the first contraction until the cervix is fully open (dilated). The cervix gradually stretches until it is large enough to let the baby pass through. (Outside a hospital setting, rescuers cannot safely check for dilation of the cervix.) The contractions usually begin as acutely aching sensations in the small of the back; in a short time, they turn into cramp-like pains recurring regularly in the lower abdomen. At first, the contractions are 10 to 15 minutes apart, are not very severe, and last less than a minute. Gradually, the intervals between contractions grow shorter, and the contractions increase in intensity. A slight, watery, bloodstained discharge from the vagina may accompany contractions or may occur before labor begins.

At the end of the first stage of labor, the amniotic sac breaks, and a pint or more of watery fluid, the amniotic fluid, discharges. Sometimes the amniotic sac breaks during the first stage of labor, which is no cause for concern because it usually does not affect labor. If the amniotic sac breaks prematurely and labor does not begin within 12 hours, the risk of infection to mother and baby is great.

The second stage lasts about 30 minutes to 2 hours. It begins when the neck of the cervix is fully open and ends with the actual birth of the baby. The baby is normally head down; as the head gets through the pelvis, the rest of the body should follow easily.

During the third stage, which lasts about 15 minutes or more, the afterbirth (placenta) is expelled.

Delivery Procedures

Ideally, you should have the following supplies for delivery:

- clean sheets, towels, and blankets to cover the mother and baby.
- a plastic bag or towel to wrap the placenta for delivery to the hospital.
- clean, unused, disposable latex gloves to reduce the likelihood of infection.
- sanitary pads.
- newspapers, plastic, or a cloth sheet to place

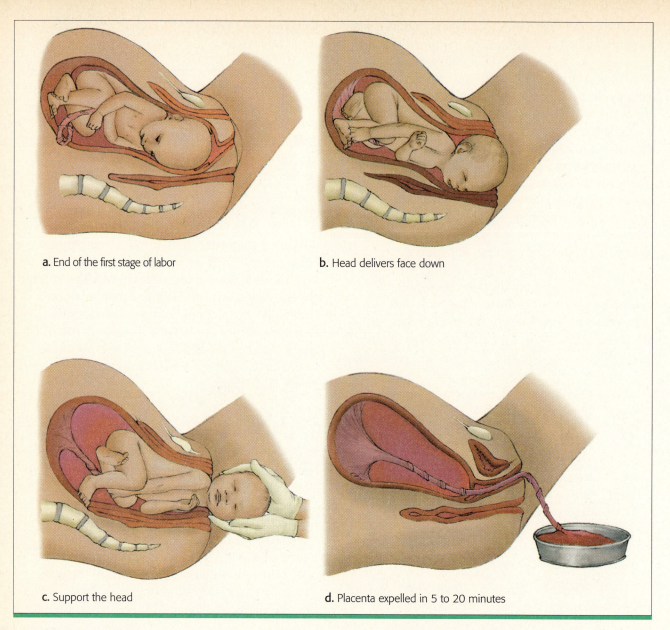

a. End of the first stage of labor

b. Head delivers face down

c. Support the head

d. Placenta expelled in 5 to 20 minutes

Normal stages of childbirth

under the woman to provide for a clean delivery area.

- rubber bulb syringe for suctioning the baby's mouth and nostrils.
- sterile gauze pads for wiping blood and mucus from the baby's mouth and nose.
- new or clean shoelaces or similar materials to tie the cord. (Do not use thread, wire, or string since they might cut through the cord.)

What to Do

If you are faced with an emergency delivery, follow these steps:

1. Take infection-control precautions by washing your hands thoroughly and wearing latex gloves. If possible, wear a mask, a gown, and eye protection.
2. Have the mother lie on her back with her knees drawn up and legs spread apart. Be prepared for vomiting by having someone with a basin or a bag near the woman's head—she could aspirate vomit while lying flat on her back. Other positions include the following:
   - Sitting up or squatting, with someone behind to support her. These two positions place less tension on the vaginal tissues, reducing the likelihood of a tear and allow the force of gravity to help.

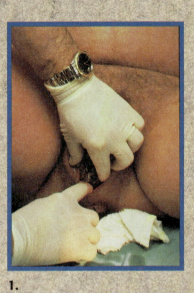

1.

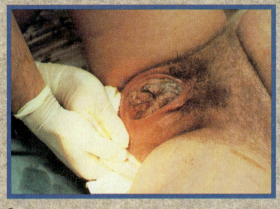

2.

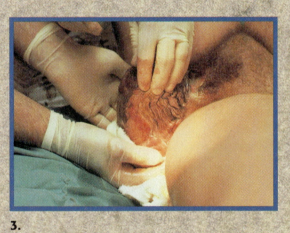

3.

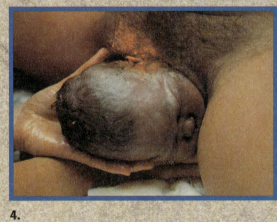

4.

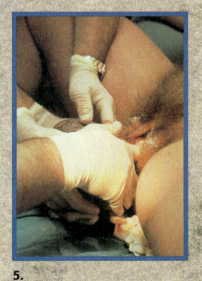

5.

1. Gentle pressure on perineum controls tearing.
2. Crowning means baby's head is visible.
3. Head leaving vagina.
4. Head delivers and turns.
5. Head and shoulders deliver.
6. Support baby's head and body.

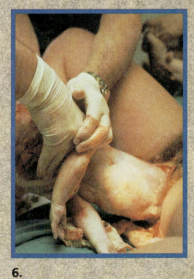

6.

- Lying on her left side, which improves blood return to her heart and prevents aspiration should she vomit. Have someone hold the woman's right leg up out of the way.
- Kneeling in a knee-chest position, which is used in less developed countries and in cases of breech presentations. This position also prevents possible aspiration if the woman vomits.

Remind the woman to take short, quick breaths during each contraction. Between contractions, she should rest and breathe deeply through her mouth.

3. Place absorbent, clean materials (sheets, towels, etc.) under the mother's buttocks.
4. Elevate her buttocks with blankets or a pillow.
5. When the baby's head appears, place the palm of your hand on top of the head and exert very gentle pressure, to prevent explosive delivery. Do not push on the fontanels (soft spots on the front and back of the infant's head).
6. If the amniotic sac does not break or has not broken, tear it with your fingers and push it away from the baby's head and mouth as they appear. The baby could suffocate if the sac is not removed.
7. As the baby's head is being born, determine if the umbilical cord is around his or her neck. If it is, try to slip the cord over the baby's shoulder. If you cannot do that, attempt to alleviate pressure on the cord or tie and cut the cord (see number *17* below for method).
8. Support the baby's head as it emerges.
9. Suction the baby's mouth and then the nostrils two or three times with the bulb syringe. Use caution to avoid contact with the back of the baby's mouth. If a bulb syringe is not available, wipe the baby's mouth and then the nose with gauze.
10. As the torso and full body are born, support the baby with both hands—he or she will be slippery.
11. Do not pull on the baby, which could cause cervical spine damage. Do not put your fingers in the baby's armpits; pressure on the nerve centers there could cause paralysis.
12. Grasp the feet as they are delivered. Keep the baby level with the vagina.
13. When the umbilical cord stops pulsating, tie it with gauze between the mother and the newborn and place the infant on the mother's abdomen for warmth.
14. Wipe blood and mucus from the baby's mouth and nose with sterile gauze; suction the mouth, then the nose again.
15. Dry the infant to reduce heat loss and help stimulate breathing. Rub the baby's back or flick the soles of its feet to stimulate breathing. The baby should breathe within 30 seconds, especially after the cord stops pulsing. (Do not hold the baby up by the feet and slap its buttocks—that could cause an increase in intracranial pressure.)
16. Wrap the infant in a warm blanket and place the baby on his or her side, head slightly lower than the trunk. Keep the infant level with the mother's vagina until the cord is cut. Raising the baby above the mother's abdomen (location of the placenta) while the umbilical cord is intact will allow the baby's blood to drain out and may put the baby in shock. Holding the baby below the mother's abdomen allows her blood to run into the baby, where the extra blood cells can cause serious problems such as jaundice.
17. If the mother is going to the hospital soon after the birth, there is no need to cut the cord in a normal delivery. Keep the infant warm and wait for the EMS personnel, who will have the proper equipment to clamp and cut the cord. If in a remote location, and after cord pulsations stop, tie the cord about 4 finger widths away from the baby and a second tie 2 inches further away from the first tie. Cut the cord between the two ties.
18. Watch for delivery of the placenta, which usually takes a few minutes, but could take as long as 30 minutes. Do not pull on the end of the umbilical cord to speed the placenta's delivery.
19. When the placenta is delivered, wrap it in a towel with three-quarters of the umbilical cord and place the towel in a plastic bag. Keep the bag at the level of the infant. Take the placenta to the hospital, where it will be examined for completeness. This procedure is necessary because pieces of placenta retained in the uterus can cause persistent bleeding or infection.
20. Place a sterile pad over the vaginal opening, lower the mother's legs, and help her hold them together.

Vaginal Bleeding Following Delivery

A woman can be expected to lose up to 300–500 ml (1–2 cups) of blood after delivery. You should be aware of this amount of blood loss so it does not cause undue psychological stress to the new mother or yourself. If blood loss continues, massage the uterus. Uterine massage stimulates the uterus to contract, thus constricting blood vessels within its walls and decreasing bleeding.

1. Use your hand with your fingers fully extended.
2. Place the palm of your hand on the lower abdomen where a grapefruit-sized mass can be felt.
3. Massage (knead) over the area.
4. If bleeding continues, check your massage technique.

Having the baby nurse following delivery of the placenta also stimulates uterine contractions and thus helps control bleeding.

Initial Care of the Newborn

Normal findings in a newborn are pulse rate greater than 100 per minute (feel the brachial artery) and a respiratory rate greater than 40 breaths per minute. The baby should be crying.

The most important care is positioning, drying, keeping warm, and stimulating the newborn to breathe. Wrap the newborn in a blanket, making sure the head is covered. Repeat suctioning if necessary and continue to stimulate the newborn if he or she is not breathing (flick soles of the feet and rub infant's back).

If the newborn does not begin to breathe within 30 seconds or continues to have difficulty breathing after one minute, you must consider the need for additional measures:

1. Ensure that the airway is open.
2. Give 1 rescue breath every 3 seconds.
3. Reassess after one minute.

Postdelivery Care of the Mother

After delivery monitor the mother's breathing and pulse. Replace any blood-soaked sheets and blankets while awaiting transport.

Abnormal Deliveries

Most childbirths are normal and natural. Sometimes, however, complications arise. It is essential that you be calm, deliberate, and gentle in a situation being made even more stressful by unforeseen problems.

Prolapsed Cord

A prolapsed cord is a condition in which the cord comes through the birth canal before delivery of the head, and the baby is in danger of suffocation.

CAUTION: DO NOT
- attempt to push the cord back into the vagina.

1. Position the woman with her head down or buttocks raised to use gravity to lessen pressure in the birth canal.
2. Insert your gloved hand into the vagina and gently push the presenting part of the fetus away from the pulsating cord. Again, do *not* push the cord back into the vagina.
3. Seek EMS transportation *immediately*.

Breech presentation and prolapsed umbilical cord are the only two cases in which the first aider should place his or her hand in the mother's vagina.

Breech Birth Presentation

A breech presentation occurs when the baby's buttocks or lower extremities will be the first part delivered. Breech presentation is the most common type of abnormal delivery, occurring in 3–4 percent of all deliveries. Place the mother in a head-down position, with her pelvis elevated, and seek medical care immediately.

CAUTION: DO NOT
- pull the baby's head out during a breech delivery.

If the baby's head is not delivered within three minutes of the body, you must act to prevent suffocation of the baby. Suffocation can occur when the baby's face is pressed against the vaginal wall or when the umbilical cord is compressed by the baby's head in the vagina. To establish an airway:

1. Place one hand in the vagina, positioning the palm toward the baby's face.
2. Form a V with your fingers on either side of the baby's nose.
3. Push the vaginal wall away from the baby's face until the head is delivered.

Limb Presentation

Limb presentation occurs when a single arm, leg, or foot of the infant protrudes from the birth canal. A foot more commonly presents when the infant is in breech presentation.

1. Place mother in head-down position with pelvis elevated. Do *not* pull on the baby or attempt to push the limb back into the vagina.
2. Call for EMS transportation *immediately*. The baby cannot be delivered in this position.

Presence of Meconium

Amniotic fluid that is greenish- or brownish-yellow rather than clear means the baby has had a bowel movement, an indication of possible fetal distress during labor.

1. Suction the mouth and nostrils thoroughly, or the baby will aspirate its own waste (meconium) with its first breath. Clear amniotic fluid, however, is harmlessly absorbed through the baby's lungs.
2. Maintain the baby's open airway.
3. Call for EMS transportation *immediately*.

Premature Birth

Any baby weighing less than 5.5 pounds or born before seven months of pregnancy is defined as premature and needs special care. Premature babies develop problems because they are so small and their organs are immature.

1. Keep the baby warm. Premature babies are always at risk for hypothermia.
2. Perform resuscitation, if necessary.

Gynecologic Emergencies

Gynecologic emergencies are reproductive-system problems that occur in nonpregnant females.

Vaginal Bleeding

For trauma-related soft-tissue injuries, use direct pressure to control bleeding. Apply an ice pack to reduce swelling and pain. Apply a diaper-type bandage to hold dressings in place. Never place or pack dressings into the vagina. Stabilize any foreign bodies in place. Seek medical attention.

Nontrauma vaginal bleeding can result from various causes, but treatment is the same. Have the victim place a sanitary pad over the vaginal opening and seek medical attention.

Hero CITATION

Adam Michael Calderon rescued Vera L. McGarrah from an attacking dog, Lake Elsinore, California, February 2, 1988. Mrs. McGarrah, 59, was knocked to the ground and repeatedly bitten by a 70-pound Doberman pinscher. She screamed for help. Adam, 17, witnessed the attack from his home and immediately ran to Mrs. McGarrah as a second fully-grown Doberman approached. Adam punched and kicked the dogs, distracting them from Mrs. McGarrah, who crawled to the safety of a fenced-in yard. After being taken to the ground and bitten several times himself by the dogs, Adam also escaped into the yard. Mrs. McGarrah was hospitalized a month for treatment of severe bite wounds to both legs. Adam required hospital treatment for less severe bite wounds, from which he recovered.

EMERGENCY CHILDBIRTH

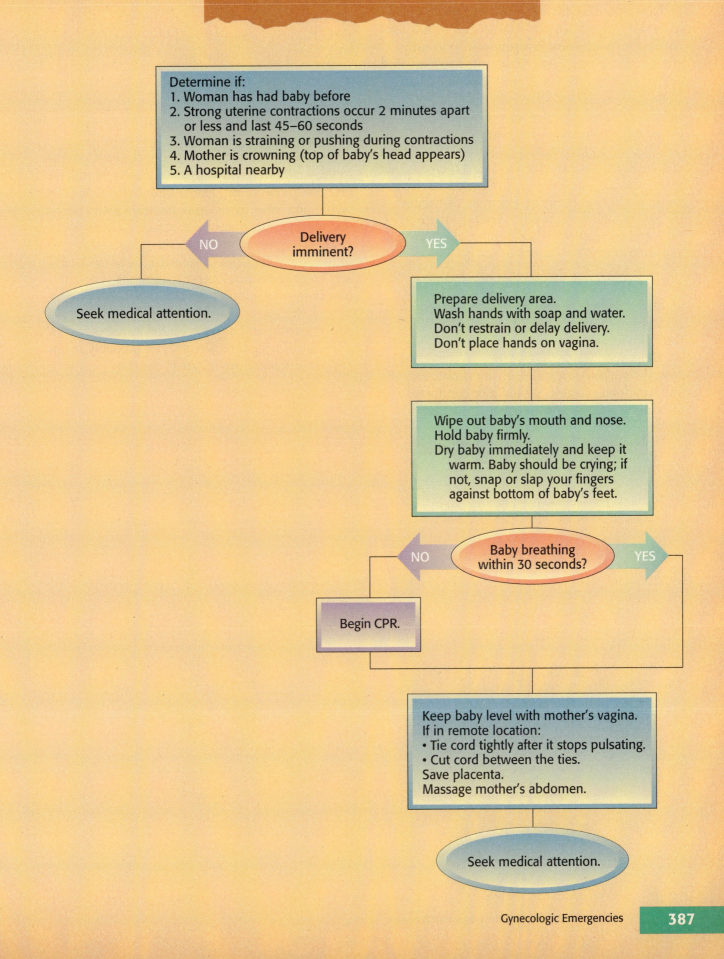

Determine if:
1. Woman has had baby before
2. Strong uterine contractions occur 2 minutes apart or less and last 45–60 seconds
3. Woman is straining or pushing during contractions
4. Mother is crowning (top of baby's head appears)
5. A hospital nearby

Delivery imminent?

NO → Seek medical attention.

YES →

Prepare delivery area.
Wash hands with soap and water.
Don't restrain or delay delivery.
Don't place hands on vagina.

Wipe out baby's mouth and nose.
Hold baby firmly.
Dry baby immediately and keep it warm. Baby should be crying; if not, snap or slap your fingers against bottom of baby's feet.

Baby breathing within 30 seconds?

NO → Begin CPR.

YES →

Keep baby level with mother's vagina.
If in remote location:
• Tie cord tightly after it stops pulsating.
• Cut cord between the ties.
Save placenta.
Massage mother's abdomen.

Seek medical attention.

Sexual Assault and Rape

Perhaps one of the most difficult emergency situations that a first aider may have to deal with is sexual assault. Rape is the fastest-growing violent crime in the United States. Authorities suspect that only a small proportion of rape cases are reported. In most cases, the victim of rape is a woman. It should be noted, however, that men, both heterosexual and homosexual, also may be raped.

There are many definitions of rape, but in general rape involves attempted or actual forced sexual intercourse, against the will of the victim. Related physical injury is common, but more damaging is the psychological trauma. It is essential that you be calm and sympathetic when dealing with a sexually assaulted victim.

Your job as a first aider is to care for the victim, not to collect evidence. Confine your questions to an assessment of the victim's injuries, not a detailed description of the events. Ask questions based on the SAMPLE survey (see Chapter 4).

Determine which injuries require immediate care. If disrobing of a female victim is necessary, and whenever possible, it should be conducted with another woman present. Also whenever possible, a same-sex first aider should do the examining.

Do not expose the genitalia unless an injury there requires immediate care (e.g., severe bleeding). Examining genitalia, except when childbirth is imminent, has serious legal implications and therefore usually should not be done.

Try, if possible, to preserve evidence but leave the actual investigation to the police. To preserve evidence, encourage the victim not to change clothes, wash, urinate, defecate, or douche. Explain to the victim in a sympathetic way that it would be best not to "clean up." Keep in mind that a rape victim, like any other victim, has the right to refuse first aid and transport to a hospital.

Even if the victim refuses aid, do not leave him or her alone. Try to have a trusted friend or relative stay with the victim. Protect the privacy of the victim. Emotional support is vital. Most large communities have rape crisis centers; furnishing the victim with the name and number of the nearest center (look in the telephone directory) is probably as important as treating any physical injuries.

Name _____ Course _____ Date _____

Case Situations

Case 1

While you are visiting your uncle and his family, a blizzard strands everyone on the uncle's farm 20 miles from town. Your pregnant aunt starts into labor. This is her first pregnancy. After about four hours of labor, you time the contractions and find they are 30 seconds in duration and about three minutes apart. You have your uncle examine his wife, and he reports no crowning.

_____ 1. Your aunt is in what stage of labor?

     a. first stage

     b. second stage

     c. third stage

_____ 2. Care of your aunt would include

     a. transport to the town's hospital

     b. calling the EMS

_____ 3. What care is considered appropriate for controlling vaginal bleeding following birth?

     a. placing a sanitary napkin into the vagina

     b. applying a warm pad over the mother's abdomen

     c. massaging the mother's lower abdomen

Case 2

A woman is expecting her first child. Her amniotic sac (bag of waters) broke one hour earlier, and her contractions are now about 10 to 12 minutes apart.

1. What stage of labor is this woman experiencing?

     _____

     _____

     _____

2. The first stage of labor typically lasts _____ hours.

3. Describe the second stage of labor and how long it typically lasts.

     _____

     _____

     _____

Case 3

The following presents an opportunity for self-evaluation and review of situations surrounding emergency childbirth.

1. When is it necessary for a first aider to assist in or perform an emergency on-site delivery of a baby?

     a. _____

     _____

     b. _____

     _____

     c. _____

     _____

2. What factors must be considered to determine if a woman is in advanced stages of labor?

     a. _____

     _____

     b. _____

     _____

     c. _____

     _____

     d. _____

     _____

3. What should you do if you have determined that an emergency on-site delivery is necessary?

     a. _____

     _____

     b. _____

     _____

     c. _____

     _____

4. When the baby's head first appears during a normal delivery, you should (check one)

_____ a. gently pull on the head to ease delivery

_____ b. support the head gently to prevent explosive delivery

5. What should you do if the umbilical cord is wrapped around the baby's neck?

     _____

     _____

     _____

     _____

Case 4

A pregnant woman lives in a rural setting approximately one hour from the closest medical facility. When you reach her home, she says she is having painful contractions three to five minutes apart and feels the urge to have a bowel movement. She informs you that she has two other children. On examination you see that the woman's vagina is bulging.

1. What would be your decision regarding moving the mother-to-be? Why?

   _____
   _____
   _____
   _____

2. What is the first thing you should do once the baby's head has been successfully delivered?

   _____
   _____
   _____

3. The umbilical cord is cut after the baby is delivered because the child no longer depends on it for oxygen and nourishment.

   _____ a. True
   _____ b. False

4. What occurs during the third stage of labor?

   _____
   _____
   _____
   _____

5. Why is it necessary to save the placenta and deliver it to the hospital with the mother and the newborn?

   _____
   _____
   _____
   _____

6. What steps should you take to care for the normal newborn child?

   a. _____
      _____

   b. _____
      _____

   c. _____
      _____

7. How does rescue breathing for a newborn differ from rescue breathing for an adult?

   a. _____
      _____

   b. _____
      _____

8. What steps are involved in caring for the umbilical cord?

   a. _____
      _____

   b. _____
      _____

9. How long after the baby is born is the placenta usually delivered?

   _____ a. 15–20 minutes
   _____ b. 30–60 minutes
   _____ c. 1–2 hours
   _____ d. More than 2 hours

10. List three types of complicated deliveries.

    a. _____
       _____

    b. _____
       _____

    c. _____

11. Describe two conditions under which a first aider should have contact with the mother's vaginal area.

    a. _____
       _____

    b. _____
       _____

12. What should you do after the baby and the placenta have been delivered?

    _____
    _____
    _____
    _____

NOTES

CHAPTER
21

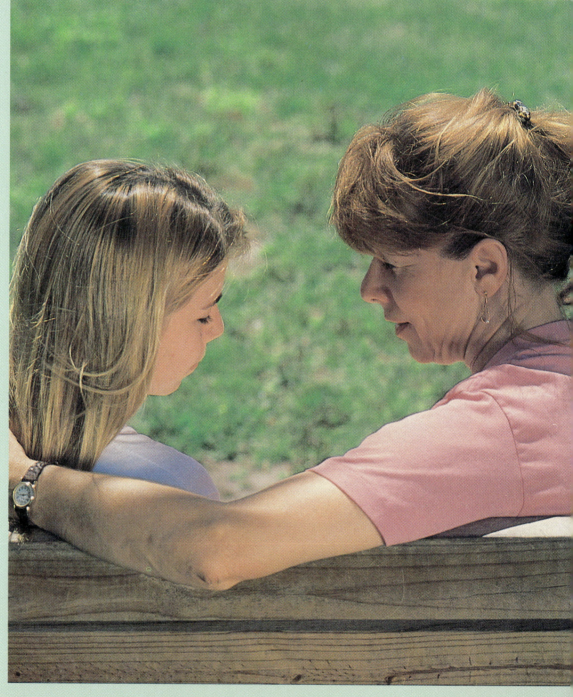

BEHAVIORAL EMERGENCIES

Behavior is how we act. Although we all act or behave differently, sometimes an individual will exhibit behavior that is unacceptable or intolerable. The abnormal behavior may be due to a psychological condition (such as a mental illness) or to a physical condition. For example, a diabetic with uncorrected low blood sugar can display aggressiveness, restlessness, or anxiety. Lack of energy in the form of blood sugar (glucose) not reaching the brain results in an altered mental status. Likewise, lack of oxygen and inadequate blood flow to the brain also cause altered mental status, resulting in similar behavior. Behavior leading to violence or other inappropriate behavior is known as a **behavioral emergency**.

Several factors can change a person's behavior, such as situational stresses, medical illnesses, psychiatric problems, alcohol, or drugs. The following are common reasons for behavior changes:

- low blood sugar in a diabetic
- lack of oxygen (known as hypoxia)
- inadequate blood flow to the brain
- head trauma
- mind-altering substances, such as alcohol, depressants, stimulants, hallucinogens, and narcotics
- psychogenic or psychiatric illness that leads to psychotic thinking, depression, or panic
- excessive cold
- excessive heat

Depression

Depression can lead to suicide; in fact, 50 percent of all suicides involve depression. Depressed persons often can be recognized by their sad appearance, crying spells, and listless or apathetic behavior. They feel worthless, guilty, and extremely pessimistic. Asserting that no one understands or cares about them and that their problems cannot be solved, they often express the desire to be left alone. Their speech may seem as if they have hardly enough energy to talk, and they may have sleeping difficulties.

Some depressed persons do not feel like talking. In such cases, saying, "You look very sad," often allows the person to talk about the depressed feelings. Such persons may burst into tears. Do not discourage their crying. Maintain a sympathetic silence and let them "cry themselves out."

A depressed person needs sympathetic attention and reassurance. He or she needs to know that the first aider is concerned. It is usually best to interview a depressed person in private, since the presence of several people may make the person uncomfortable. Tell the depressed person that many people have periods of unhappiness, but they can be helped to feel better. Mention community resources where such help can be found.

Suicide

Suicide is defined as any willful act that ends one's own life. Each year, a reported 25,000 to 30,000 Americans commit suicide; it is the tenth leading cause of death in the United States. Many experts, however, believe that suicide is vastly underreported. Suicide in the United States is increasingly a problem of adolescents, college-age students, and the very old.

The male rate for suicides is more than three times that for females. It is most common in men who are single, widowed, or divorced. Slightly more than half of all suicides—both men and women—use firearms. The next most common method is hanging. Poisoning by solids or liquids is the most common method used by women who attempt but do not complete suicide. Jumping from high places, carbon monoxide poisoning by auto exhaust, drowning, and self-inflicted wounds are less common methods.

The frequency of suicide peaks during spring months, rises again in the fall, and is lowest in December. Suicide rates are lowest in the Northeast and highest in the West, which may reflect the greater availability of firearms in the western states.

Suicide attempts are eight times more common than completed suicides. In addition, it is known that while males complete suicide three times more often than females, females are reported to attempt suicide three times more often. It is not known whether males are more reluctant to seek help and therefore less likely to report their attempts. It also is not known whether the lower rate of suicide among females results from their choice of less lethal methods despite an equal desire to die.

Despite its role as a major cause of death, suicide is a rare event. Except in the case of suicide clusters (three or more completed suicides closely

Table 21-1: Suicide Risk Factors

The SAD PERSONS scale is a mnemonic list of known suicide high-risk characteristics. A score of 9 or greater indicates the probable need for psychiatric consultation.

Mnemonic		Characteristics	Score
S	**S**ex	Male	1
A	**A**ge	<19 or >45	1
D	**D**epression or hopelessness	Admits to depression or decreased concentration, appetite, sleep, libido	2
P	**P**revious attempts or psychiatric care	Previous inpatient or outpatient psychiatric care	1
E	**E**xcessive alcohol or drug use	Chronic addiction or recent frequent use	1
R	**R**ational-thinking loss	Organic brain syndrome or psychosis	2
S	**S**eparated, widowed, or divorced		1
O	**O**rganized or serious attempt	Well-thought-out plan or "life-threatening" display	2
N	**N**o social support	No close family, friends, job, or active religious affiliation	1
S	**S**tated future intent	Determined to repeat attempt	2

Determining if high-risk factors are involved will help you maintain objectivity. It is important that the first aider maintain a nonjudgmental approach. Knowing the seriousness by using the SAD PERSONS mnemonic reminds the first aider that ridicule, demeaning comments, or ignoring the person is neither helpful nor proper.

Take precautions by keeping the person under close observation, removing any potentially dangerous items from the immediate area (e.g., glass, razors, medicines), and not allowing the person to go *anywhere* (e.g., bathroom) unaccompanied.

Source: R. S. Hockberger and R. J. Rothstein, "Assessment of Suicide Potential by Non-psychiatrists Using the SAD PERSONS Score," *Journal of Emergency Medicine* 99:6 (1988).

Fables and Facts about Suicide

These statements are not true:

Fable: People who talk about suicide do not commit suicide.

Fable: Suicide happens without warning.

Fable: Suicidal people are fully intent on dying.

Fable: Once a person is suicidal, he or she is suicidal forever.

Fable: Improvement following a suicidal crisis means that the suicidal risk is over.

Fable: Suicide strikes more often among the rich—or, conversely, it occurs more frequently among the poor.

Fable: Suicide is inherited or "runs in a family" (i.e., is genetically determined.)

Fable: All suicidal individuals are mentally ill, and suicide is always the act of a psychotic person.

Source: U.S. Department of Health and Human Resources.

These statements are true:

Fact: Of every 10 people who kill themselves, 8 have given definite warnings of their suicidal intentions. Suicide threats and attempts *must* be taken seriously.

Fact: Studies reveal that the suicidal person gives many clues and warnings regarding suicidal intentions. Alertness to these cries for help may prevent suicidal behavior.

Fact: Most suicidal people are undecided about living or dying, and they gamble with death, leaving it to others to save them. Almost no one commits suicide without letting others know how he or she is feeling. Often this cry for help is given in code. Decoding these distress signals can be used to save lives.

Fact: Fortunately, individuals who wish to kill themselves are suicidal only for a limited period of time. If they are saved from self-destruction, they can go on to lead useful lives.

Fact: Most suicides occur within three months after the beginning of improvement, when the individual has the energy to put morbid thoughts and feelings into effect. Relatives and physicians should be especially vigilant during this period.

Fact: Suicide is neither the rich man's disease nor the poor man's curse. Suicide is democratic and is represented proportionately at all levels of society.

Fact: Suicide does *not* run in families. It is an individual matter, and can be prevented.

Fact: Studies of hundreds of genuine suicide notes indicate that although a suicidal person is extremely unhappy, he or she is not necessarily mentally ill. The overpowering unhappiness may result from a temporary emotional upset, a long and painful illness, or a complete loss of hope. It is circular reasoning to say that suicide is an insane act; therefore, all suicidal people are psychotic.

related in time and place), no community is likely to experience many suicides.

Suicide is often attempted by depressed persons and alcoholics. At least 60 percent of all suicide victims previously attempted suicide, and 75 percent gave clear warning that they intended to kill themselves. Typically, a suicide attempt occurs when an individual's close emotional attachments are in danger or when he or she loses a significant family member or friend. Suicidal people often feel unable to manage their lives. Frequently, they lack self-esteem.

CAUTION: DO NOT

- ignore a suicide threat. Every suicidal act or gesture should be taken seriously and the person referred to a professional counselor.

Many suicidal people make last-minute attempts to communicate their intentions. When an individual phones to threaten suicide, someone should stay on the line until the EMS reaches the scene.

If you encounter a person who is attempting or threatening suicide, discreetly remove any dangerous articles. Talk quietly with the person. Encourage him or her to discuss the situation. Ask the following: *Have you attempted suicide before? Have you made any concrete plans concerning a method of suicide? Has any family member ever committed suicide?*

Persons who have made a previous suicide attempt, who have detailed suicide plans, or who have a close relative who committed suicide are more likely to try to kill themselves. These persons must be reassured and taken to medical help, usually at a hospital. Do *not* leave them alone under any circumstances.

When a person has attempted suicide, first aid care has priority. Drug overdoses must be managed. Bleeding from slashed wrists must be controlled. As you render first aid, try to encourage the person to talk about the situation. If a drug overdose is involved, collect any medication containers, pills, or other drugs found on the scene and bring the items to the hospital emergency department with the victim. In many cases, law enforcement authorities should be contacted.

Emotional Injury

First aid for an emotional injury really means nothing more than being supportive of people with emotional injuries, whether those injuries are from physical injury or from excessive or unbearable strain on the victim's emotions.

Emotional first aid often goes hand in hand with physical first aid, because a physical injury and the circumstances surrounding it may actually cause emotional injury. On the other hand, emotional injury may occur even when there is no physical injury. Emotional injuries usually are not as obvious as physical injuries, but both can be severe and require first aid.

Although most emotional reactions are temporary, lasting only minutes, hours, or, at the most, a few days, they are seriously disabling and may upset others. It is important to know that first aid can be applied to emotional as well as physical injuries.

Typical Reactions

With few exceptions, all people experience fear in the face of an emergency. Feeling shaky, perspiring profusely, and becoming a little nauseated are com-

mon. Such reactions are normal and no cause for concern. Most people are able to collect themselves reasonably quickly.

Extensive training is not needed to recognize severe, abnormal reactions. To determine whether a person needs help, find out if the person is doing something that makes sense and is able to take care of himself or herself.

For the most part, emotional first aid measures are simple and easy to understand. However, improvisation often is in order, just as it is in splinting a fracture. Whatever the situation, you will have your own emotional reactions toward the victim. These reactions are important—they can either enhance or hinder your ability to help the person. Especially when you are tired or worried, you may easily become impatient with the victim who seems to be "making a mountain out of a molehill." You may even feel resentful toward the victim for being a burden. Be on guard against becoming impatient, intolerant, or resentful. Victims who can see the first aider's calmness, confidence, and competence will be reassured.

On the other hand, do not be overly sympathetic or overly solicitous. Excessive sympathy for an incapacitated person can be as harmful as negative feelings. The victim needs strong help but does not need to be overwhelmed with pity.

Aggressive, Hostile, and Violent Behavior

When you are faced with aggressive, hostile, or violent behavior, size up the situation before you do anything. It may be unsafe for you and for others. The person may be standing or sitting in a threatening position. For example, the person may have clenched fists or be holding a lethal object. Is the person yelling or verbally threatening harm to anyone? If the scene appears unsafe, do not enter. If needed, contact law enforcement officers.

The angry, violent person is ready to fight with anyone who approaches and may be difficult to control. Remember that anger may be a response to illness and that aggressive behavior may be a person's way of coping with feelings of helplessness. Avoid responding with anger. Many angry or violent persons can be calmed by someone who is trained and who appears confident that the person will behave well. Encourage the person to speak directly about the cause of his or her anger. A statement like "I'm not sure I understand why you are

Table 21-2: Psychological First Aid for Emergency Reactions

Reaction	Symptoms	Do	Don't
Normal	Trembling Muscular tension Perspiration Nausea Mild diarrhea Urinary frequency Pounding heart Rapid breathing Anxiety	Give reassurance. Provide group identification. Motivate. Talk with victim. Observe to see that individual is gaining composure, not losing it.	Don't show resentment. Don't overdo sympathy.
Individual Panic (flight reaction)	Unreasoning attempt to flee Loss of judgment Uncontrolled weeping Wild running about	Try kindly firmness at first. Give something warm to eat or drink. Get help to isolate if necessary. Be empathetic. Encourage victim to talk. Be aware of your own limitations.	Don't use brutal restraint. Don't strike. Don't douse with water. Don't give sedatives.
Depression (underactive reactions)	Stands or sits without moving or talking Vacant expression Lack of emotional display	Make contact gently. Secure rapport. Get victim to tell you what happened. Be empathetic. Recognize feelings of resentment in victim and yourself. Give simple, routine task. Give warm food, drink.	Don't tell victim to "snap out of it." Don't overdo pity. Don't give sedatives. Don't act resentful.
Overactive	Argumentative Talks rapidly Jokes inappropriately Makes endless suggestions Jumps from one activity to another	Let victim talk about it. Find victim jobs that require physical effort. Give warm food, drink. Supervision necessary. Be aware of own feelings.	Don't suggest that victim is acting abnormally. Don't give sedatives. Don't argue with victim.
Physical (conversion reaction)	Severe nausea and vomiting Can't use some part of the body	Show interest in victim. Find small job for victim to make him/her forget. Make comfortable. Get medical help if possible. Be aware of own feelings.	Don't tell victim that there's nothing wrong with him/her. Don't blame. Don't ridicule. Don't ignore disability openly.

Source: Modified from M 51-400-603-1, Department of Nonresident Instruction, Medical Field Service School, Brooke Army Medical Center, Fort Sam Houston, Texas.

angry" often brings results. Reassure the person that you are there to help.

A person who is violent and out of control presents a special problem. Notify the police if you are unable to communicate with a person who is dangerous to himself or herself or to others.

Calming a Person

Confronting a person who is experiencing a behavioral emergency can be a trying and frustrating experience. Use these guidelines when you are trying to calm a person who is upset:

- Acknowledge that the person seems upset and reiterate that you are there to help.
- Maintain a comfortable distance.
- Encourage the person to state what is troubling him or her.
- Do not make quick moves.
- Respond honestly to the person's questions.
- Do not threaten, challenge, or argue with a disturbed person.
- Tell the truth—do not lie.
- Do not "play along" with any of a disturbed person's visual or auditory disturbances.
- Involve trusted family members or friends.
- Be prepared to stay with the person for a long time. Never leave the person alone.
- Avoid unnecessary physical contact.
- Use good eye contact.

Sexual Assault and Rape

The definitions of rape and sexual assault vary widely. Rape is generally defined as forcible sexual intercourse without the consent of one participant. Categories of rape include the following:

- **Acquaintance rape** involves individuals who knew each other prior to the rape, including relatives, neighbors, or friends.
- **Date rape** takes place within a relationship but without the consent of one person and when harm or the threat of harm is used by the other.
- **Marital rape** occurs when the victim and the offender are married to each other.
- **Stranger rape** occurs when the victim and the offender have no relation to each other.

The victim may hesitate to report a rape for various reasons, such as shame, guilt, fear of retaliation, or reluctance to deal with law enforcement officials or the judicial system. The victim may even begin to have doubts about whether a "real" rape occurred.

Rape is a traumatic crisis that disrupts the physical, psychological, social, and sexual aspects of the victim's life. The most common physical injuries are bruises, black eyes, and cuts.

As a first aider, you must be tactful and sensitive with the victim. The victim may find it extremely difficult to discuss what happened and may feel fear or hostility toward a first aider of the opposite sex. Every effort should be made to understand the victim's feelings and to respond with kindness and reassurance. The emotional trauma of rape is usually more prolonged and severe than the physical trauma. The attitude shown toward the victim during the initial care can have a serious influence, for good or ill, on future psychological and physical recovery. Convince the victim to seek counseling through community resources (e.g., a rape crisis center) and to report the crime to the police. Ask the victim not to change clothes or to bathe since doing so can alter legal evidence. For the same reason, suggest that the victim not urinate, douche, defecate, or wash before being examined by a physician. Care for any injuries incurred during the attack.

Child Abuse and Neglect

Because child abuse and neglect usually occur in the privacy of the home, no one knows exactly how many children are affected. One estimate is that 3 million children are physically abused and over 1 million are victims of sexual abuse each year. Child abuse and neglect can cause permanent damage to a child's physical, emotional, and mental development. The physical effects often are damage to the brain, vital organs, eyes, ears, arms, or legs, which, in turn, can result in mental retardation, blindness, deafness, or loss of a limb. At its most serious, abuse or neglect can result in a child's death.

Child abuse and neglect are usually divided into four major categories: physical abuse, neglect, sexual abuse, and emotional maltreatment. Each has recognizable characteristics, and all may be encountered by a first aider.

The National Center on Child Abuse and Neglect has set forth physical and behavioral indicators of child abuse and neglect. Their list is not intended to be exhaustive; many more indicators

Type of Child Abuse/Neglect	Physical Indicators	Behavioral Indicators
Physical Abuse	Unexplained bruises and welts: 　on face, lips, mouth, 　on torso, back, buttocks, thighs 　in various stages of healing 　clustered, forming regular patterns 　reflecting shape of articles used to 　　inflict (electric cord, belt buckle) 　on several different surface areas 　regularly appearing after absence, weekend, 　　or vacation 　especially about the trunk and buttocks Be particularly suspicious if there are old bruises 　in addition to fresh ones. Unexplained burns: 　cigar, cigarette burns, especially on soles, 　palms, back, or buttocks Immersion burns (socklike, glovelike, doughnut- 　shaped on buttocks or genitalia) Patterned like electric burner, iron, etc. Rope burns on arms, legs, neck, or torso Unexplained fractures (particularly if multiple): 　to skull, nose, facial structure 　in various stages of healing 　multiple or spiral fractures Unexplained lacerations or abrasions: 　to mouth, lips, gums, eyes 　to external genitalia	Wary of adult contacts Apprehensive when other children cry Behavioral extremes: 　aggressiveness or withdrawal Frightened of parents Afraid to go home Reports injury by parents Acts apathetic and does not cry despite injuries Has been seen by emergency personnel re- 　cently for related complaints Was injured several days before medical atten- 　tion was sought
Physical Neglect	Consistent hunger, poor hygiene, inappropriate 　dress Consistent lack of supervision, especially in dan- 　gerous activities or for long periods Unattended physical problems or medical needs Abandonment	Begs, steals food Extended stays at school (early arrival and late 　departure) Constant fatigue, listlessness, or falling asleep in 　class Alcohol or drug abuse Delinquency (e.g., thefts) States there is no caretaker
Sexual Abuse	Difficulty in walking or sitting Torn, stained, or bloody underclothing Pain or itching in genital area Bruises or bleeding in external genitalia, vaginal, 　or anal areas Venereal disease, especially in preteens Pregnancy	Unwillingness to change for gym or participate in 　physical education class Withdrawal, fantasizing, or infantile behavior Bizarre, sophisticated, or unusual sexual behavior 　or knowledge Poor peer relationships Delinquency or truancy Reports sexual assault by caretaker

Table 21-3: Physical and Behavioral Indicators of Child Abuse and Neglect (continued)

Type of Child Abuse/Neglect	Physical Indicators	Behavioral Indicators

Emotional Maltreatment	Speech disorders
	Lags in physical development
	Failure to thrive
		Habit disorders (sucking, biting, rocking, etc.)
		Conduct disorders (antisocial, destructive, etc.)
		Neurotic traits (sleep disorders, inhibition of play)
		Psychoneurotic reactions (hysteria, obsession,
		    compulsion, phobias, hypochondria)
		Behavior extremes:
		    compliant, passive-aggressive, demanding
		Overly adaptive behavior:
		    inappropriately adult
		    inappropriately infantile
		Developmental lags (mental, emotional)
		Attempted suicide

Source: National Center on Child Abuse and Neglect.

exist than can be included. The presence of a single indicator does not necessarily prove that child abuse or neglect has occurred. However, the repeated occurrence of an indicator, the presence of several indicators in combination, or the appearance of serious injury should alert the first aider to the possibility of child abuse. Every state has child abuse and neglect reporting laws.

First aid for an abused child's injuries is similar to the care for non-abuse injuries.

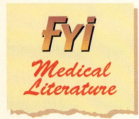

Shaken Baby Syndrome: The Shake That Can Break Physical abuse is the main cause of serious head injury in infants. But some parents who shake a baby "to stop it from crying" or just in anger may not realize the damage they are causing. Babies have very weak neck muscles, so any shaking severely jars the head, causing blood vessel breakage and internal bleeding. Some infant victims immediately fall into a coma and die. Others suffer mental retardation and motor disorders that become apparent years later. In short, *never* shake a baby.

Source: R. D. Krugman et al., *Pediatrics* 92:872 (Dec. 1993).

Spouse Abuse

Abuse may be the single most common source of serious injury to women. Physical domestic violence includes slapping, punching, kicking, and choking. Women also report being shot, stabbed, and bludgeoned. Injuries tend to be on the head, neck, chest, breast, abdomen, and perineum rather than the extremities.

First aid includes calling the police and the EMS and treating any injuries.

Elder Abuse

The types of physical abuse of elders vary from passive neglect to active assault. Some physically abused elderly report having had something thrown at them; some are pushed, grabbed, or shoved; others are slapped, bitten, or kicked.

First aid includes calling the police and the EMS, if warranted, and treating any injuries.

STUDY QUESTIONS 21

Name _____ Course _____ Date _____

Activities

Activity I

1. List eight common reasons for behavior changes:

   a. _____
   b. _____
   c. _____
   d. _____
   e. _____
   f. _____
   g. _____
   h. _____

___ 2. The term *child abuse* encompasses which of the following?

   a. physical or sexual abuse
   b. psychological or emotional abuse
   c. neglect
   d. all the above

___ 3. Who usually deliberately injures a child?

   a. a parent
   b. older siblings
   c. a teacher
   d. a stranger

___ 4. What is the speech of a depressed person like?

   a. faint, as if there is barely enough energy to speak
   b. incoherent
   c. repeats same words in conversations
   d. agitated and rambling

___ 5. Depressed persons can be recognized by their

   a. hostility and anger
   b. uncontrollable and erratic behavior
   c. energy and vivaciousness
   d. listless or apathetic behavior

___ 6. When giving psychological first aid to a depressed person, the first aider should

   a. tell the person to "snap out of it"
   b. give the person sedatives
   c. be empathetic
   d. all the above

___ 7. Which is the most common method of suicide for both men and women?

   a. hanging
   b. drug overdose
   c. firearms
   d. carbon monoxide poisoning

___ 8. Which region in the United States has the highest suicide rate?

   a. West
   b. Midwest
   c. South
   d. East

___ 9. For every suicide completion, there are how many attempts?

   a. 2
   b. 4
   c. 6
   d. 8

___ 10. Identify the correct statement about suicide.

   a. The majority of suicide victims gave clear warning that they intended to kill themselves.
   b. Most suicide victims had previously attempted suicide.
   c. Suicidal people frequently lack self-esteem.
   d. All the above.

___ 11. How should you react when faced with a person who is threatening suicide?

   a. Take the suicidal act or gesture seriously.
   b. Talk quietly with the individual.
   c. Encourage the person to discuss his or her situation.
   d. All the above.

___ 12. A rape victim may hesitate to report rape for which reasons?

a. feelings of shame and guilt

b. reluctance to deal with law enforcement officials

c. questioning whether a "real" rape occurred

d. all the above

____ 13. To preserve legal evidence, the rape victim should not

a. change clothes until after medical evaluation

b. urinate or defecate until after medical evaluation

c. wash or douche until after medical evaluation

d. all the above

Activity 2

1. What are the four major categories of child abuse?

a. _____

b. _____

c. _____

d. _____

2. Give several signs of possible child abuse:

a. _____

b. _____

c. _____

3. How should a suspected child abuse situation be handled?

a. _____

b. _____

c. _____

d. _____

4. How should every suicide attempt be taken?

_____

5. What signs indicate that a person is likely to attempt a suicide?

a. _____

b. _____

c. _____

6. What are the four categories of rape?

a. _____

b. _____

c. _____

d. _____

7. You should try to convince a victim of rape to seek _____.

Case Situations

Case 1

A 45-year-old male has attempted suicide by cutting both wrists. Blood is flowing from several slits across his wrists.

1. This victim is experiencing _____ bleeding.

a. arterial

b. capillary

c. venous

____ 2. To control the bleeding, you should apply

a. tourniquets to both arms at the elbows

b. direct pressure over the wounds

c. pressure to the brachial arteries

d. constricting bands at the wrists

e. elastic bandages around both wrists

Case 2

A 22-year-old female has taken an overdose of aspirin. She responds to your questions about what, when, and how much was taken.

____ 1. What is the first step for this victim's care?

a. Call the poison control center.

b. Call the local emergency telephone number (usually 911).

c. Call the victim's physician.

d. Call the hospital emergency department.

e. Call your physician.

STUDY QUESTIONS 21

Name _____ Course _____ Date _____

____ 2. Which is the more likely treatment
for a swallowed-poison victim?
   a. syrup of ipecac
   b. two glasses of water
   c. epsom salts
   d. activated charcoal

Case 3
You are an elementary school teacher with a class-room full of seemingly happy and well-adjusted children. One day one of your students returns to school after a two-day absence. You notice bruises on his face and mouth. He seems wary when you get near him. He definitely has changed.

1. What do you suspect?

_____

____ 2. What should you do?
   a. report your suspicions to the proper authorities
   b. confront the parent(s)
   c. question the child about what happened
   d. nothing, it is none of your business

____ 3. How many states have child abuse and neglect reporting laws?
   a. one-fourth
   b. one-half
   c. three-fourths
   d. all states

____ 4. No one knows exactly how many children are abused.
   a. true
   b. false

____ 5. Child abuse can result in a child's death.
   a. true
   b. false

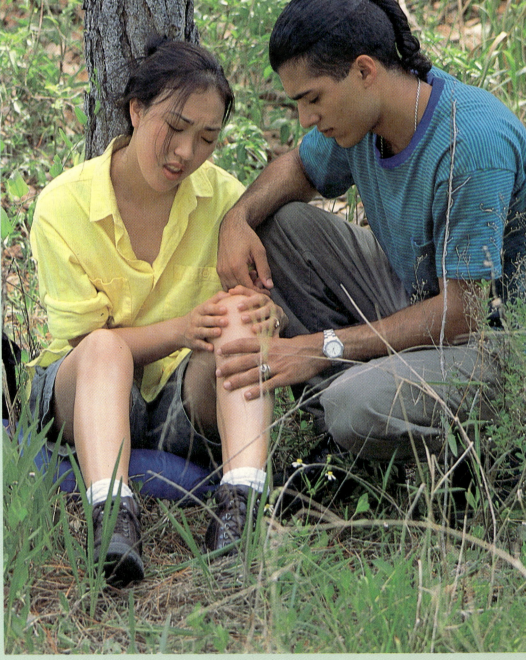

WILDERNESS FIRST AID

Anyone living, working, traveling, or recreating in the wilderness will probably encounter, at some time, dangers unfamiliar to most people. Regardless of precautions, injuries and illnesses happen.

Wilderness, as defined by the Wilderness Medical Society (WMS), is a "remote geographical location more than one hour from definitive medical care." According to that definition, "wilderness" could describe a variety of situations, including

- recreation (e.g., fishing, camping, hiking, hunting)
- occupations in remote areas (e.g., farming, forestry, fishing)
- urban areas with overwhelmed emergency medical services (EMS) after a natural or manmade disaster
- residences in remote communities, farms, ranches, vacation homes
- developing countries

The millions of people in the so-called wilderness should be as medically prepared as possible to manage a problem either for others or for themselves. The need for first aid with a wilderness focus appears indispensable for the following circumstances:

- injuries and illnesses in the outdoors where adverse environmental conditions (e.g., heat, cold, altitude, rain, snow) may be a major concern
- definitive medical care delayed for hours or days because of location, bad weather, lack of transportation, or lack of communication
- injuries and illnesses not commonly seen in urban or suburban areas (e.g., altitude illness, frostbite, wild animal attacks)
- the need to give some advanced medical care (e.g., reduction of some dislocations, wound cleansing)
- a limited amount of first aid supplies and equipment
- making a decision about giving unrealistic care (e.g., CPR) in a remote setting

Most first aid books and training courses describe situations in which the EMS response is expected within 10 to 20 minutes. In these cases the first aider usually helps for only a few minutes before an ambulance arrives. When the victim is transported, the first aider's job is finished.

Wilderness first aid is similar to that needed in urban situations, except that extra or extended skills are needed. Consideration must be given to time, distance, and availability of medical care. A first aider in the wilderness may

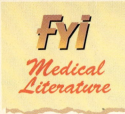
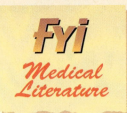
have to remain many hours or days with a sick or injured person.

Cardiac Arrest

Because a cardiac arrest victim's heart activity must be restored within a short time (which requires defibrillation and medications) for survival, CPR has limited use in a wilderness or remote setting. That is especially true if severe trauma (e.g., massive head or chest injury, severe blood loss, severed spinal cord) accompanies the cardiac arrest. In addition, CPR is difficult to continue during a wilderness evacuation.

Rescue breathing can be continued for hours when there is a pulse, but chest compressions cannot support circulation for very long. The National Association of Emergency Medical Services Physicians (NAEMSP) gives the following guidelines for treating victims with normal core body temperatures or mild hypothermia (core body temperature above 90°F):

- If the victim is not breathing, give rescue breathing; if no pulse can be felt, give CPR.
- If the victim has been in cardiac arrest for more than 30 minutes without prior resuscitation efforts, do not start CPR.
- If CPR is given for more than 30 minutes without success, stop CPR (see exceptions below).

The NAEMSP recommends starting and continuing CPR for more than 30 minutes in the following situations:

- cold-water immersion of less than one hour (Hypothermia slows metabolism.)
- avalanche burial
- hypothermia
- lightning strike

The NAEMSP says that CPR has no effect on recovery and therefore should not be started if

- The victim's core temperature is less than 60°F.
- The victim's chest is frozen.
- The victim has been submerged in water for more than 60 minutes.
- The procedures will place the rescuer at risk.
- An obvious lethal injury is present.

CPR for Hypothermia Victims

For the profoundly hypothermic victim, CPR should not delay evacuation to a location for rewarming and advanced cardiac life support. Rough handling of a hypothermic victim or CPR chest compressions when the heart is beating can cause a form of heart attack (ventricular fibrillation). Therefore, be sure there is no pulse before starting CPR. The American Heart Association recommends that a first aider take 30 to 45 seconds, instead of the usual 5 to 10, to feel for a pulse in an unresponsive hypothermic victim. Determining the existence of a pulse is difficult in cold environments because of the victim's very slow pulse rate and because of the rescuer's cold fingers. Hypothermia is one of the cases in which CPR should be continued for more than 30 minutes. See Chapter 18.

CPR for Avalanche Victims

It is suffocation and/or blunt trauma that kills avalanche victims. For pulseless victims, stabilize the cervical spine and start CPR immediately, continuing for more than 30 minutes if necessary.

CPR for Lightning-Strike Victims

Start CPR on unresponsive and pulseless victims immediately. In the case of multiple victims, treat the unresponsive ones first. Continue CPR for more than 30 minutes.

Dislocations

In a wilderness situation, reduction of some dislocated joints is recommended. The WMS gives the following reasons for reducing a joint dislocation quickly after it happens:

- Reduction is easier immediately after the injury, before swelling has developed.
- It is easier to transport a victim after reduction.

- Dramatic relief of pain results. (It is inhumane to leave a joint dislocated for several hours.)
- The joint can be stabilized and protected better.
- Reduction lessens the possibility of jeopardizing circulation in the extremity. (If the blood supply is cut off, gangrene could develop, which could result in amputation.)
- Several simple dislocations can be reduced through simple and safe techniques.

Stop any attempts to reduce a simple dislocation if doing so increases the victim's pain or if you feel resistance in the joint.

A dislocation is considered **simple** if it involves the anterior shoulder, a finger, or the patella (the kneecap, *not* the knee itself). Do *not* attempt to reduce a dislocated elbow or hip. Elbow and hip dislocations resemble fractures; reduction techniques for those joints are painful and can cause further injury.

Shoulder Dislocation

Anterior shoulder joint dislocations account for over 90 percent of shoulder dislocations. Because the problem often recurs, the victim usually can readily identify the dislocation. The upper arm is held away from the body in various positions and cannot be brought next to the body into a sling-type position. The victim is unable to reach the hand of the injured extremity to touch the unin-

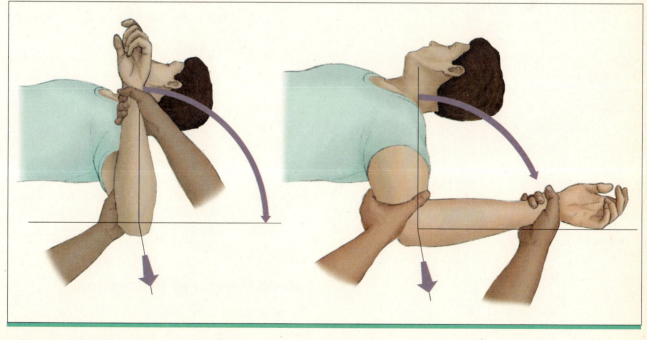

Applying traction (left) and external rotation (right) to anterior shoulder dislocation

jured shoulder. Compare the injured shoulder to the uninjured one. Check CSM (circulation, sensation, and movement) of the hand.

There are two methods for reducing a shoulder dislocation. Do *not* try pulling on the victim's arm with your foot in the victim's armpit. With either method, stop if pain increases or resistance is met.

Traction and External Rotation

This is the easiest and most effective method for reducing an anterior shoulder dislocation.

1. Gently but steadily pull the arm out to the side while another rescuer provides countertraction against the chest wall, just below the armpit, using straps, a sleeping bag, clothing, or a flotation vest.
2. Tell the victim to relax. Massage may help.
3. While pulling, gently and slowly (take 5 to 15 minutes) rotate the arm into a baseball-throwing position. Keep the arm in that position; the muscles will fatigue within 15 minutes, allowing the joint to slip back into place.
4. After successful reduction, stabilize the arm with a sling and swathe.

Simple Hanging Traction

1. Lay the victim face down on a surface high enough so the injured arm can hang over the side.
2. Attach a 10- to 15-pound weight to the victim's wrist. Keep the victim's palm facing inward.
3. It may take up to 60 minutes to stretch and tire the muscles, allowing the joint to pop back in.

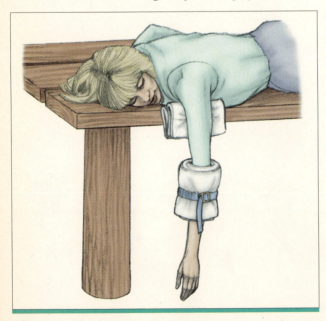

Simple hanging traction to reduce anterior shoulder dislocation

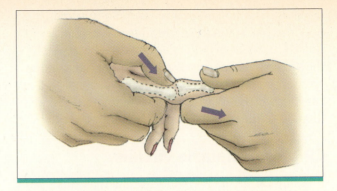

Reducing a finger dislocation

4. After successful reduction, stabilize the arm with a sling and swathe.

Finger Dislocation

Deformity and loss of use identify a dislocated finger. Often, persons with this injury can reduce the finger dislocation themselves. In a remote location, you should try to reduce a finger dislocation only once. Do *not* attempt to reduce a dislocation at the base of the index finger or at the base of the thumb—those areas require surgery for reduction. To reduce a finger dislocation, use one of two methods:

1. Hold the finger in a slightly flexed position (use a cloth to prevent slipping).
2. Apply traction to the tip of the finger while you push the end of the dislocated bone back into place.
3. Whether or not the reduction is successful, stabilize the joint in the **position of function** (fingers and hand in a cupping shape, as though holding a baseball).

or

1. Hold the end of the finger with one hand and the rest of the finger in the other.
2. Pull the end of the finger first in the direction it is pointing; then, while maintaining traction, swing it back in normal anatomical position.
3. Whether or not the reduction is successful, stabilize the joint in the position of function (fingers and hand in a cupping shape, as though holding a baseball).

Patella (Kneecap) Dislocation

When dislocated, the patella is displaced on the outside, with the leg bent for comfort. The problem often recurs, and the victim usually can identify the dislocation. For most dislocated kneecaps, you should only apply an ice pack and use a splint to stabilize the leg in place as you found it. For remote locations, however, always consider reducing a dislocated kneecap using the following method. All dislocations, whether successfully reduced in the field or not, should be seen by a physician.

1. Bend the hip toward the chest to relax the quadriceps muscle.
2. At the same time, slowly straighten the knee while gently pushing the kneecap back into its normal position. Straightening alone may replace the kneecap.
3. Stabilize the leg straight. The victim usually can walk on the injured leg.

With the knee extended (straight) and stabilized, the victim may be able to walk well enough for self-evacuation. Because of the heavy physical demands, often at high altitude, carrying a victim out of the backcountry can take 8 to 16 rescuers rotating the task. In the wilderness, a ski pole or a tree branch makes a good walking aid. Helicopter evacuation usually is not justified for a kneecap dislocation.

Spine Injury

The necessity of stabilizing the spine after trauma is well known. An unconscious victim with a cervical spine injury who is moved without stabilization may become quadriplegic or die. In urban settings, spine stabilization is almost always automatically applied for survivors of violent accidents, such as automobile crashes or falls from a height.

In the wilderness, full-spine stabilization may not always be necessary—such a procedure can be difficult, impractical, impossible, or even dangerous during prolonged evacuation in severe environments. For example, an injured climber far above timberline could wait for hours, even days, depending on the distance someone has to go for help. The injured climber would have to wait in a hostile environment and risk death from avalanche, rockfall, or hypothermia. If the victim were cleared of a spine injury, he or she could self-evacuate.

Spine fractures can be difficult to determine, even by physicians reading x-rays. One study found that all the spine fractures reviewed had at least one of the following findings: midline neck tenderness, altered mental status, evidence of intoxication, or a separate painful injury away from the neck.

Assessing a Possible Spine-Injury Victim

Assessment of a spine injury can be made by a process of elimination. First, ask these four questions:

- Is the victim alert and oriented?
- Does the victim have any major painful injury? Distracting injuries include fractures, deep lacerations, severe contusions, or large burns.
- Is the victim complaining of neck pain?
- Does the victim have tingling, numbness, weakness in the extremities?

Next, perform these physical exams:

- Check for neck tenderness by pressing firmly on the bony part of the spine. This is a safe procedure, and there is little chance of injuring the spinal cord by feeling the bony spinal column as long as movement of the spine is prevented.
- Determine if the victim has sensation in the hands or feet and if he or she can move fingers or toes.

A simple protocol for clearing a spine injury in the wilderness is as follows: The victim does not need to be stabilized in one position if he or she is completely alert, not intoxicated, has no distracting injuries, does not complain of neck pain, can feel normal touch and can move the fingers and toes.

Follow these guidelines to assess a suspected spine injury:

- Victim is responsive:
  - Determine if mechanism of injury was a violent-impact force capable of damaging the bony spinal column. Examples are a fall from 20 feet, a high-velocity gunshot wound near the spine, and a high-velocity vehicle crash.
  - Ask questions: *Does your neck or back hurt? What happened? Can you move your hands and feet? Can you feel me touching your fingers and toes?*
  - Look and feel for DOTS (deformity, open wounds, tenderness, swelling) along the bony spinal column.
  - Assess equality of strength of extremities: Have victim grip your hand and push his or her feet against your hands.

- Victim is unresponsive:
  - Determine mechanism of injury.

- Look for deformity, open wounds, and swelling on the bony spinal column.
- Feel for deformity and swelling along the bony spinal column.
- Obtain information from others at the scene to determine information relevant to mechanism of injury and victim's mental status prior to your arrival.

Stabilizing a Spine Injury

Providing effective spine stabilization in the wilderness often requires you to improvise methods. Initially, you can use your hands or knees to hold the victim's head in place. While kneeling at the victim's head, use your hands or thighs to stabilize the victim's neck in relation to the long axis of the spine.

Improvised cervical collars (e.g., a blanket, an Ensolite® pad, SAM Splint®) alone are inadequate. Improvise supports by placing dirt or sand in garbage bags, stuff sacks, or roll up extra articles of clothing. Place them on both sides of the victim's head and secure them in place.

Leave the victim on the ground and avoid movement. If necessary to prevent heat loss, log roll the victim, keeping the spine straight, and place insulating materials underneath.

For spine injury procedures when EMS response time is less than one hour, see page 202.

Spine Injury

Question: Should a suspected broken neck or back be stabilized as found or moved to an in-line position?

Answer: The National EMT curriculum says that the head can be placed in an in-line position unless the victim complains of pain or the head is not easily moved into that position. The anatomical (normal) position is the most stable position for all bony structures, including the spine, and movement toward that position from the position found generally is considered to be safe. Therefore, in wilderness settings, it is best to reposition suspected spine injuries into the normal, anatomical ("eyes forward") position. If movement causes increased pain or if there is resistance to movement, it is best to splint the spine in the position found.

Splinting Femur Fractures

Victims with a femur fracture can easily lose more than a quart of blood in the thigh and develop massive swelling.

Because EMS personnel have the training, the experience, and the equipment, it is best to let them apply traction splints, if possible. However, first aiders can use the methods on page 257 to stabilize a femur.

Femur Fracture

Question: Do improvised traction splints work?

Answer: While the advantages of stabilizing a broken femur by applying a traction splint are clear, there are dissenting opinions about the effectiveness of improvised traction splints. For example, Outward Bound says, "Improvised traction splints for field use employing ski poles, canoe paddles, and other pieces of equipment are usually more architecturally interesting than medically useful. The simplest, safest, and most universal splint is firm immobilization on a long board or litter without traction."

Avalanche Burial

Avalanches are falling masses of snow that may also contain rocks, soil, or ice. Since the early 1970s, the number of deaths caused by avalanches has increased rapidly, as a result of the tremendous growth in backcountry winter mountain travel (skiing, mountaineering, snowmobiling). Recent statistics show that the average annual number of deaths is about 14 per year in the United States and 7 in Canada.

Avalanches kill in two ways. The first is from serious injury the victim acquires while tumbling down an avalanche path. Trees, rocks, cliffs, and the wrenching action of snow are hazards. About one-third of all deaths are related to trauma, especially trauma to the head and neck. The second way is snow burial, which causes suffocation in the other two-thirds of avalanche deaths. Inhaled snow clogs the mouth and nose, and suffocation happens quickly if the victim is buried with the airway already blocked.

Snow sets up solid after an avalanche. It is almost impossible for victims to dig themselves out, even if they are buried under less than a foot of snow. The pressure of several feet of snow sometimes is so great that victims are unable to expand their chests to breathe.

A completely buried victim has a poor chance of survival. In the first 15 minutes, more persons are found alive than dead. Between 16 and 30 minutes after an avalanche, an equal number are found dead and alive (50 percent chance of survival). After 30 minutes, more are found dead than alive.

In the absence of fatal injuries, speed of extrication from the avalanche and existence of an air pocket are the main factors that determine survival of a buried victim. There are no documented reports of anyone surviving a burial of seven feet or more.

Avalanche Rescue

If you survive an avalanche, follow these steps to find other victims:

1. With a piece of equipment, clothing, or tree branch, mark the spot where a victim was last seen.
2. Search the area below the last-seen point for any clues of the victim. Make shallow probes into likely burial spots with a ski, ski pole, or tree limb.
3. If beacons were being used, all survivors must immediately switch their units to the receive mode and listen for a beeping sound from buried beacons.
4. If a second avalanche is possible, place one person in a safe location to shout a warning so rescuers can flee to safety.
5. Send a person to notify the ski patrol immediately if you are near a ski area and there are several rescuers. If you are the only rescuer, do a fast surface search for clues before leaving to notify the ski patrol. In remote backcountry, all survivors should remain and search until they cannot or should not continue.

Rescue transceivers or beacons are an efficient way of locating victims. Organized probe lines have found more victims than any other method, but because of the time involved, most of the victims were dead. Trained search dogs can locate buried victims quickly, but they often are brought to the scene only after long periods of burial. One trained dog can search more effectively than 30 searchers.

What to Do

After you have first checked for further avalanche danger and then found a victim (see page 410 for rescue procedures), follow these steps:

1. Quickly free the victim's head, chest, and stomach.
2. Send for help.
3. Clear the victim's airway and check the ABCs.
4. If a pulse is present but breathing is not, begin rescue breathing.
5. If no pulse is found, begin CPR.
6. Check for severe bleeding.
7. Examine for and stabilize a spine injury.
8. Treat for hypothermia.

Altitude Sickness

If you live in or visit mountainous regions, you need to know about altitude sickness. Altitude sickness is not simply an exotic affliction of mountaineers but a common environmental risk to which millions of people are exposed, often without adequate knowledge.

Also called acute mountain sickness, this condition affects about one in four people from lower elevations who visit areas 6,000 to 12,000 feet above sea level. Such elevations are common at ski resorts and on mountain hiking trails.

Altitude illnesses actually are a spectrum of a single problem, hypoxia. **Hypoxia** occurs when the body's tissues do not have enough oxygen. Altitude illnesses include **acute mountain sickness** (AMS), **high-altitude pulmonary edema** (HAPE), and **high-altitude cerebral edema** (HACE).

The actual incidence of altitude illness varies with rate of ascent and altitude attained. About 67 percent of climbers on Mt. Rainier in Washington suffer at least mild AMS because of rapid ascent to a moderately high altitude. The incidence of AMS in a study of Colorado skiers at lower altitudes (usually one day's ascent from Denver or lower) was only 15 to 40 percent.

Although anyone can get altitude sickness, certain factors increase the risk. Different people under similar conditions sometimes respond quite differently to altitude. For most people, at least four factors determine whether they will be sick or well after going to a higher altitude: (1) the speed of ascent (the slower the climb, the fewer the symptoms); (2) the altitude reached (the higher one goes, the more likely are problems); (3) one's health at the time (malnutrition, dehydration, fatigue, and any of several illnesses increase the risk); and (4) individual differences and genetic influences.

Altitude sickness occurs because oxygen levels decrease as elevation increases, and it takes a few days to adapt to the "thinner" air. At 11,500 feet, the amount of oxygen in the air is about 65 percent the amount at sea level, so the body has to struggle to maintain normal levels of oxygen.

What to Look For

Altitude illness typically strikes in the first 12 hours, and a headache is the most common problem. Other symptoms include loss of appetite, nausea, insomnia, fatigue, and shortness of breath with exertion. Three-fourths of all people who go from sea level to above 8,000 feet have at least one symptom (usually a headache), and the other fourth have three or more symptoms. Many people mistake the symptoms for a cold, the flu, or a hangover and wonder why it had to happen on their long-awaited mountain vacation.

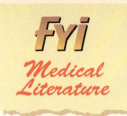

Acute Mountain Sickness Rapid ascent from low to high altitude is often followed by headaches, fatigue, shortness of breath, sleeplessness and loss of appetite—symptoms of acute mountain sickness. Acute mountain sickness affects climbers who ascend above 12,000 feet, but it was not thought to be common at lower altitudes. In a study of 3,158 adult visitors to Rocky Mountain elevations of 6,300 to 9,700 feet, more than 70 percent had at least one symptom of mountain sickness. One out of every four developed three or more symptoms, usually within 12 hours after arriving. Symptoms were most common in people age 18 to 19, people in poor physical condition or with a history of lung problems, and those whose permanent homes were at sea level. To reduce the risk of sickness, stop at an intermediate altitude for at least 36 hours and limit activities on arrival at the higher altitude.

Source: B. Honigman, et al., "Acute Mountain Sickness in a General Tourist Population at Moderate Altitudes," *Annals of Internal Medicine* 118:587–592 (March 1993).

Table 22-1: Characteristics of Altitude Illnesses

	AMS	HAPE	HACE
Elevation	Above 8,000 ft.	Usually above 10,000 ft.	Above 12,000 ft.
Time after ascent	1–2 days	3–4 days, possibly later	4–7 days, possibly later
Symptoms	Result from hypoxia and include headache, sleep disturbance, fatigue, shortness of breath, dizziness, loss of appetite, vomiting	Caused by pulmonary fluid and include shortness of breath, dry cough, mild chest pain, weakness, insomnia, rapid pulse, cyanosis, rales (crackles) or gurgling sounds	Caused by intracranial pressure on brain and include severe headache (unrelieved), vomiting, Cheynes-Stokes breathing (irregular breathing pattern followed by breathing stops), ataxia (inability to walk straight line), unconsciousness
First aid	• Stop ascending or go down. • Drink fluids. • Rest. • Take aspirin or ibuprofen. • Get prescription for Diamox™.	• Descend at least 2,000 ft. • Seek medical attention *immediately.*	• Descend 4,000 ft. • Seek medical attention *immediately.*

Notes: AMS = acute mountain sickness; HAPE = high-altitude pulmonary edema; HACE = high-altitude cerebral edema. HAPE and HACE occur when reduced oxygen causes capillary leakage and body-tissue swelling. Both conditions are life threatening.

Preventing Altitude Illness

You can take several measures to lower your risk of getting altitude sickness. First, start slowly and avoid overexerting yourself. By going easy, you allow your body to acclimatize, that is, adjust to different conditions. Simply put, your body becomes more efficient at using less oxygen. Unfortunately, it does not appear that the effects of acclimatization last once you return to your normal altitude. You must repeat the process for every subsequent return to higher elevations.

If you can't or won't take the time, then protective medications are available by prescription. Diamox™ (acetazolamide) has been effectively used to prevent AMS for more than 30 years. Diamox also seems to prevent HAPE and HACE, although that is almost impossible to prove because those two conditions are rare. The simplest explanation of the benefits of Diamox is that it enables the body to blow off more carbon dioxide while decreasing the alkalosis that results.

Side effects of Diamox include increased urination and tingling or numbness in the fingers and toes. If you are allergic to sulfa drugs, you may be allergic to Diamox. Also, you should wear a sunscreen with an SPF of at least 15 while taking the drug.

Diamox is effective for most lowlanders going to moderate altitude and perhaps for high-altitude residents returning after a short stay at low altitude. It has been called an artificial acclimatizer. Just how much Diamox to take and when to take it are still debated. Most experts suggest half a tablet (125 mg) in the morning and the evening of the ascent and twice a day for two more days.

Because dehydration can be a factor at high altitude, drink plenty of fluids like water and juice. Mountain air is drier than air at lower elevations. You are drinking enough fluid when your urine is clear. Tea, coffee, and alcohol cause more frequent urination and may lead to dehydration. Eat lightly for a few days.

Avoid taking sleeping pills because they tend to cause shallow breathing while you sleep, which can make it harder for your body to get enough oxygen. Likewise, do not smoke because it increases carbon monoxide levels in the blood, which diminishes the body's ability to use oxygen.

What to Do

It is important to recognize the symptoms of altitude sickness and take steps to treat it. In a small number of people, simple altitude sickness can progress to pulmonary edema (HAPE), in which fluid builds up in the lungs, or cerebral edema (HACE), in which fluid collects in the brain. Although uncommon, both conditions can be fatal in less than 12 hours. Seek medical help if any of the following, more serious symptoms happen: persistent cough, shortness of breath while resting, noisy breathing, loss of balance, confusion, or vomiting.

Most people who have altitude sickness get better with rest as the body acclimatizes. But anyone who has recently ascended to above 6,000 feet, is feeling ill, and does not improve in one to two days should see a physician. If that is not possible, the victim should descend 2,000 to 3,000 feet, rest, and drink plenty of fluids. Aspirin or a similar pain reliever can be taken for a mild headache. If rest and over-the-counter medication do not provide relief, a physician may have to administer oxygen or prescribe medication.

People with mild altitude illness usually improve even at altitude after a few days of rest and can continue with what they came to do (ski, hike, hunt, etc.). As long as the condition does not worsen and the victim can be carefully watched, a day or two of rest at altitude may be sufficient.

All forms of altitude illness are improved simply by descending a few thousand feet. If HACE is suspected, early descent is wise, because it is more serious. The next best step after descent is breathing additional oxygen to raise the inspired oxygen pressure to that at sea level. Both those steps relieve the headache rapidly and completely and make breathing easier.

At 18,000 feet, humans reach their ceiling if they stay for more than a few weeks. Any sea-level person taken quickly to 20,000 feet will be almost incapacitated in less than half an hour, and death will occur soon thereafter.

Lightning

Lightning is an awesome and frightening event. Lightning kills about 150 people and injures about 250 more in the United States each year (the actual numbers may be much higher). About 30 percent of lightning strikes to humans result in death. Lightning claims more lives in the United States than any other natural disaster, including earthquakes, blizzards, tornadoes, floods, hurricanes, and volcanic eruptions.

In the past, farmers, sailors, and other outdoor

workers in isolated areas tended to be the most frequently injured. Today, a larger proportion of victims are hikers, campers, golfers, and others who are outdoors for recreational purposes.

Almost 70 percent of lightning deaths involve just one person. Fifteen percent of victims are killed in groups of two, and another 15 percent are fatally injured in groups of three or more. Lightning deaths happen more often during daytime hours when people are active and outdoors. Most occur in the summer months of June through September, when thunderstorms are most frequent. There are more thunderstorm days in the South than in any other region of the United States. Thunderstorms occur frequently over high mountains. People are better protected in urban areas where high buildings have metal frames and lightning devices.

How Lightning Injures

Lightning injures in five ways. A **direct strike** is actually being struck by lightning and is most likely to hit a person in the open who has been unable to find shelter. Any conductor of electricity that the victim carries, especially if it is metal and carried above shoulder level (e.g., umbrella, golf clubs) increases the chances of a direct hit.

A more frequent cause of injury is from a **splash**, which happens when lightning that has hit a tree or a building "splashes" onto a victim who may be seeking shelter nearby. The electrical current, seeking the path of least resistance, may jump to a person whose body has less resistance than the tree or object that the lightning initially contacted. Frequently, groups of animals are killed as they stand near a fence or seek shelter under trees.

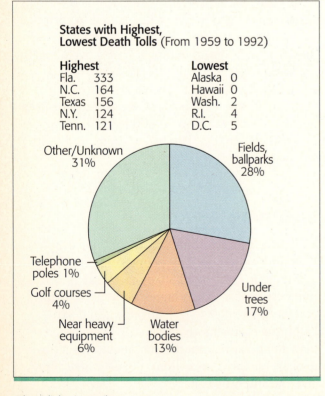

States with Highest, Lowest Death Tolls (From 1959 to 1992)

Highest		Lowest	
Fla.	333	Alaska	0
N.C.	164	Hawaii	0
Texas	156	Wash.	2
N.Y.	124	R.I.	4
Tenn.	121	D.C.	5

Other/Unknown 31%
Fields, ballparks 28%
Under trees 17%
Water bodies 13%
Near heavy equipment 6%
Golf courses 4%
Telephone poles 1%

Where lightning strikes

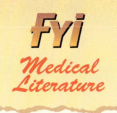

FYI

Medical Literature

Lightning Strikes: You Are Not Immune Indoors

Most lightning strike injuries occur outdoors—at golf courses, swimming pools, lakes, and open fields. Many victims make the error of standing under a tree, which is a common target for lightning. According to one report, it is better to take refuge under a shelter or in a closed automobile. If it is not possible to go inside, it is safer to seek shelter in a thick forest or grove of several trees, rather than under an isolated tree. Also, avoid contact with metal objects such as golf clubs and carts, fishing rods, bicycles, and umbrellas. But even if you are indoors, you are not fully protected. Lightning can travel through phone lines and grounded water pipes. So during lightning storms, do not use the phone and stay out of the shower or bathtub.

Source: M. Cherington, "Lightning Injuries," *Annals of Emergency Medicine* 25:516 (April 1995).

Contact injury happens when a person is holding onto an object that is either directly hit or splashed by lightning.

Ground current is produced when lightning hits the ground or an object nearby. The current spreads like a wave in a pond. Although ground current is less likely to produce fatalities than direct hits or splashes, it often creates multiple victims and injuries. Large groups have been injured on baseball fields, hiking paths, and military maneuvers.

People can be injured by the explosive force of the shock wave produced as lightning hits nearby. Victims are actually thrown by this **blast effect**.

Differences between Injuries from High-Voltage Electricity and from Lightning

Lightning contact with the body is almost instantaneous, leading to **flashover.** The current flashes over the body instead of going through it, so there are seldom burns of any magnitude. Exposure to high-voltage electricity tends to be much more prolonged, because the victim freezes to the circuit. The electrical energy surges through the tissues with little resistance to flow, causing massive internal thermal injury, with major amputations resulting.

Avoid Lightning Injury

- Be alert about weather conditions and predictions before going outdoors.
- Do not stand underneath a natural lightning rod such as a tall, isolated tree in an open area.
- Avoid projecting above the surrounding landscape, as you would do if you were standing on a hilltop, in an open field, on the beach, or fishing from a small boat.
- Get out of and away from open water.
- Get away from tractors and other metal farm equipment.
- Get off and away from motorcycles, scooters, golf carts, and bicycles. Put down golf clubs.
- Stay away from wire fences, clotheslines, metal pipes, rails, and other metallic paths that could carry lightning to you from some distance away.
- Avoid standing in small, isolated sheds or other small structures in open areas.
- In a forest, seek shelter in a low area under a thick growth of small trees. In open areas, go to a low place such as a ravine or valley.
- If you are hopelessly isolated in a level field or prairie and you feel your hair stand on end—indicating lightning is about to strike—drop to your knees and bend forward, putting your hands on your knees. *Do not lie flat on the ground.* You want as small an area of your body as possible touching the ground to minimize the possibility of your body acting as a conductor.
- While indoors during a thunderstorm, avoid open doors and windows, fireplaces, and metal objects such as pipes, sinks, and plug-in electrical appliances. Avoid using the telephone.
- If you are in an automobile (without a cloth top), stay in it. The vehicle will diffuse the current around you to the ground. It is a myth that the rubber tires will provide insulation, but true that the metal body affords protection.
- If a group of people is exposed, they should spread out and stay several yards apart. That way, should a strike hit, the least number will be seriously injured.

Causes of Death and Injuries

The most common cause of death in a lightning victim is cardiopulmonary arrest. It is highly unlikely for a victim to die unless cardiac arrest is suffered as an immediate effect of the strike. Until recently, nearly 75 percent of those who suffered cardiac arrest from lightning injuries died, often because CPR was not attempted.

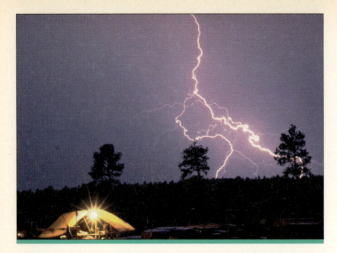

Lightning strike

The second major cause of death and injury is central nervous system damage. When electrical current traverses the brain, brain damage can occur. Seizures, paralysis, loss of consciousness, and amnesia can result.

Most people believe that a lightning victim will be severely burned. However, due to the flashover effect, most victims suffer only minor burns. The entrance and exit burn points common with electrical burns are rare with lightning. The types of burns seen with lightning strikes are punctate

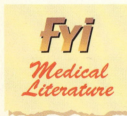

FYi
Medical Literature

Lightning Strikes Lightning strikes cause about 150 to 300 fatalities per year and 1,500 injuries. The majority of deaths are due to immediate cardiac arrest, while 74 percent of survivors sustain significant injury. Compared to electrical shock, lightning has a much higher voltage but much shorter duration of exposure (100 million to 2 billion volts for .01 to .001 second). This results in less energy delivered internally and, therefore, much less internal injury compared to electrical shock. Lightning may flash over the victim and only a small amount of current actually enter.

Lightning strikes may involve more than one victim up to 30 percent of the time. A person sustaining a lightning strike who does not go into cardiac arrest is unlikely to die. Therefore, a victim who appears dead should be treated before other victims who show obvious signs of life.

Source: P. Fontanarosa, "Electric Shock and Lightning Strike," *Annals of Emergency Medicine* 22(2):378–387 (February 1993).

FYi
World Record

Lightning Strike Survivals The only person in the world to be struck by lightning seven times and survive is ex-park ranger Roy C. Sullivan, of Virginia. His attraction to lightning began in 1942 (he lost his big toenail) and recurred in July 1969 (lost eyebrows), in July 1970 (left shoulder seared), on April 16, 1972 (hair set on fire), in August 1973 (hair set on fire again and legs seared), and on June 5, 1976 (ankle injured). He was sent to Waynesboro Hospital with chest and stomach burns on June 25, 1977, after being struck while fishing. In September 1983 he died by his own hand, reportedly rejected in love.

Source: The Guinness Book of Records (New York: Bantam Books, 1995), p. 167.

burns (small circular injuries resembling cigarette burns), feathering or ferning burns, linear burns, and ignited clothing and heated-metal burns. On rare occasions, clothing is ignited by lightning. A victim wearing metal, such as a necklace or a belt buckle, or carrying coins in a pocket may suffer burns as the objects become heated.

What to Do

1. If more than one victim has been struck by lightning at the same time, go to the quiet and motionless one first, check the ABCs, and treat accordingly.
2. If the victim is in cardiac arrest, start CPR. Persistent care is crucial for such victims.
3. Since spine injuries can occur with lightning strikes, precautions should be taken to stabilize the spine.
4. Raise the legs and keep the victim warm.

Wild Animal Attacks

Despite the fact that few large wild animals remain in the United States (bears, bison, cougars, and alligators), attacks on humans still occur. Wild animal attacks outside the United States are more common. Attacks, especially fatalities, are often reported and sensationalized in the media.

The incidence of injuries from wild animal attack is not known. Reporting is not mandatory, and many attacks are not recorded. Perhaps one or two deaths occur each year in the United States. Outside the United States, animal attacks by crocodiles, elephants, cape buffalo, lions, and tigers are a much greater cause of injury and death.

Wild animal attacks occur most often in rural or wilderness settings, a long distance from medical care.

Prevention of wild animal attacks is largely common sense and awareness. An increasing number of parks and wilderness areas are posting warning signs. Recreationalists should be aware of and knowledgeable about the animal habitats through which you travel and take precautions in food handling that attracts some animals.

Generally, if you encounter a large wild animal, try to remove yourself from the scene quietly and slowly. Running will elicit a predatory response. In most cases, a general rule is if attacked, fight back. Vigorous resistance with physical fighting, including striking the attacking animal with fists, a weapon, or any other object has been effective in repelling attacks by cougars, lions, tigers, brown and black bears, even crocodiles. An exception to this recommendation is the grizzly bear and a mother black bear with cubs. In these cases you should lie down and play dead.

Wilderness Evacuation

Determining the best mode of victim evacuation (e.g., helicopter evacuation versus walking the victim out or carrying the victim on a litter) must be based on several factors:*

- the severity of the illness or injury
- the rescue and medical skill of the rescuers
- the physical and psychological condition of the rescuers and the victims
- the availability of equipment and aid for the rescue
- the time, determined by distance, terrain, weather, and other conditions, it would take to evacuate the victim by other means
- the cost

When requesting outside assistance, you must consider the safety of incoming rescuers, their time commitment, and the cost of the rescue.

As a general rule, you should delay travel plans

*The recommendations presented here regarding wilderness evacuation are adapted from WMS guidelines.

or start evacuation of a victim from the wilderness for any of the following reasons:

- The victim is not improving.
- The victim is experiencing debilitating pain.
- The victim is unable to travel at a reasonable pace due to a medical problem.
- The victim is passing blood by the mouth or rectum (not from an obviously minor source).
- The victim has signs and symptoms of serious altitude illness.
- Infections are not improving.
- Chest pain is not from a rib cage injury.
- The victim's dysfunctional psychological status is impairing the safety of others.

When to Evacuate

Use these guidelines to decide if a victim should be evacuated.

Fractures

Rapidly evacuate the following types of fractures:

- open fractures
- extremity injuries in which circulation is absent
- spine injuries with no sensation in the fingers or toes or inability of victim to move fingers or toes

Do not rapidly evacuate these types of injuries:

- finger or toe injuries
- minimal injuries to joints

Wounds

In the wilderness, all bleeding should be controlled and all wounds cleaned and irrigated under pressure. The standard rule is not to remove blood-soaked dressings, but to place new dressings on top. In the wilderness, you should remove blood-soaked dressings, locate the bleeding vessels, and reapply pressure directly over the bleeding vessels. Do not close a wound with adhesive strips, butterfly bandages, staples, or sutures.

Evacuate a wounded victim for physician suturing of a wound within 6 hours for hand or foot injuries and within 24 hours for head or trunk injuries. (If necessary, closure can be done by a physician up to about the fourth day.)

Hypothermia

Do not evacuate a victim of mild hypothermia if the victim has a normal mental status.

Evacuate hypothermic victims who have profound hypothermia. It is impossible to rewarm a profoundly hypothermic victim in a wilderness or remote location. See Chapter 18.

Guidelines for Ground Evacuation

If the victim is walking out, at least two people should accompany the victim. If the victim is being carried out, one or two people should be sent to notify authorities that assistance is needed and to give them specifics about the problem.

During a litter evacuation, at least four, preferably six, bearers should carry the litter at all times. Over rough terrain, eight carriers (six over smooth trail) should carry the litter 100 yards and then rest or rotate with eight other carriers. It is very demanding to carry a loaded litter for more than 15 minutes without a break.

Guidelines for Helicopter Evacuation

Helicopters can reduce the time to medical care. Evacuate by helicopter only if the following conditions apply:

- The victim's life will be saved, or the victim will have a significantly better chance for full recovery.
- The pilot believes conditions are safe enough for helicopter evacuation.
- Ground evacuation would be unusually dangerous or excessively prolonged, or not enough rescuers are available for ground evacuation.

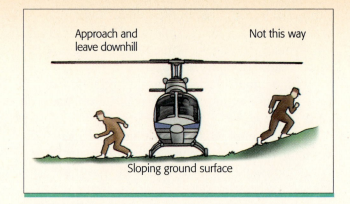

Helicopter safety

CAUTION: DO NOT

- approach a helicopter until a signal has been given by one of the aircraft personnel.
- approach a helicopter from the rear, where the fast-spinning tail rotor is invisible and dangerous. Many people walk into spinning rotors each year.
- forget to protect against windchill in the winter from the rotor blades or to protect eyes against flying dirt and debris.
- approach from the uphill side. The rotor is closer to the ground on the uphill side.
- stand up when approaching a helicopter. Keep as low as possible in a crouched position. Because the blade is flexible, it may dip as low as four feet off the ground.

STUDY QUESTIONS 22

Name _____ Course _____ Date _____

Activities

Activity 1

Mark each statement as true (T) or false (F).

T F 1. Most first aid books and training courses focus on situations in which EMS response time is quick.

T F 2. The wilderness setting may require you to use some advanced first aid methods.

T F 3. First aid supplies and equipment in a wilderness setting usually are limited.

T F 4. Environmental conditions such as heat, cold, and precipitation can become major concerns.

T F 5. CPR has limited use in remote locations.

T F 6. Attempt to reduce all finger and thumb dislocations.

T F 7. Straightening the leg can sometimes reduce a patella dislocation.

T F 8. Four rescuers can easily carry a victim out of the backcountry.

T F 9. In wilderness settings, wounds need to be closed by adhesive strips, butterfly bandages, stapling, or sutures.

T F 10. The most common cause of death from lightning is from the electrical current traveling to the brain.

T F 11. Entrance and exit burn points are common in those struck by lightning.

T F 12. During most animal attacks, the victim should fight back.

Activity 2

_____ 1. The Wilderness Medical Society defines *wilderness* as

    a. a remote geographical location

    b. an area or situation more than one hour from medical care

    c. both a and b

2. List five situations that would fit the WMS definition of *wilderness*:

    a. _____

    b. _____

    c. _____

    d. _____

    e. _____

3. List six reasons for wilderness first aid training:

    a. _____

    b. _____

    c. _____

    d. _____

    e. _____

    f. _____

_____ 4. In the wilderness, how long may a first aider have to remain with a sick or injured person before medical attention becomes available?

    a. many hours

    b. few minutes

    c. days

    d. both a and c

_____ 5. In a remote location, with a few exceptions, CPR can be stopped after how many minutes?

    a. 30

    b. 60

    c. 120

_____ 6. How long should you take to check an unconscious hypothermic victim's pulse?

    a. 3–5 seconds

    b. 5–10 seconds

    c. 30–45 seconds

    d. 2 minutes

7. Ordinarily, first aiders should never reduce dislocations. The Wilderness Medical Society, however, gives six reasons for reducing a joint dislocation quickly after it happens.

    a. _____

    b. _____

    c. _____

    d. _____

    e. _____

    f. _____

8. In wilderness locations, what three simple dislocations can a first aider attempt to reduce?

    a. _____

    b. _____

    c. _____

9. How can you identify an anterior shoulder dislocation?
    a. Upper arm is held away from the body.
    b. Arm cannot be brought next to the body.
    c. Hand of affected arm cannot touch the uninjured shoulder.
    d. All the above.

10. Name and describe the two methods of reducing an anterior shoulder dislocation:
    a. _____
    b. _____

11. What four questions should you ask to assess a suspected spine injury in the wilderness?
    a. _____
    b. _____
    c. _____
    d. _____
    What two physical exams should you perform?
    a. _____
    b. _____

12. List six factors influencing your decision to call for a helicopter evacuation.
    a. _____
    b. _____
    c. _____
    d. _____
    e. _____
    f. _____

13. What precautions should you take around a helicopter?
    a. _____
    b. _____
    c. _____
    d. _____
    e. _____

14. In what two ways do avalanches kill?
    a. _____
    b. _____

____ 15. About what percent of people from lower elevations who visit areas 6,000 to 12,000 feet above sea level experience acute mountain sickness?
    a. 25
    b. 50
    c. 66
    d. 75

____ 16. Hypoxia—the biggest factor in altitude illnesses—refers to
    a. low blood sugar
    b. anemia
    c. insufficient oxygen
    d. lactic acid

17. List the three types of altitude illness:
    a. _____
    b. _____
    c. _____

____ 18. The single best way to care for altitude illness is to
    a. carry and use oxygen
    b. descend to a lower elevation
    c. take aspirin
    d. rest and sleep

19. List the five ways that lightning injures people:
    a. _____
    b. _____
    c. _____
    d. _____
    e. _____

20. List four large wild animals in North America that attack humans.
    a. _____
    b. _____
    c. _____
    d. _____

Case Situations

Case 1

You take a summer job at Yellowstone National Park. During your first day, you experience a headache, fatigue, and shortness of breath. You have no appetite for food.

____ 1. What are you experiencing?
    a. heartbeat irregularity
    b. hypothermia
    c. acute mountain sickness
    d. excitement about your job and the surroundings.

Name _____ Course _____ Date _____

2. Check the statements below that are recommended for your condition:

_____ rest

_____ take a short walk

_____ take aspirin or ibuprofen

_____ drink fluids

_____ avoid drinking water

_____ see a physician for medication

Case 2

During a campout at a national forest, a thunderstorm unexpectedly develops. Everyone runs for shelter from the wind and rain, but a sudden lightning strike hits two of your companions at the same time. One is motionless while the other is mumbling and asking what happened.

_____ 1. Who do you check first?

    a. responsive victim

    b. unresponsive victim

_____ 2. If needed, should you start CPR in a wilderness location?

    a. yes

    b. no

Case 3

A mountain bike slipped on gravel while descending a trail causing the 19-year-old rider to fall on his outstretched arm. He complains of severe pain in his shoulder and tingling in his fingers. He has no other complaints. He is holding his upper arm away from the body.

_____ 1. You suspect a

    a. fractured clavicle

    b. fractured scapula

    c. anterior shoulder dislocation

    d. fractured sternum

Check the other indicators of what you suspect in question 1:

_____ 2. Victim may have experienced the injury before.

_____ 3. Victim is unable to reach across and touch the opposite uninjured shoulder.

CHAPTER

23

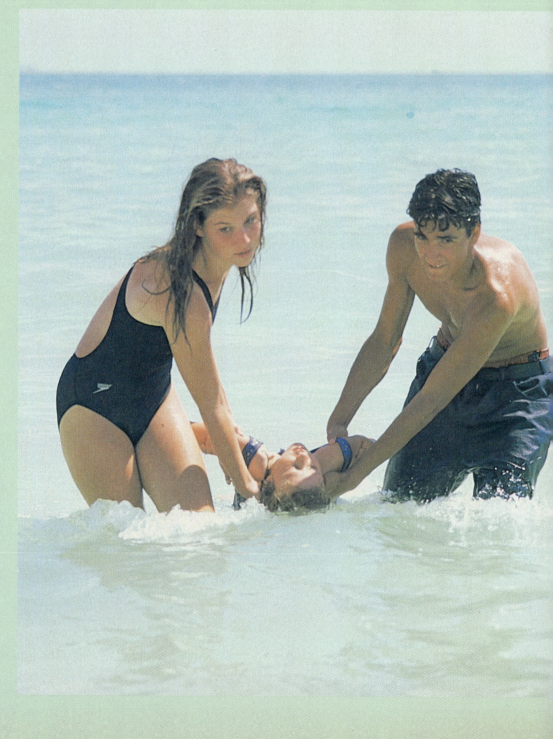

RESCUING AND MOVING VICTIMS

Victim Rescue

Water Rescue

Reach-throw-row-go identifies the sequence for attempting a water rescue. The first and simplest rescue technique is to **reach** for the victim. Reaching requires a lightweight pole, ladder, long stick, or any object that can be extended to the victim. Once you have your "reacher," secure your footing and have a bystander grab your belt or pants for stability. Secure yourself before reaching for the victim.

You can **throw** anything that floats—empty picnic jug, empty fuel or paint can, life jacket, floating cushion, piece of wood, inflated spare wheel—whatever is available. If there is a rope handy, tie it to the object to be thrown so you can pull the victim in, or, if you miss, you can retrieve the object and throw it again. The average untrained rescuer has a throwing range of about 50 feet.

> **"**
> *It is chance chiefly that makes heroes.*
> **"**
>
> Carlyle

If the victim is out of throwing range and there is a rowboat, canoe, motor boat, or boogie board nearby, you can try to **row** to the victim. Maneuvering these craft requires skill learned through practice. Wear a personal flotation device (PFD) for your own safety. To avoid capsizing, never pull the victim in over the side of a boat but over the stern (rear end).

If the three techniques are impossible and you are a capable swimmer trained in water lifesaving procedures, you can **go** to the drowning victim by swimming. Entering even calm water to make a swimming rescue is difficult and hazardous. All too often a would-be rescuer becomes a victim as well.

 CAUTION: DO NOT
- swim to and grasp a drowning person unless you are trained in lifesaving.

Near-Drowning

In the United States there are about 4,000 fatalities each year from drowning. In addition to the drownings, there are many cases of extreme, permanent disability that result from near-drowning. It is estimated that for every 10 children

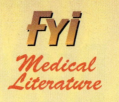

Near-Drowning: Quick Treatment Saves Lives

About 4,000 people die each year in the United States as a result of drowning. Reportedly, for every drowning case, there are about 500 to 600 near-drownings. Quick action can make the difference between life and death. The outcome is usually good for victims who are submerged less than five minutes and if CPR is started less than 10 minutes after submersion. Near-drowning victims often have spine injuries, so care should be taken when positioning the head and neck during rescue breathing. More important, preventive measures can avoid such life-threatening events: supervise infants and toddlers, install fencing around home swimming pools, and do not use alcohol before swimming or playing water sports.

Source: M. H. Bross and J. L. Clark, *American Family Physician* 51:1545 (May 1995).

near-drowning without aspiration is easier to resuscitate because water has not entered the airway.

Eighty-five percent of near-drownings are **wet drownings,** that is, water, vomitus, or foreign bodies are aspirated into the lungs. Fresh water in the lungs enters the bloodstream and has a profound effect on blood cells, resulting in their destruction (they swell and burst) and subsequent cardiac arrest (ventricular fibrillation). In saltwater drownings, water is taken from the bloodstream and goes into the lungs. As much as one-quarter the total blood volume is lost as fluids move into the lungs. The victims drown in their own fluids as much as in the saltwater itself.

A **secondary drowning** is one in which a victim who is resuscitated dies within 96 hours. Aspiration pneumonia is a late complication of near-drownings occurring 48 to 72 hours after the episode. Near-drowning victims should be hospitalized or at least closely monitored.

What to Do

1. Survey the scene (see Chapter 2), then carry out a water rescue.
2. If the victim was diving (or it is unknown if he or she was diving), suspect a possible spine injury. Keep the victim in-line floating on the water surface until properly trained rescuers arrive with a backboard.

who drown, 36 are admitted to hospitals and 140 are treated in emergency rooms for near-drowning.

Drowning means suffocation by immersion in water or other liquid. **Near-drowning** occurs when a victim survives an immersion incident. About two-thirds of drowning victims are less than 30 years old. Most of them are males.

Usually, the initial reaction of drowning persons is panic. Then violent struggling occurs. Frequently, as they become short of breath, victims swallow water during attempts to breathe. That water is often vomited. Further attempts at breathing may then result in aspiration of water, vomitus, or foreign bodies into the lungs. Sometimes the vocal cords (larynx) close and will not allow any water to enter the lungs. A seizure may occur and then death.

Drownings can be classified into three basic types. Ten to 15 percent are **dry drownings** because no water passes the vocal cords. Presumably, in these cases, when water touches the cords, they shut tightly (laryngospasm). Other things being equal, a

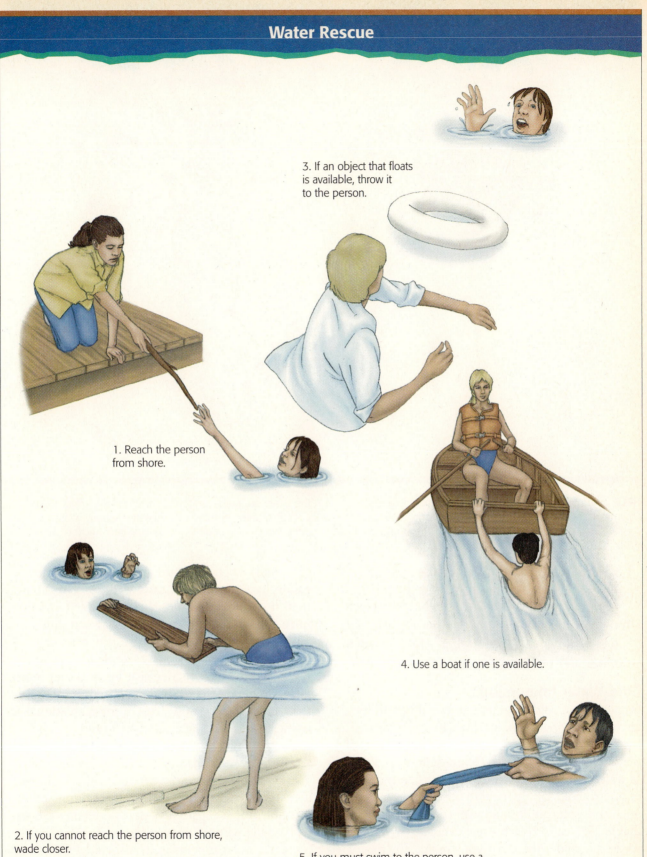

3. If an object that floats is available, throw it to the person.

1. Reach the person from shore.

4. Use a boat if one is available.

2. If you cannot reach the person from shore, wade closer.

5. If you must swim to the person, use a towel or board for him or her to hold onto. Do not let the person grab you.

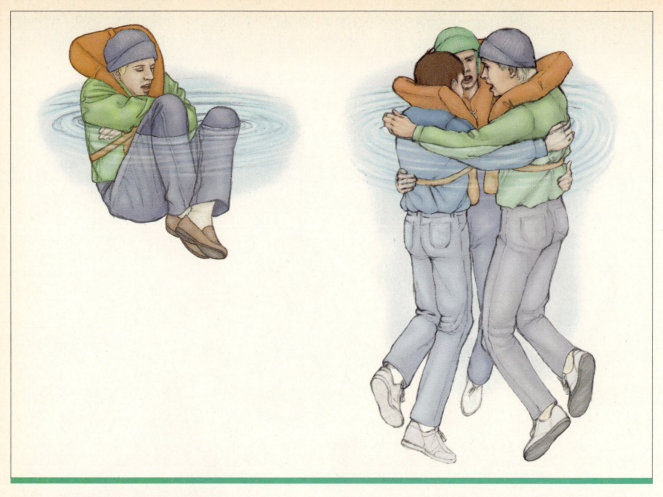

HELP or Huddle A person wearing a flotation device can minimize heat loss and increase chances of survival by assuming the Heat Escape Lessening Position, or HELP (left), in which the knees are pulled up to the chest and the arms crossed. Groups of three or more can conserve heat by wrapping their arms around one another and pulling into a tight circle (right).

3. Check the ABCs and treat accordingly. Any pulseless, nonbreathing victim who has been submerged in cold water should be resuscitated.
4. If no spine injury is suspected, place the victim on his or her side to allow fluids to drain from the airway.

Cold-Water Immersion

Immersion in cold water is a potential hazard for anyone participating in activities in the oceans, lakes, and streams of all but the tropical regions of the world. The U.S. Coast Guard defines cold water as water below 70°F. However, water does not need to be that cold for a person to become hypothermic. A person can become hypothermic in water that is 77°F. Most North American lakes, rivers, and coasts are colder than that year-round. The risk of immersion hypothermia in North America is nearly universal most of the year. A person immersed in cold water loses heat about 25 times faster than someone exposed to cold air.

The U.S. Coast Guard and other rescue organizations recommend that survivors get as much of their bodies out of the water as possible to minimize cooling rate and maximize survival time. A widespread misunderstanding of the concept of windchill often causes many people to conclude that survivors have higher heat losses if they are exposed to wind, especially if they are wet, than if they are immersed in water. During recreational activities at beaches, lakes, and swimming pools, most people have experienced feeling colder after leaving the water than they do while swimming. That reinforces the misunderstanding, which has sometimes led accident victims to abandon a safe position atop a capsized vessel and reenter the water, usually with tragic results.

Cold-water immersion is associated with two potential medical emergencies: drowning and hypothermia. Numerous case histories and statistical evidence document the prominence of cold-water immersion as a cause of drowning and hypothermia.

American Academy of Pediatrics Recommendations for Preventing Childhood Drowning (by Age Group)

4 years and younger
- Never leave them alone in bathtubs, spas, or wading pools—or near nearly filled buckets, toilets, irrigation ditches, or other standing water.
- Recognize that swimming lessons do not "drownproof" them.
- Fence entire pool so that it is separated from the house. Pool covers are not a substitute for fences.
- Learn CPR and keep a telephone and emergency equipment—such as life preservers and a shepherd's crook—poolside.

5 to 12 years
- Provide them with swimming lessons that include safety rules.
- Never let them swim alone or without adult supervision.
- Make sure they wear approved flotation devices when playing in or near a body of water.
- Teach them the dangers of jumping or diving into water and of being on thin ice.

13 to 19 years
- In addition to relaying the safety tips above, counsel them about the dangers of substance abuse combined with swimming, diving, or boating.
- Teach them CPR.

Source: American Academy of Pediatrics, "Drowning in Infants, Children, and Adolescents," *Pediatrics* 92(2): 292–294 (1993).

Perhaps the most famous occurrence of cold-water immersion was the sinking of the *Titanic* on April 14, 1912. After striking an iceberg, the ship sank in calm seas. Of the 2,201 people on board, only 712 were rescued, all from the ship's lifeboats. The remaining 1,489 people died in the water, despite the arrival of a rescue vehicle within two hours. Nearly all those victims were wearing life preservers, yet the cause of death was officially listed as drowning. More likely, the cause of death was immersion hypothermia.

A person's cooling depends on several factors:

- *Body fat.* The fatter a person is, the slower cooling occurs. More fat increases survival chances.
- *Body type.* Big people cool slower than smaller people. Children cool faster than adults.

Women have more fat but are usually smaller, so they cool at the same rate as men.

- *Physical fitness.* Cardiovascular fitness can help meet the stress of cold-water immersion, but physically fit people usually have less subcutaneous fat for insulation.
- *Water temperature.* The colder the water, the faster a person cools.
- *Clothing.* Clothing can insulate, and some types of fabric, such as wool, are better than others.
- *Alcohol.* Drunks are more likely to get into dangerous situations. Alcohol impairs judgment and coordination. Research studies have found alcohol to be implicated in 10 to 50 percent of all drownings. Alcohol dilates the skin's blood vessels, which allows more body heat to escape.
- *Behavior.* Swimming and treading water increase the flow of warm blood from the body's core to the muscles, thus increasing the cooling rate. The swimmers often die first, since they are more likely to try to tread water or swim rather than float. Likewise, so-called drownproofing, a technique of bobbing in the water (like a jellyfish), markedly increases heat loss as water circulates around the head.

A heat escape lessening position (HELP) has been devised, in which the victim draws the knees up close to the chest, presses the arms to the sides and remains as quiet as possible. For two or more people, huddling quietly and closely together (huddle position) will decrease heat loss from the groin and the front of the body. Both of these positions require personal flotation devices (life jackets).

Table 23-1: Effect of Flotation Devices on Survival Times

Situation (50° Water)	Predicted Survival Time (Hours)
No Flotation Device	
Drownproofing	1.5
Treading water	2.0
With Flotation Device	
Swimming	2.0
Holding still	2.7
HELP position	4.0
Huddle position	4.0

Surviving long periods of submersion has been explained by the **diving reflex** found in mammals. Some say that the diving reflex slows the heart rate, shunts blood to the brain, and closes the airway. Recent research, however, suggests that the diving reflex is present in marine mammals (e.g, seals, porpoises, whales, walruses) but not in humans. If the diving reflex is discounted, the most likely explanation for prolonged submersion survival is that cold water produces hypothermia, which reduces the body's demand for oxygen and protects the brain.

Ice Rescue

If a person has fallen through the ice near the shore, extend a pole or throw a line with a floatable object attached to it. When the person has a hold, pull him or her toward the shore or the edge of the ice.

If the person is through the ice away from the shore and you cannot reach him or her with a pole or a throwing line, lie flat and push a ladder, plank, or similar object ahead of you. If you have nothing but a spare wheel, tie a rope to the wheel and the other end to an anchor point, lie flat, and push the wheel ahead of you. Pull the person ashore or to the edge of the ice.

CAUTION: DO NOT
- go near broken ice without support.

Electrical Emergency Rescue

Electrical injuries are devastating. Even just a mild shock can cause serious internal injuries. A current of 1,000 volts or more is considered high voltage, but even the 110 volts of household current can be deadly.

When a person gets an electric shock, electricity enters the body at the point of contact and travels along the path of least resistance (nerves and blood vessels). The current travels rapidly, generating heat and causing destruction.

Most indoor electrocutions are caused by faulty electrical equipment or careless use of electrical appliances. Before you touch the victim, turn off the electricity at the circuit breaker, fuse box, or outside switch box or unplug the appliance if the plug is undamaged.

If the electrocution involves high-voltage *power lines,* the power must be turned off before anyone approaches a victim. If you approach a victim and

CAUTION: DO NOT
- touch an appliance or the victim until the current is off.
- try to move downed wires.
- use *any* object, even dry wood (e.g., broomstick, tools, chair, stool) to separate the victim from the electrical source.

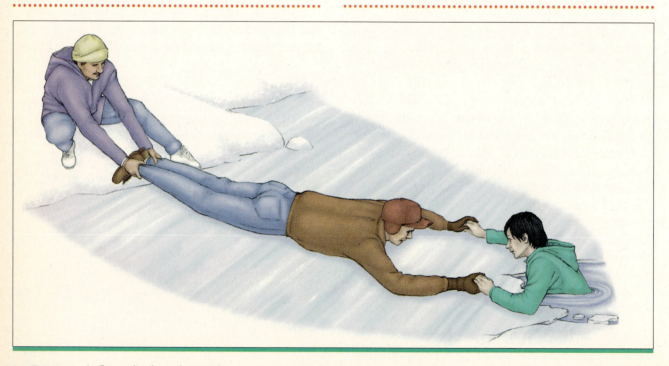

Ice Rescue   Lie flat to distribute the weight.

feel a tingling sensation in your legs and lower body, stop. You are on energized ground, and an electrical current is entering one foot, passing through your lower body, then leaving through the other foot. If that happens, raise one foot off the ground, turn around, and hop to a safe place. Wait for trained personnel with the proper equipment to cut the wires or disconnect them.

If a power line has fallen over a car, tell the driver and passengers to stay in the car. A victim should try to jump out of the car *only* if an explosion or fire threatens, and then without making contact with the car or the wire.

Hazardous Materials Incidents

At almost any highway accident scene, there is the potential danger of hazardous chemicals. Clues that indicate the presence of hazardous materials include

- signs on vehicles (e.g., "explosive," "flammable," "corrosive")
- spilled liquids or solids
- strong, unusual odors
- clouds of vapor

Stay well away and upwind from the area. Only persons who are specially trained in handling hazardous materials and who have the proper equipment should be in the area.

Motor Vehicle Accidents

In most states, you are legally obligated to stop and give help when you are involved in a motor vehicle accident. If you come on an accident shortly after it happens, the law does not require you to stop, although it might be argued that you have a moral responsibility to render any aid you can.

1. Stop your vehicle in a safe place. If the police have taken charge, do not stop unless you are asked to do so.
2. Turn on your flashing hazard lights.
3. Direct bystanders to warn other drivers and to set up warning flares.
4. Try to enter an involved vehicle through a door. If the doors are jammed, try to get someone inside the car to roll down a window. As a last resort, break a window to gain access. Once inside, place the vehicle in park, turn off the key, and set the parking brake.

CAUTION: DO NOT
- rush to get victims out of a car that has been in an accident. Contrary to opinion, most vehicle crashes do not involve fire, and most vehicles stay in an upright position.

5. For any unconscious victims and those who might have broken necks, use your hands to stabilize their heads and necks.
6. Treat any life-threatening injuries.
7. Whenever possible, wait for EMS personnel to extricate the victims because of their training and having the proper equipment. In most cases, keep the victims stabilized inside the vehicle.

Fires

Should you encounter a fire, you should

1. Get all the people out fast.
2. Call the emergency telephone number (usually 911).

Then—and *only* then—if the fire is small and if your own escape route is clear should you fight the fire yourself with a fire extinguisher. You may be able to put out the fire or at least hold damage to a minimum. Fire fighting during the first five minutes of a fire is worth more than the work of the next several hours.

If clothing catches fire, tear it off away from the face. Keep the victim from running, since that fans the flames. Wrap a rug or a woolen blanket around the victim's neck to keep the fire from the face or throw a blanket on the victim. In some cases, you may be able to smother the flames by throwing the victim to the floor and rolling him or her in a rug.

To use a fire extinguisher, aim directly at whatever is burning and sweep across it. Extinguishers expel their contents quickly, in 8 to 25 seconds for most home models containing dry chemicals.

CAUTION: DO NOT
- let a victim run if clothing is on fire.
- get trapped while fighting a fire. Always keep a door behind you so you can exit if the fire gets too big.

Threatening Dogs

When you enter any emergency scene, look for signs of a dog and ignore it if the animal is not threatening. Ask the owner to control a threatening dog. If you cannot be delayed, consider using a fire extinguisher, water hose, or pepper spray. For a vicious dog, call the police for assistance.

Farm Animals

Emergencies involving farm animals can be dangerous to rescuers. Horses kick and bite. Cattle kick, bite, gore, or squeeze people against a pen or barn. Pigs can deliver severe bites.

- Approach a situation involving animals with caution.
- Do not frighten an animal. Speak quietly to reassure it.
- If food is available, use it to lure the animal away from the victim.

Confined Spaces

A confined space is any area not intended for human occupancy that also has the potential for containing or accumulating a dangerous atmosphere. Examples of confined spaces are tanks, vessels, vats, bins, vaults, trenches, and pits.

An accident in a confined space demands immediate action. If an entrant into a confined space signals for help or becomes unconscious, follow these steps to help:

1. Call for immediate help.
2. Do *not* rush in to help.
3. If you are the attendant, do *not* enter the confined space unless you are relieved by another attendant *and* you are part of the rescue team.
4. When help arrives, try to rescue the victim without entering the space.
5. If rescue from the outside cannot be done, allow trained and properly equipped (respiratory protection plus safety harnesses or lifelines) rescuers to enter the space and remove the victim.
6. Activate the local EMS.
7. Give first aid, rescue breathing, or CPR if necessary and if you are trained.

Triage: What to Do with Multiple Victims

You may encounter emergency situations in which there are two or more victims. This often is the case in multiple-car accidents or disasters. After making a quick scene survey, decide who must be cared for and transported first. This process of prioritizing or classifying injured victims is called triage. *Triage* is a French word meaning *to sort*. The goal is to do the greatest good for the greatest number of victims.

Finding Life-Threatened Victims

A variety of systems are used to identify care and transportation priorities. To find those needing immediate care for life-threatening conditions, first tell all victims who can get up and walk to move to a specific area. Victims who can get up and walk rarely have life-threatening injuries. These victims ("walking wounded") are classified as delayed priority (see below). Do not force a victim to move if he or she complains of pain.

Find the life-threatened victims by performing only the primary survey on all remaining victims. Go to motionless victims first. You must move rapidly (spend less than 60 seconds with each victim) from one victim to the next until all have been assessed. Classify victims according to the following care and transportation priorities:

1. **Immediate care.** Victim has life-threatening injuries but can be saved.
   - airway or breathing difficulties (not breathing or breathing rate faster than 30 per minute)
   - weak or no pulse
   - uncontrolled or severe bleeding
   - unresponsive or unconscious
2. **Urgent care.** Victims not fitting into the immediate or delayed categories. Care and transportation can be delayed up to one hour.
3. **Delayed care.** Victims with minor injuries. Care and transportation can be delayed up to three hours.
4. **Dead.** Victims are obviously dead, mortally wounded, or unlikely to survive because of the extent of their injuries, age, and medical condition.

Do not become involved in treating the victims at this point, but ask knowledgeable bystanders to care for immediate life-threatening problems (i.e., rescue breathing, bleeding control).

Reassess victims regularly for changes in their condition. Only when the immediate life-threatening conditions receive care should those with less serious conditions be given care.

Later, you will usually be relieved when more highly trained emergency personnel arrive on the scene. You may then be asked to provide first aid, to help move, or to help with ambulance or helicopter transportation.

Moving Victims

A victim should not be moved until he or she is ready for transportation to a hospital, if required. All necessary first aid should be provided first. A victim should be moved only if there is an immediate danger:

- There is a fire or danger of fire.
- Explosives or other hazardous materials are involved.
- It is impossible to protect the accident scene from hazards.
- It is impossible to gain access to other victims in the situation (e.g., a vehicle) who need life-saving care.

CAUTION: DO NOT

- move a victim unless you absolutely have to. That might happen if the victim is in immediate danger or must be moved to shelter while waiting for the EMS to arrive.
- make the injury worse by moving the victim.
- move a victim who could have a spine injury.
- move a victim without stabilizing the injured part.
- move a victim unless you know where you are going.
- leave an unconscious victim alone.
- move a victim when someone could be sent for help. Wait with the victim and send someone else for help.
- try to move a victim by yourself if other people are available to help.

Principles of Lifting

- Know your capabilities. Do not try to handle too heavy or awkward a load—seek help.
- Use a safe grip. Use as much of your palms as possible.
- Keep your back straight. Tighten the muscles of your buttocks and abdomen.
- Bend your knees to use the strong muscles of the thighs and buttocks.
- Keep your arms close to your body and elbows flexed.
- Position your feet shoulder width apart for balance, one in front of the other.
- When lifting, keep and lift the victim close to your body.
- While lifting, do not twist your back; pivot with the feet.
- While lifting and carrying, do so slowly, smoothly, and in unison with other helpers.
- Before you move a victim, tell him or her what you are doing.

A cardiac arrest victim is usually moved unless he or she is already on the ground or floor, because CPR must be performed on a firm surface.

Emergency Moves

The major danger in moving a victim quickly is the possibility of aggravating a spine injury. In an emergency, every effort should be made to pull the victim in the direction of the long axis of the body to provide as much protection to the spinal cord as possible. If victims are on the floor or ground, you can drag them away from the scene by one of various techniques.

Nonemergency Moves

All injured parts should be stabilized before and during moving. If rapid transportation is not needed, it is helpful to practice on another person about the same size as the injured victim.

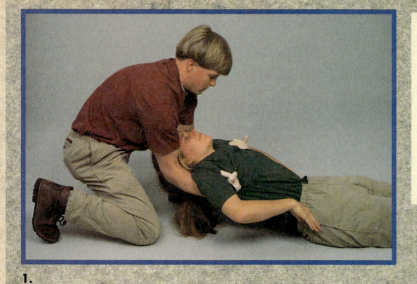

1. *Shoulder drag.* For short distances over a rough surface, stabilize victim's head with your forearms.
2. *Ankle drag.* The fastest method for a short distance on a smooth surface.
3. *Blanket pull.* Roll the victim onto a blanket and pull from behind the victim's head.

1.

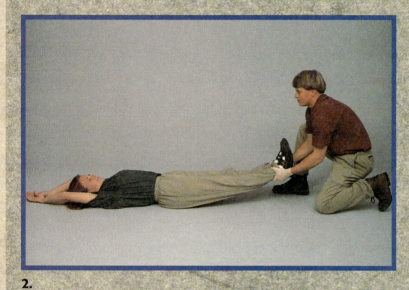

2.

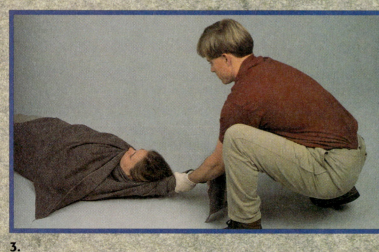

3.

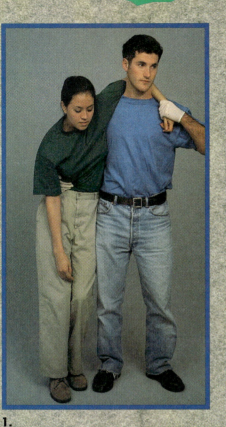

1.

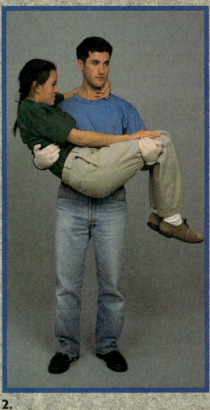

2.

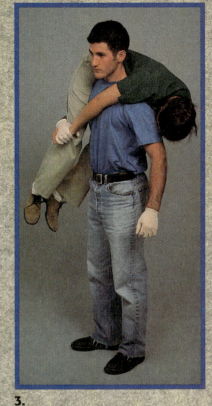

3.

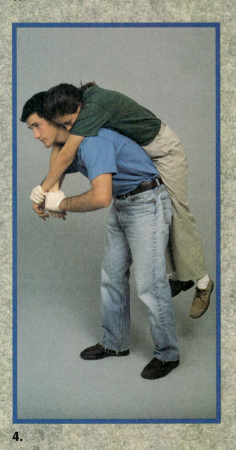

4.

1. *Human crutch* (*one person helps victim to walk*). If one leg is injured, help the victim to walk on the good leg while you support the injured side.
2. *Cradle carry*. Use for children and lightweight adults who cannot walk.
3. *Fireman's carry*. If the victim's injuries permit, longer distances can be traveled if the victim is carried over your shoulder.
4. *Pack-strap carry*. When injuries make the fireman's carry unsafe, this method is better for longer distances.
5. *Piggyback carry*. Use this method when the victim cannot walk but can use the arms to hang onto the rescuer.

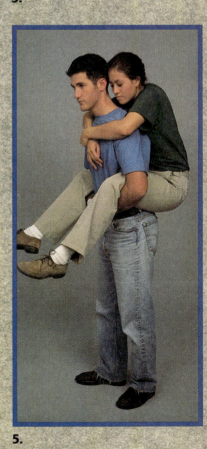

5.

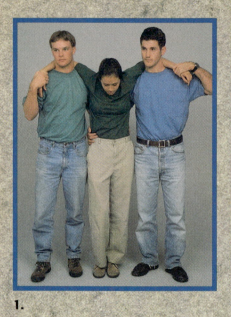

1.

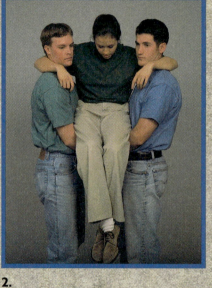

2.

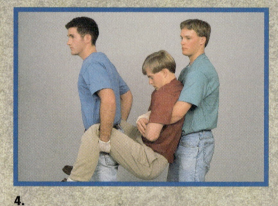

3.

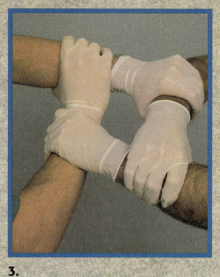

4.

1. *Two-person assist.* Similar to human crutch.
2. *Two-handed seat carry.*
3. *Four-handed seat carry.* The easiest two-person carry when no equipment is available, and the victim cannot walk but can use the arms to hang onto the two rescuers.
4. *Extremity carry.*
5. *Chair carry.* Useful for a narrow passage or up or down stairs. Use a sturdy chair that can take the victim's weight.
6. *Hammock carry.* Three to six people stand on alternate sides of the injured person and link hands beneath the victim.

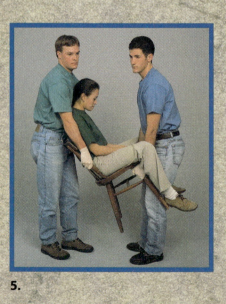

5.

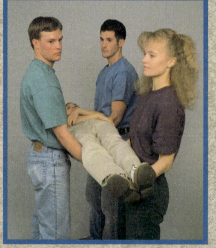

6.

Stretcher or Litter

The safest way to carry an injured victim is on some type of stretcher or litter, which can be improvised. Before using it, test an improvised stretcher by lifting a rescuer about the same size as the victim.

- *Blanket-and-pole improvised stretcher.* If the blanket is properly wrapped, the victim's weight will keep it from unwinding.
- *Blanket with no poles.* The blanket is rolled inward toward the victim and grasped for carrying by four or more rescuers.
- *Board improvised stretcher.* Sturdier than a blanket-and-pole stretcher but heavier and less comfortable. Tie the victim on to prevent rolling off.

Commercial stretchers and litters usually are not available except through the EMS.

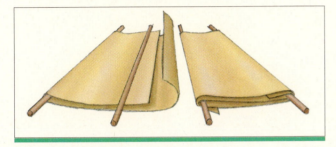

Blanket-and-pole improvised stretcher

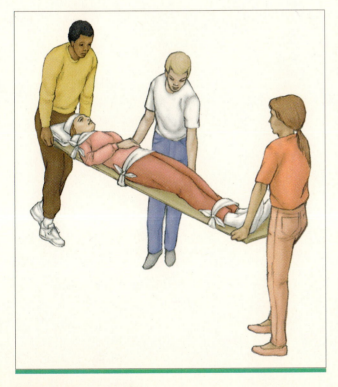

Board improvised stretcher

Hero CITATION

David M. Nyman saved James P. Sweeney from exposure and avalanche, Denali National Park, Alaska. On April 19, 1989, Sweeney, 33, was climbing Mt. Johnson, near Ruth Glacier, when he fell, fracturing and dislocating a hip. His climbing partner, Nyman, 31, lowered him to the base of the mountain, where they spent the night. The following day, Nyman skied to a lodge several miles away and dispatched rescuers, but they could not reach Sweeney. Nyman immediately returned, alone, to Sweeney, believing that evacuation by air was forthcoming. A snowstorm caused avalanches, which buried Nyman and Sweeney despite Nyman's repeated efforts to secure refuge. On April 25, their supplies nearly depleted, Nyman began to remove Sweeney singlehandedly. Nyman painstakingly covered almost a mile over terrain that descended 1,200 feet to the glacier. On April 26, they were evacuated by helicopter from the glacier and taken to a hospital. Sweeney was detained 6 weeks for his injuries. Nyman recovered from marked dehydration and frostbite.

Moving Victims   **435**

Many injuries and sudden illnesses can be cared for without medical attention. For these situations and for situations requiring medical attention later, it is a good idea to have useful supplies on hand for emergencies.

A first aid kit's supplies should be customized to include those items likely to be used on a regular basis. For example, a kit for a home will be different from one at a workplace or one found on a boat.

The list here includes nonprescriptive (over-the-counter) medications. Some drug products lose their potency over time, especially after they have been opened. Other drugs change in consistency. Buying the large "family size" of a product infrequently used may seem like a bargain, but it is poor economy if the product has to be thrown out before the contents are used. Note every medication's expiration date.

Keep all medicines out of the reach of children. Read and follow all directions for properly using medications.

Keep your first aid supplies in either a fishing tackle box or a tool box. Boxes with an O-ring gasket around the cover are dustproof and waterproof.

Equipment

Scissors
- Regular
- Bandage (blunt-tip prevents injury while cutting next to skin)
- EMT shears (to cut through metal, leather, heavy clothing)

Tweezers (to remove splinters, ticks, small objects from wounds)

Pocket knife, folding

Disposable gloves, latex (protection against disease)

Mouth-to-barrier device, face mask with 1-way valve, or face shield (protection against disease during rescue breathing)

Thermometer (to measure body temperature)

Penlight, battery or disposable

Light stick

Resealable plastic bags, pint and quart (for ice

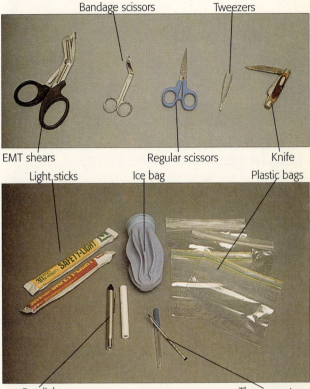

Bandage scissors — Tweezers — EMT shears — Regular scissors — Knife

Light sticks — Ice bag — Plastic bags — Pen lights — Thermometer

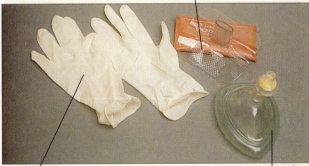

Face shield — Latex gloves — Face mask

packs, amputation care, barrier against blood)

Ice bag (ice pack)

Cotton-tipped swabs (to remove small objects from eye, evert eyelid, apply ointment)

Extractor, from Sawyer Products (to suction snakebite venom)

SAM splint (to stabilize almost any part of the body)

Emergency blanket (to protect victim from heat loss and weather)

Safety pins, size 3 (to hold bandages in place, improvise slings)

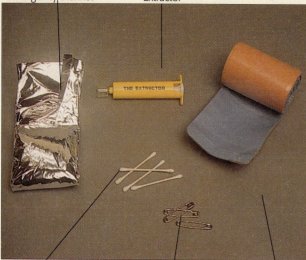

Emergency blanket   Extractor™

Cotton-tipped swabs   Safety pins   SAM Splint™

Bandages and Dressings

Gauze pads, 2-inch by 2-inch, 3-inch by 3-inch, 4-inch by 4-inch (to stop bleeding and cover wounds)

Nonstick pads, 2-inch by 3-inch, 3-inch by 4-inch

Adhesive strip bandages, various sizes and materials (to cover small wounds)

Trauma dressings, 5-inch by 9-inch, 8-inch by 10-inch (to cover large wounds)

Gauze roller bandages, 1-inch, 2-inch (to hold dressings in place)

Conforming, self-adhering roller bandages, 2-inch, 3-inch (to hold dressings in place)

Elastic roller bandages, 2-inch, 3-inch, 4-inch, 6-inch (for compression on sprains and strains)

Adhesive tape, ½-inch or 1-inch (to hold dressings in place, secure end of roller bandages)

Gauze pads

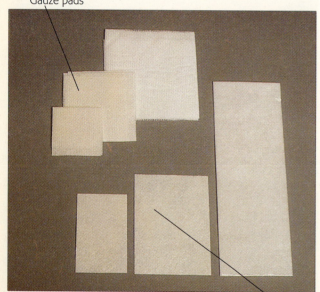

Nonstick pads

Hypoallergenic paper tape (to hold dressings in place; prevents skin reactions)

Waterproof tape (to hold dressings in place)

Knuckle bandages

Fingertip strips

Eye pads

Triangular bandages (for arm sling and to form cravat bandages for holding splints and dressings in place)

Moleskin and molefoam (blister prevention and care)

Duct tape, roll (blister prevention, to hold splints in place)

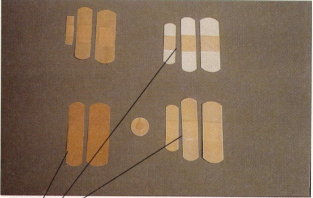

Adhesive strip bandages

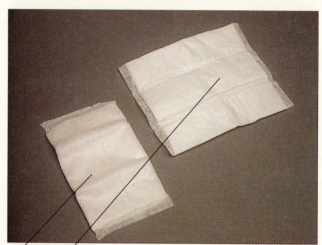

Trauma dressings

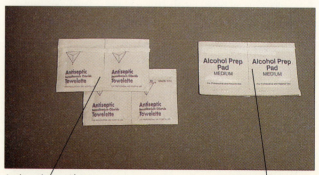

Antiseptic towelettes   Alcohol prep pads

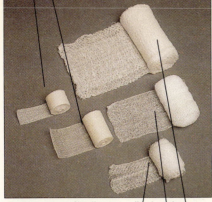
Gauze rollers

Conforming, self-adhering roller bandages

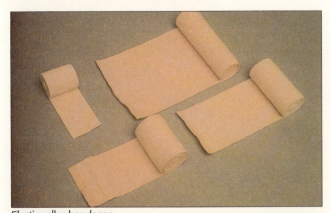
Elastic roller bandages

Ointments and Topicals

Antiseptic towelettes (to clean hands and skin around wounds)

Alcohol prep pads (to clean skin around wounds)

Antibiotic ointment (for minor cuts, abrasions, burns)

Hydrocortisone cream, 1 percent (for skin irritation and itching)

Antifungal cream

Calamine lotion (anti-itch and drying agent for poison ivy/oak/sumac and skin rashes)

Sting-relief swabs (to relieve pain from insect bites and stings)

Instant ice pack (to use when ice is not available)

Spenco Second Skin Pads (for blister care)

Aloe vera gel, 100 percent (for minor burns, frostbite)

Sunscreen (SPF 15)

Lip balm with sunscreen (to protect lips)

Insect repellent, containing less than 30 percent DEET (less than 10 percent for children under 5 years of age)

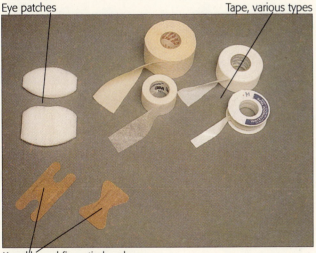
Eye patches   Tape, various types

Knuckle and fingertip bandages

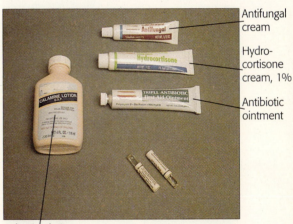
Antifungal cream

Hydro-cortisone cream, 1%

Antibiotic ointment

Calamine lotion

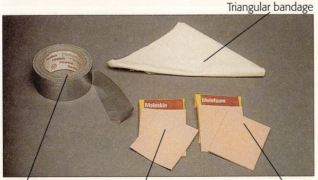
Triangular bandage

Duct tape   Moleskin   Molefoam

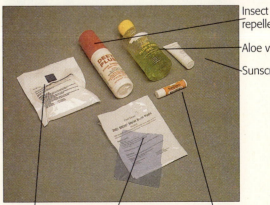
Insect repellent

Aloe vera gel

Sunscreen

Instant ice pack   Spenco Second Skin™   Lip balm

Over-the-Counter Internal Medicines

Aspirin (for pain, swelling, fever)

Ibuprofen (for pain, swelling, fever)

Acetaminophen (for pain)

Antihistamine (for allergy)

Decongestant, tablets and nasal spray

Antacid (for gas)

Antidiarrhea, antinausea, antivomiting preparation

Anticonstipation preparation

Motion sickness preventative

Glucose gel (for insulin reaction)

Oil of cloves (for toothache)

Activated charcoal, premixed liquid (for swallowed poisoning)

Ipecac syrup (use only when medical authority directs for swallowed poisoning)

Cough suppressant

Powdered electrolyte drink mix (for heat stress)

Pencil and small notebook (to record information and send messages) and National Safety Council *First Aid Guide*.

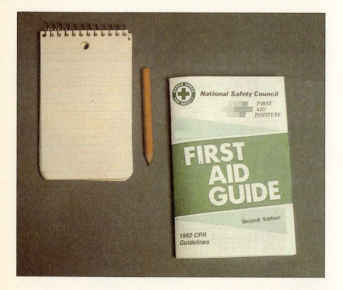

As a first aider, you may be in a situation that requires you to give a victim certain medications (or to assist a victim in taking his or her own medication). A knowledgeable first aider should be familiar with the following medications:

Over-the-counter pain relievers

- acetaminophen
- aspirin
- ibuprofen
- naproxen

Victim's physician-prescribed medications

- metered-dose inhaler
- nitroglycerin
- epinephrine

Over-the-counter medications carried in a first aid kit or available from the victim

- oral glucose
- activated charcoal

Pros and Cons of Popular Pain Relievers

Acetaminophen. Brand names: Tylenol, Datril.
Advantages: Relieves pain and fever, does not irritate stomach.
Disadvantages: Heavy or prolonged use may damage liver and kidneys.

Aspirin. Brand names: Bufferin, Anacin.
Advantages: Relieves pain, fever, inflammation; prevents heart attacks
Disadvantages: Interferes with blood clotting; may trigger stomach bleeding; may cause Reye's syndrome in children with viral infections.

Ibuprofen. Brand names: Advil, Nuprin.
Advantages: Relieves pain, fever, inflammation.
Disadvantages: Interferes with clotting; may cause stomach bleeding, ulcers, irritation; heavy or prolonged use may damage liver and kidneys.

Naproxen. Brand name: Aleve.
Advantages: Relieves pain and fever; one dose lasts 8–12 hours.
Disadvantages: May cause stomach bleeding, ulcers, irritation; prolonged use may harm kidneys.

Nitroglycerin

Give victim nitroglycerin (trade name Nitro-stat™) if *both* of the following conditions apply:

- Victim has chest pain.
- Victim has physician-prescribed sublingual tablets or spray.

Do *not* give a victim nitroglycerin if *any* of the following conditions applies:

- Victim has a head injury.
- Victim is an infant or a child.
- Victim has already taken three doses.

Medication forms: tablet (about one-half the size of an aspirin); sublingual spray

Dosage: One dose, then repeat in 3–5 minutes. If no relief, repeat again (maximum of three doses).

Procedure

1. Check expiration date of nitroglycerin.
2. Ask victim about last dose taken.
3. Ask victim to lift tongue. Place tablet or spray dose under tongue or have victim do so. Do not touch the tablet—wear gloves because your skin will absorb nitroglycerin and affect your heart rate.
4. Have victim keep mouth closed, with tablet under tongue (without swallowing) until it has been dissolved and absorbed.

Actions

- relaxes blood vessels
- decreases workload of heart

Side effects

- lowered blood pressure (victim should sit or lie down)
- headache
- pulse-rate changes

Epinephrine Auto-Injector

Give victim epinephrine (trade name Adrenaline™) if *both* of the following conditions apply:

- Victim exhibits signs of a severe allergic reaction (includes breathing distress or shock).
- Victim has physician-prescribed medication.

Medication form: liquid from automatic needle-and-syringe injection system

Dosage

- Adult: One adult auto-injector (0.3 mg)
- Child/infant: One infant/child auto-injector (0.15 mg)

Procedure

1. Obtain victim's physician-prescribed auto-injector.
2. Remove safety cap.
3. Place tip of auto-injector against victim's thigh.
4. Push injector firmly against the thigh to inject medication.
5. Hold injector in place for 10 seconds.

Actions

- dilates the bronchioles (small tubes in lungs)
- constricts blood vessels

Side effects

- increased heart rate
- dizziness
- headache
- chest pain
- nausea
- vomiting
- anxiety

Reassessment: Monitor ABCs. If victim worsens, give an additional dose; treat for shock; prepare to give CPR.

A mnemonic is a combination of letters or words that helps you recall facts or procedures quickly during an emergency. The mnemonics in this book include the following:

ABCD: First steps in assessing a victim for life-threatening conditions. Sometimes **E** is added, for Exposure and Exam.
- A Airway open?
- B Breathing?
- C Circulation (pulse, major bleeding, and skin condition)?
- D Disability?

RAP ABC: Sequence of action for starting adult CPR
- R Responsive?
- A Activate EMS
- P Position victim on back

- A Airway open?
- B Breathing?
- C Circulation (pulse)?

ESP ABC: Sequence of action for starting child/infant CPR
- E Establish responsiveness
- S Send bystander for help
- P Position victim on back

- A Airway open?
- B Breathing?
- C Circulation (pulse)?

LAF: Procedure used to determine injuries
- L Look at the area for deformity, open wounds, swelling
- A And
- F Feel for deformity, tenderness, swelling

DOTS: Signs of injury
- D Deformity
- O Open wounds
- T Tenderness
- S Swelling

PEARL: Victim's pupil status
- P Pupils
- E Equal
- A And
- R React to
- L Light

SAMPLE: Critical information about the victim
- S Symptoms (chief complaint)?
- A Allergies?
- M Medications?
- P Pertinent medical history?
- L Last oral intake?
- E Events leading to injury/illness?

AVPU: Level of consciousness
- A Alert victim
- V Voice (victim responds to voice)
- P Pain (victim responds only to painful stimulus)
- U Unresponsive victim

AEIOU TIPS: Causes of altered mental status unresponsiveness/unconsciousness
- A Alcohol; Airway blocked; Anaphylaxis
- E Epilepsy; Electrocution
- I Insulin reaction (diabetes)
- O Oxygen (lack of); Overdose of drugs
- U Underdose of insulin

- T Trauma (brain); Temperature (hyper-, hypo-)
- I Infection (meningitis)
- P Psychogenic fainting; Poisoning
- S Stroke; Seizure; Shock

RICE: First aid for musculoskeletal injuries
- R Rest injured part
- I Ice applied
- C Compression using elastic bandage
- E Elevation

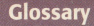
Glossary

abandonment: A termination of a helping relationship by a first aider without consent of the victim and without replacement care to the victim by qualified medical personnel.

ABCs: Airway, Breathing, and Circulation; the first three steps in the examination of any victim; basic life support.

abdomen: The large body cavity below the diaphragm and above the pelvis.

abnormal: Nor normal; malformed.

abrasion: An injury consisting of the loss of a partial thickness of skin from rubbing or scraping on a hard, rough surface; also called brush burn, friction burn.

acetone: A chemical compound found normally in small amounts in the urine; diabetic victims are said to produce a fruity odor when larger amounts are produced in blood and urine.

activated charcoal: Powdered charcoal that has been treated to increase its powers of absorption; used in a slurry to absorb ingested poison.

acute: Having rapid onset, severe symptoms, and a relatively short duration.

acute abdomen: A serious intra-abdominal condition causing irritation or inflammation of the peritoneum, attended by pain, tenderness, and muscular rigidity (boardlike abdomen).

acute myocardial infarction (AMI): The acute phase of a heart attack, in which a spasm or blockage of a coronary artery produces a spectrum of signs and symptoms, commonly including chest pain, nausea, diaphoresis, anxiety, pallor, and lassitude.

Adam's apple: The projection on the anterior surface of the neck, formed by the thyroid cartilage of the larynx.

addiction: The state of being strongly dependent on some agent, for example, drugs or tobacco.

adjunct: An accessory or auxiliary agent or measure; an oropharyngeal airway is an airway management adjunct.

Adrenalin: The proprietary name for epinephrine.

afterbirth: The placenta and membranes expelled after the birth of a child.

air: The gaseous mixture that makes up the Earth's atmosphere; composed of approximately 21 percent oxygen, 79 percent nitrogen, plus trace gases.

air embolism: The presence of air bubbles in the heart or blood vessels, causing an obstruction.

air splint: A double-walled plastic tube that immobilizes a limb when sufficient air is blown into the space between the walls of the tube to cause it to become almost rigid.

airway: An air passage.

allergic reaction: A local or general reaction to an allergen, usually characterized by hives or tissue swelling or dyspnea.

allergy: Hypersensitivity to a substance, causing an abnormal reaction.

AMI: Abbreviation for *acute myocardial infarction.*

amnesia: Loss or impairment of memory.

amniotic fluid: The fluid surrounding the fetus in the uterus, contained in the amniotic sac.

amniotic sac: A thick, transparent sac that holds the fetus suspended in the amniotic fluid.

amputation: Complete removal of an appendage.

analgesic: A pain-relieving drug; a class of drugs used to reduce pain.

anaphylaxis: An exaggerated allergic reaction, usually caused by foreign proteins.

anatomic position: The presumed body position when referring to anatomical landmarks; upright, facing the observer, with hands and arms at sides, thumbs pointing away from the body, legs and feet pointing straight ahead.

anesthesia: A partial or complete loss of sensation with or without loss of consciousness; can result from drug administration or from injury or disease.

aneurysm: A permanent blood-filled dilation of a blood vessel resulting from disease or injury of the blood vessel wall.

Adapted from National Highway Traffic Safety Administration, *Emergency Medical Care* (Washington, D.C.: U.S. Government Printing Office).

angina pectoris: A spasmodic pain in the chest, characterized by a sensation of severe constriction or pressure on the anterior chest; associated with insufficient blood supply to the heart, aggravated by exercise or tension, and relieved by rest or medication.

angulation: The formation of an angle; an abnormal angle in an extremity or organ.

anoxia: Without oxygen; a reduction of oxygen in body tissues below required physiology levels.

ante-: A prefix meaning *before* in time or place.

anterior: Situated in front of, or in the forward part of; in anatomy, used in reference to the ventral, or belly, surface of the body.

anti-: A prefix that shows a negative or reversal of the word root placed after it.

antibody: A substance produced in the body in response to an antigen that destroys or inactivates the antigen.

antidote: A substance to counteract or combat the effect of poison.

antigen: A substance that causes the formation of antibodies.

antihistamine: A substance capable of counteracting the effects of histamine.

antipyretic: A class of drugs that reduces fever.

antiseptic: Any preparation that prevents the growth of bacteria.

antivenin: An antiserum containing antibodies against reptile or insect venom.

arm: The upper extremity, specifically that segment between the shoulder and hand.

arterial blood: Oxygenated blood.

artery: A blood vessel, consisting of three layers of tissue and smooth muscle, that carries blood away from the heart.

artificial ventilation: Movement of air into and out of the lungs by artificial means.

asphyxia: Suffocation.

aspirate: To inhale foreign material into the lungs; to remove fluid or foreign material from the lungs or elsewhere by mechanical suction.

aspirin: Salicylic acid acetate; a drug known for its analgesic, fever-reducing, and anti-inflammatory properties.

asthma: A condition marked by recurrent attacks of dyspnea with wheezing, due to spasmodic constriction of the bronchi, often as a response to allergens or to mucous plugs in the bronchioles.

avulsion: An injury that leaves a piece of skin or other tissue either partially or completely torn away from the body.

axilla: The armpit.

axillary temperature: Body temperature measured by placing a thermometer in the axilla while holding the arm close to the body for a period of 10 minutes.

Babinski reflex: A reflex response of movement of the big toe; positive reflex is determined when, as the sole is stroked, the toe turns upward; negative is determined by a downward movement or no movement of the toe.

bag of waters: The amniotic sac and the fluid it contains.

ball-and-socket joint: A joint wherein the distal bone has a rounded head (ball) that fits into the proximal bone's cuplike socket; the hip and shoulder joints, for example.

bandage: A material used to hold a dressing in place.

basal skull fracture: A fracture involving the base of the cranium.

basic life support: Maintenance of the ABCs (airway, breathing, and circulation) without adjunctive equipment.

Battle's sign: A contusion on the mastoid area of either ear; sign of a basal skull fracture.

biological death: A condition present when irreversible brain damage has occurred, usually from 3 to 10 minutes after cardiac arrest.

blanch: To become white or pale.

blister: A collection of fluid under or within the epidermis.

blood: The fluid that circulates through the heart, arteries, capillaries, and veins carrying nutriment and oxygen to the body cells and removing waste products such as carbon dioxide and various metabolic products for excretion.

blood clot: A soft, coherent, jellylike mass resulting from the conversion of fibrinogen to fibrin, thereby entrapping red blood cells and other formed elements in the fibrinic web.

bone: The hard form of connective tissue that constitutes most of the skeleton in a majority of vertebrates.

bowel: See *intestine*.

brachial artery: The artery of the arm that is the continuation of the axillary artery that in turn branches at the elbow into the radial and ulnar arteries. Used to determine an infant's pulse.

brain: The soft, large mass of nerve tissue that is contained in the cranium.

breech birth (breech delivery): Delivery during which the presenting part of the fetus is the buttocks or a foot instead of the head.

bronchial asthma: The common form of asthma.

bruise: An injury that does not break the skin but causes rupture of small underlying blood vessels, with resulting tissue discoloration; a contusion.

burn: An injury caused by heat, electrical current, or a chemical of extreme acidity or alkalinity.

> **first-degree burn:** A burn causing only reddening of the outer layer of skin; sunburn is usually a first-degree burn.

second-degree burn: A burn extending through the outer layer of skin, causing blisters and edema; a scald is usually a second-degree burn.

third-degree burn: A burn extending through all layers of skin, at times through muscle or connective tissue, having a white, leathery look and lacking sensation; grafting is more often necessary with a third-degree burn; a flame burn is usually third-degree.

burn center: A medical facility especially designed, equipped, and staffed to treat severely burned patients.

capillary: Any one of the small blood vessels that connect arteriole and venule and through whose walls various substances pass into and out of the interstitial tissues and thence on to the cells.

carbon monoxide (CO): A colorless, odorless, and dangerous gas formed by incomplete combustion of carbon; it combines four times more quickly with hemoglobin than oxygen; when in the presence of heme, replaces oxygen and reduces oxygen uptake in the lungs.

cardiac arrest: The sudden cessation of cardiac function, with no pulse, no blood pressure, unresponsiveness.

cardiopulmonary arrest: The cessation of cardiac and respiratory activity.

cardiopulmonary resuscitation (CPR): The application of artificial ventilation and external cardiac compression in victims with cardiac arrest to provide adequate circulation to support life.

carotid artery: The principal artery of the neck, palpated easily on either side of the thyroid cartilage.

carpals: The eight small bones of the wrist.

cartilage: A tough, elastic, connective tissue that covers opposite surfaces of movable joints and also forms parts of the skeleton, such as the ear and nose.

caustic: Corrosive; destructive to living tissue.

centigrade scale: The temperature scale in which the freezing point of water is 0° and the boiling point at sea level is 100°.

cerebral contusion: A bruise of the brain, causing a characteristic symptomatic response.

cerebral hemorrhage: Bleeding into the cerebrum; one form of stroke or cerebrovascular accident.

cerebrospinal fluid (CSF): The fluid contained in the four ventricles of the brain and the space around the brain and spinal cord.

cerebrovascular accident (CVA): The sudden cessation of circulation to a region of the brain due to thrombus, embolism, or hemorrhage; also, a stroke or apoplexy.

cervical: Pertaining to the neck.

cervical collar: A device used to immobilize and support the neck.

chief complaint: The problem for which a person seeks help, stated in a word or short phrase.

chills: A sensation of cold, with convulsive shaking of the body.

circulatory system: The body system consisting of the heart and blood vessels.

clammy: Damp and usually cool.

clavicle: The collarbone; attached to the uppermost part of the sternum at a right angle and joined to the scapular spine to form the point of the shoulder.

clinical death: A term that refers to the lack of signs of life, when there is no pulse and no blood pressure; occurs immediately after the onset of cardiac arrest.

clot: A semisolid mass of fibrin and cells.

closed fracture: A fracture in which there is no laceration in the overlying skin.

closed wound: A wound in which there is no tear or cut in the epidermis.

coffee grounds vomitus: A vomitus having the appearance and consistency of coffee grounds; indicates slow bleeding in the stomach and represents the vomiting of partially digested blood.

coma: A state of unconsciousness from which the victim cannot be aroused even by powerful stimulation.

comminuted fracture: A fracture in which the bone ends are broken into many fragments.

communicable disease: A disease that is transmissible from one person to another.

compound fracture: An open fracture; a fracture in which there is an open wound of the skin and soft tissues leading down to the location of the fracture.

compress: A folded cloth or pad used for applying pressure to stop hemorrhage or as a wet dressing.

concussion: A violent jar or shock that injures the central nervous system.

conscious: Capable of responding to sensory stimuli and having subjective experiences.

consent: An agreement by a patient or victim to accept treatment offered as explained by medical personnel or first aiders.

implied consent: An assumed consent given by an unconscious adult when emergency lifesaving treatment is required.

informed consent: A consent given by a mentally competent adult who understands what the treatment will involve; it can also be given by the parent or guardian of a child, as defined by the state, or for a mentally incompetent adult.

constrict: To be made smaller by drawing together or squeezing.

constricting band: A band used to restrict the lymphatic flow of blood back to the heart.

contagious: A term that refers to a disease that is readily transmitted from one person to another.

contagious disease: An infectious disease transmissible by direct or indirect contact; now synonymous with *communicable disease.*

contaminated: A term used in reference to a wound or other surface that has been infected with bacteria; may also refer to polluted water, food, or drugs.

contusion: A bruise; an injury that causes a hemorrhage in or beneath the skin but does not break the skin.

convulsion: A violent involuntary contraction or series of contractions of the voluntary muscles; a fit or seizure.

core temperature: Body temperature measured centrally, from within the esophagus or rectum.

coronary: A term applied to the cardiac blood vessels that supply blood to the walls of the heart.

coronary artery: One of the two arteries arising from the aortic sinus to supply the heart muscle with blood.

CPR: Abbreviation for *cardiopulmonary resuscitation.*

cramp: A painful spasm, usually of a muscle; a gripping pain in the abdominal area; colic.

cravat: A type of bandage made from a large triangular piece of cloth and folded to form a band; used as a temporary dressing for a fracture or wound.

crepitus: A grating sound heard and the sensation felt when the fractured ends of a bone rub together.

crowning: The stage of birth when the presenting part of the baby is visible at the vaginal orifice.

CVA: Abbreviation for *cerebrovascular accident.*

cyanosis: A blueness of the skin due to insufficient oxygen in the blood.

defibrillation: Direct current electrical shock applied to stop fibrillation of the heart.

dehydration: Loss of water and electrolytes; excessive loss of body water.

depressed fracture: A skull fracture with impaction, depression, or sinking in of the fragments.

diabetes: A general term referring to disorders characterized by excessive urine excretion, excessive thirst, and excessive hunger.

diabetes mellitus: A systemic disease marked by lack of production of insulin, which causes an inability to metabolize carbohydrates, resulting in an increase in blood sugar.

diabetic coma: Loss of consciousness due to severe diabetes mellitus that has not been treated or to treatment that has not been adequately regulated.

diarrhea: The frequent passage of watery or loose stools.

digestive tract: The passages of tubes leading from the mouth and pharynx to the anus; the alimentary tract; mouth, pharynx, esophagus, stomach, small intestine, large intestine, rectum, and anus.

dilated pupil: A pupil enlarged beyond its normal size.

dilation: The process of expanding or enlarging.

dispatcher: One who transmits calls to service units and vehicles and personnel on assignments.

distal: Farthest from any point on the center or median line; in extremities, farthest from the point of junction of the trunk of the body.

drag: A general term referring to methods of moving victims without a stretcher or litter, usually employed by a single rescuer.

> **blanket drag:** A method by which one rescuer encloses a victim in a blanket and then drags the victim to safety.
>
> **clothes drag:** A method by which one rescuer can drag a victim to safety by grasping the victim's clothes and pulling him away from danger.
>
> **fireman's drag:** A method by which one rescuer crawls with a victim, looping the victim's tied wrists over the rescuer's neck to support the victim's weight.

dressing: A protective covering for a wound; used to stop bleeding and to prevent contamination of the wound.

-ectomy: Suffix meaning surgical removal, as in *appendectomy.*

edema: A condition in which fluid escapes into the body tissues from the vascular or lymphatic spaces and causes local or generalized swelling.

electrocution: Death caused by passage of electrical current through the body.

embolism: The sudden blocking of an artery or vein by a clot or foreign material that has been brought to the site of lodgement by the blood current.

emesis: Vomiting.

EMS: Emergency medical services.

EMT: Emergency medical technician.

epidermis: The outermost and nonvascular layer of the skin.

epiglottis: The lidlike cartilaginous structure overhanging the superior entrance to the larynx and serving to prevent food from entering the larynx and trachea during swallowing.

epilepsy: A chronic brain disorder marked by paroxysmal attacks of brain dysfunction, usually associated with some alteration of consciousness, abnormal motor behavior, psychic or sensory disturbances; may be preceded by an aura.

epinephrine: A hormone released by the adrenal medulla that stimulates the sympathetic nervous system, producing vasoconstriction, increased heart rate, and bronchodilation.

epistaxis: Nosebleed.

esophagus: The portion of the digestive tract that lies between the pharynx and the stomach.

exhalation: The act of breathing out; expiration.

extremity: A limb; an arm, or a leg.

extrication: Disentanglement; freeing from entrapment.

Fahrenheit scale: The temperature scale in which the freezing point is 32° and the boiling point at sea level is 212°.

fainting: A momentary loss of consciousness caused by insufficient blood supply to the brain; syncope.

feces: The product expelled by the bowels; semisoft waste products of digestion.

femoral artery: The principal artery of the thigh, a continuation of the iliac artery; supplies blood to the lower abdomen wall, the external genitalia, and the lower body extremities; pulse may be palpated in the groin area.

femur: The bone that extends from the pelvis to the knee; the longest and largest bone of the body; the thighbone.

fever: An elevation of body temperature beyond normal.

fibrillation: Ineffective contractions of the heart muscles.

fibula: The smaller of the two bones of the lower leg; the most lateral bone of the lower leg.

first aid: Immediate care given to the injured or suddenly ill person. First aid does not take the place of proper medical treatment. It consists only of furnishing temporary assistance until competent medical care, *if needed,* is obtained, or until the chance for recovery without medical care is assured.

first-degree burn: A burn causing only reddening of the outer layer of skin; sunburn usually is a first-degree burn.

first responder: A person who has been trained to provide emergency care before the EMTs arrive; usually police or fire fighters.

flail chest: A condition in which several ribs are broken, each in at least two places; a sternal fracture or separation of the ribs from the sternum producing a free floating segment of the chest wall that moves paradoxically on respiration.

forearm: The part of the upper extremity between the elbow and the wrist.

fracture: A break or rupture in a bone.

> **closed fractrue:** A fracture that does not cause a break in the skin; a simple fracture.

> **comminuted fracture:** A fracture in which the bone is shattered.

> **compound fracture:** A fracture in which the bone ends pierce the skin; an open fracture.

> **greenstick fracture:** An incomplete fracture (the bone is not broken all the way through); seen most often in children.

> **impacted fracture:** A fracture in which the ends of the bones are jammed together.

> **oblique fracture:** A fracture in which the break crosses the bone at an angle.

> **open fracture:** A fracture in which the skin is open; a compound fracture.

> **simple fracture:** A fracture in which the skin is not broken; a closed fracture.

> **spiral fracture:** A fracture in which the breakline twists around and through the bone.

> **transverse fracture:** A fracture in which the breakline extends across the bone at a right angle to the long axis.

fracture of the hip: A fracture that occurs at the upper end of the femur, most often at the neck of the femur.

frostbite: The damage to tissues as a result of prolonged exposure to extreme cold.

frostnip: The superficial local tissue destruction caused by freezing; it is limited in scope and does not destroy the full thickness of skin.

gangrene: Local tissue death as the result of an injury or inadequate blood supply.

gastrointestinal tract: The digestive tract, including stomach, small intestine, large intestine, rectum, and anus.

glucose: Blood sugar.

glycogen: Carbohydrates stored in the liver and muscle tissue.

grand mal seizure: A type of epileptic attack; characterized by a short-term, generalized, convulsive seizure.

gullet: The esophagus; the passage from the pharynx to the stomach.

half-ring splint: A traction splint with a hinged half-ring at the upper end that allows the splint to be used on either the right or the left leg.

heart: The hollow muscular organ that receives blood from the veins, sends it through the lungs to be oxygenated, then pumps it to the arteries.

heart attack: Lay term for a condition resulting from blockage of a coronary artery and subsequent death of part of the heart muscle; an acute myocardial infarction; sometimes called simply a "coronary."

heat cramp: A painful muscle cramp resulting from excessive loss of salt and water through sweating.

heat exhaustion: A prostration caused by excessive loss of water and salt through sweating; characterized by clammy skin and a weak, rapid pulse.

hematoma: A localized collection of blood in an organ, tissue, or space as a result of injury or a broken blood vessel.

heme: The deep red, iron-containing group of hemoglobin.

hemiplegia: Paralysis of one side of the body.

hemoglobin: The oxygen-carrying substance of the red blood cells.

hemophilia: An inherited blood disease occurring mostly in males, characterized by the inability of the blood to clot.

hemorrhage: Abnormally large amount of bleeding.

hemorrhagic shock: A state of inadequate tissue perfusion due to blood loss.

hemothorax: Bleeding into the thoracic cavity.

hives: Red or white raised patches on the skin, often attended by severe itching; a characteristic reaction in allergic responses.

humerus: The bone of the upper arm.

hyper-: Prefix meaning *excessive* or *increased*.

hyperglycemia: An abnormally increased concentration of sugar in the blood.

hypertension: High blood pressure, usually in reference to a diastolic pressure greater than 90–95 mm Hg.

hyperthermia: An abnormally increased body temperature.

hyperventilation: An increased rate and depth of breathing resulting in an abnormal lowering of arterial carbon dioxide, causing alkalosis.

hyphema: Hemorrhage in the anterior chamber of the eye.

hypo-: A prefix meaning *less than, lack of;* a deficiency.

hypoglycemia: An abnormally diminished concentration of sugar in the blood; insulin shock.

hypothermia: Decreased body temperature.

hypovolemic shock: Shock caused by a reduction in blood volume, such as caused by hemorrhage.

hypoxia: A low oxygen content in the blood; lack of oxygen in inspired air.

immobilize: To hold a part firmly in place, as with a splint.

impaled object: An object that has caused a puncture wound and remains embedded in the wound.

incision: A wound usually made deliberately in connection with surgery; a clean cut as opposed to a laceration.

infarction: The death (*necrosis*) of a localized area of tissue caused by the cutting off of its blood supply.

infection: An invasion of a body by disease-producing organisms.

inferior: Anatomically, situated below or the lower surface or part of a structure.

inflammation: A tissue reaction to disease, irritation, or infection; characterized by pain, heat, redness, and swelling.

ingestion: Intake of food or other substances through the mouth.

inhalation: The drawing of air or other substances into the lungs.

insulin: A hormone secreted in the pancreas; essential for the proper metabolism of blood sugar.

insulin shock: Not a true form of shock; hypoglycemia caused by excessive insulin dosage, characterized by sweating, tremor, anxiety, unusual behavior, and vertigo; may cause death of brain cells.

intestine: The portion of the alimentary canal extending from the stomach to the anus.

intoxicate: To poison; commonly, to cause diminished control by means of drugs or alcohol.

ipecac syrup: A medication used to induce vomiting.

-itis: A suffix meaning *inflammation.*

jaw-thrust maneuver: A procedure for opening the airway in which the jaw is lifted and pulled forward to keep the tongue from falling back into the airway.

joint: The point at which two or more bones articulate; also, commonly, a marijuana cigarette.

jugular: Pertaining to the neck; large vein on either side of the neck, draining the head via the *external jugular* or draining the brain via the *internal jugular.*

kidneys: The paired organs that filter blood and produce urine; they also act as adjuncts to keep a proper acid-base balance.

knee: The hinge joint between the femur and the tibia.

labor: The process or period of childbirth; especially, the muscular contractions of the uterus designed to expel the fetus from the mother.

laceration: A wound made by tearing or cutting of body tissues.

ladder splint: A flexible splint consisting of two stout parallel wires and finer crosswires; resembles a ladder.

laryngospasm: A severe constriction of the vocal cords, often in response to allergy or noxious stimuli.

larynx: The organ of voice production.

lateral: Of or toward the side; away from the midline of the body.

leg: The lower limb generally, specifically, that part of the lower limb extending from the knee to the ankle.

lesion: A distinct area of pathologically altered tissue; an injury or wound.

lethal: Fatal.

lethargy: A lack of activity; drowsiness; indifference.

ligament: A tough band of fibrous tissue that connects bone to bone or that supports any organ.

limb presentation: A delivery in which the presenting part of a fetus is an arm or a leg.

linear fracture: A fracture running parallel to the long axis of the bone.

linear skull fracture: A skull fracture that runs in a straight line.

litter: A stretcher.

liver: The large organ in the right upper quadrant of the abdomen that secretes bile, produces many essential proteins, detoxifies many subtances, and stores glycogen.

log roll: A method for placing a person on a carrying device, usually a long spineboard or a flat litter; the person is rolled onto his or her side, then back onto the litter.

lungs: The paired organs in the thorax that effect ventilation and oxygenation.

lymph: A straw-colored fluid that circulates in the lymphatic vessels and interstitial space.

mastoid: A portion of the temporal bone that lies behind the ear and contains spongy bone tissue.

medial: Toward the midline of the body.

metacarpal bones: The five cylindrical bones of the hand extending from the wrist to the fingers.

metatarsal bones: The five cylindrical bones of the foot extending from the ankles to the toes.

morbidity: A synonym for illness; generally used to refer to an untoward effect of an illness or injury.

mortality: Refers to death from a given disease or injury; generally thought of as a statistic to state the ratio of death to recovery.

motion sickness: A sensation induced by repetitive motion, characterized by nausea and lightheadedness.

mottled: Characterized by a patchy, discolored appearance.

mouth-to-mouth ventilation: The preferred emergency method of artificial ventilation when adjuncts are not available.

mouth-to-nose ventilation: An emergency method of artificial ventilation when mouth-to-mouth cannot be used.

mucus: A viscid, slippery secretion that lubricates and protects various body structures.

muscle: A tissue composed of elongated cells that have the ability to contract when stimulated, thus causing bone and joints to move or other anatomical structures to be drawn together.

myocardial infarction: The damaging or death of an area of the heart muscle resulting from a lack of blood supplying the area; a heart attack.

nausea: An unpleasant sensation, vaguely referred to the epigastrium and abdomen, often culminating in vomiting.

necrosis: The death of an area of tissue, usually caused by the cessation of blood supply.

nerve: A cordlike structure composed of a collection of fibers that conveys impulses between a part of the central nervous system and some other region.

nervous system: The brain, spinal cord, and nerve branches from the central, peripheral, and autonomic systems.

nitroglycerin: A drug used in the treatment of angina pectoris.

noxious: Injurious.

oblique fracture: A fracture that runs diagonally to the long axis of the bone.

occipital: Pertaining to the back of the head.

ointment: A semisolid preparation for external application to the body, usually containing a medicinal substance.

open fracture or dislocation: A fracture or dislocation exposed to the exterior; an open wound lies over the fracture or dislocation.

open wound: A wound in which the affected tissues are exposed by an external opening.

oral: Pertaining to the mouth.

-otomy: A suffix meaning surgical incision into an organ, as in *tracheotomy*.

oxygen: A colorless, odorless, tasteless gas that is essential to life and that makes up 21 percent of the atmosphere; chemical formula: O_2.

pallor: A paleness of the skin.

palpation: The act of palpating; the act of feeling with the hands for the purpose of determining the consistency of the part beneath.

palpitation: A sensation felt under the left breast when the heart "skips a beat" because of premature ventricular contractions.

paralysis: Loss of impairment of motor function of a part due to a lesion of the neural or muscular mechanism.

paraplegia: The loss of both sensation and motion in the lower extremities, most commonly due to damage to the spinal cord.

patella: A small, flat bone that protects the knee joint; the kneecap.

pediatrics: The medical specialty devoted to the diagnosis and treatment of diseases of children.

penetrate: To pierce; to pass into the deeper tissues or into a cavity.

perfusion: The act of pouring through or into; the blood suffusing the cells in order to exchange gases, nutrients, etc., with the cells.

petit mal seizure: A type of epileptic attack characterized by a momentary loss of awareness but not accompanied by loss of motor tone.

pharynx: The portion of the airway between the nasal cavity and the larynx.

placenta: The vascular organ attached to the uterine wall that supplies oxygen and nutrients to the fetus; also called *afterbirth*.

pneumothorax: An accumulation of air in the pleural cavity usually entering after a wound or injury that causes a penetration of the chest wall or laceration of the lung.

point tenderness: An area of tenderness limited to two or three centimeters in diameter; point tenderness can be located in any area of the body; usually associated with acute inflammation, as in peritonitis (abdominal point tenderness).

posterior: Situated in the back of or behind a surface.

presenting part: The part of the baby that emerges first during delivery.

pressure dressing: A dressing with which enough pressure is applied over a wound site to stop bleeding.

pressure point: One of several places on the body where the blood flow of a given artery can be restricted by pressing the artery against an underlying bone.

pressure splints: An inflatable plastic circumferential splint that can be applied to an extremity and inflated to achieve stability after a fracture.

prognosis: The probable outcome of a disease based on assumptive knowledge.

prolapsed cord delivery: A delivery in which the umbilical cord appears at the vaginal opening before the head of the infant.

prone: A position of lying face down.

psychogenic shock: A fainting spell resulting from transient generalized cerebral ischemia; not a true shock condition.

psychosomatic: An indication of an illness in which some part of the cause is related to emotional factors.

pulse rate: The heart rate determined by counting the number of pulsations occurring in any superficial artery.

pump failure: A partial or total failure of the heart to pump blood effectively.

pupil: The small opening in the center of the iris.

quadrant: One of the four quarters of the abdomen.

quadriplegia: Paralysis of both the arms and the legs.

radial artery: One of the major arteries of the forearm; the pulse is palpable at the base of the thumb.

radiation sickness: The condition that follows excessive irradiation from any source.

radius: The bone on the thumb side of the forearm.

rape: Sexual intercourse by force.

rash: An eruption of the skin, either localized or generalized.

rectal temperature: The core body temperature obtained by inserting a thermometer into the rectum and retaining it for a minute; normally 1°F higher than oral temperature.

regurgitation: A backward flowing, as the casting up of undigested food from the stomach to the mouth.

respiration: The act of breathing; the exchange of oxygen and carbon dioxide in the tissues and lungs.

respiratory arrest: The cessation of breathing.

respiratory system: The system of organs that controls the inspiration of oxygen and the expiration of carbon dioxide.

resuscitation: The act of reviving an unconscious victim.

rib: One of the 24 bones forming the thoracic cavity wall.

rigid splint: A splint made of a firm material that can be applied to an injured extremity to prevent motion at the site of a fracture or dislocation.

roller dressing: A strip of rolled-up material used for dressings.

Rothberg position: Heart attack victim placed in sitting position with legs up and bent at the knees.

saliva: The clear, alkaline fluid secreted by the salivary glands.

scab: A crust formed by the coagulation of blood, pus, serum, or any combination of these on the surface of an ulcer, erosion, abrasion, or any other type of wound.

scapula: The shoulder blade.

sclera: The white, opaque, outer layer of the eyeball.

second-degree burn: A burn penetrating beneath the superficial skin layers, producing edema and blisters.

seizure: A sudden attack or recurrence of a disease; a convulsion; an attack of epilepsy.

semiconscious: Stuporous; partially conscious.

shell temperature: The temperature of the extremities and surface of the body.

shivering: A trembling from cold or fear; it produces heat by muscular contractions.

shock: A state of inadequate tissue perfusion that may be a result of pump failure (cariogenic shock), volume loss or sequestration (hypovolemic shock), vasodilation (neurogenic shock), or any combination of these.

> **anaphylactic shock:** A rapidly occurring state of collapse caused by hypersensitivity to drugs or other foreign materials (insect venom, certain foods, inhaled allergens); symptoms may include hives, wheezing, tissue edema, bronchospasm, and vascular collapse.

> **septic shock:** A shock developing in the presence of, and as a result of, severe infection.

sign: Any objective evidence of physical manifestation of a disease.

simple fracture: A fracture that is not compound; the skin is not broken over the break in the bone.

skeleton: The hard, bony structure that forms the main support of the body.

skin: The outer integument or covering of the body, consisting of the dermis and the epidermis; the largest organ of the body, it contains various sensory and regulatory mechanisms.

skull: The bony structure surrounding the brain; it consists of the cranial bones, the facial bones, and the teeth.

sling: A triangular bandage applied around the neck to support an injured upper extremity; any material long enough to suspend an upper extremity by passing the material around the neck; used to support and protect an injury of the arm, shoulder, or clavicle.

sling and swathe: A bandage in which the arm is placed in a sling and is bound to the body by another bandage placed around the chest and arm to hold the arm close to the body.

small intestine: The portion of the intestine between the stomach and the colon.

snowblindness: Obscured vision caused by sunlight reflected off snow.

spasm: A sudden, violent, involuntary contraction of a muscle or group of muscles attended by pain and interference with function; a sudden but transitory constriction of a passage, canal, or orifice.

spineboard: A wooden or metal device primarily used for extrication and transportation of victims with actual or suspected spine injuries.

spiral fracture: A fracture in which the line of break runs diagonally around the long axis of the bone.

spleen: The largest lymphatic organ of the body; located in the left upper quadrant of the abdomen.

splint: Any support used to immobilize a fracture or to restrict movement of a part.

sprain: A trauma to a joint that injures the ligaments.

sputum: Expectorated matter, especially mucus or matter resulting from diseases of the air passages.

status asthmaticus: A severe, prolonged asthmatic attack that cannot be broken with epinephrine.

status epilepticus: The occurrence of two or more seizures with a period of complete consciousness between them.

sterile: Free from living organisms, such as bacteria.

sterilize: To render sterile or free from bacterial contamination; to make an organism unable to reproduce.

sternum: The long, flat bone located in the midline in the anterior part of the thoracic cage; articulates above with the clavicles and along the sides with the cartilages of the first seven ribs.

stomach: A hollow digestive organ in the epigastrium that receives food from the esophagus.

stool: Feces; the matter discharged at defecation.

stove-in chest: See *flail chest.*

strain: An injury to a muscle caused by a violent contraction or an excessive, forcible stretching.

stretcher: A carrying device that enables two or more persons to lift and carry a person who is lying down.

stroke: A cerebrovascular accident of sudden onset.

sublingual: Under the tongue.

sucking chest wound: An open pneumothorax.

suffocate: To impede breathing; to asphyxiate.

suicide: The act of deliberately taking one's own life.

sunstroke: A form of heatstroke due to prolonged sun exposure.

superior: In anatomy, used to refer to an organ or part that is located above another organ or part.

supine: Lying in a face-upward position.

suture: The material used to close a surgical wound or to repair a gaping wound.

swathe: A cravat tied around the body to decrease movement of a part.

symptom: A subjective sensation or awareness of disturbance of bodily function.

syncope: Fainting; a brief period of unconsciousness.

syndrome: A complex of symptoms and signs characteristic of a condition.

synovial fluid: A clear fluid that lubricates joints; it is secreted by the synovial membrane.

tachycardia: Abnormally rapid heart rate, over 100 beats per minute.

tarsal: Pertaining to the tarsus (the ankle).

temperature: The degree of heat of a living body; varies in cold-blooded animals with environmental temperature and is constant, within a narrow range, for warm-blooded animals; 98.6°F oral temperature and 99.6°F rectal are considered normal for humans.

tendon: A tough band of dense, fibrous, connective tissue that attaches muscles to bone and other parts.

tetanus: An infectious disease caused by the bacteria *Clostridium tetani* that is usually introduced through a wound, characterized by extreme body rigidity and spasms of voluntary body muscles.

thermal: Pertaining to heat.

thigh: The portion of the lower extremity between the hip and the knee.

third-degree burn: A full-thickness burn destroying all skin layers and underlying tissue; has a charred or white, leathery appearance and is insensitive.

thoracic: Pertaining to the chest.

thrombosis: Formation of a blood clot, or *thrombus.*

tibia: The larger of the two bones in the leg; the shinbone.

tissue: An aggregation of similarly specialized cells and their intercellular substance, united in the performance of a particular function.

tourniquet: A constrictive device used on the extremities to impede venous blood return to the heart or obstruct arterial blood flow to the extremities.

toxin: Any poison manufactured by plant or animal life.

trachea: The cartilaginous tube extending from the larynx to its division into the primary bronchi; the windpipe.

traction: The act of exerting a pulling force.

transient ischemic attack (TIA): Symptoms of a stroke lasting from several minutes to several hours, with a return to normal neurological function.

triage: A system used for sorting victims to determine the order in which they will receive medical attention.

triangular bandage: A piece of cloth cut in the shape of a right-angle triangle; used as a sling or folded for a cravat bandage.

trunk: The body excluding the head and limbs; the torso.

ulcer: An open lesion of the skin or mucous membrane.

ulna: The larger bone of the forearm, on the side opposite that of the thumb.

umbilical cord: The flexible structure that connects the fetus to the placenta.

umbilicus: The navel.

unconscious: Without awareness; comatose.

universal access number: A telephone number that can be called in emergency situations and that ties in with the police, fire, and emergency medical services; in most areas the number is 9-1-1.

universal dressing: A large (9-in. by 36-in.) dressing of multilayered material that can be used open, folded, or rolled to cover most wounds, to pad splints, or to form a cervical collar.

uterus: The muscular organ that holds and nourishes the fetus, opening into the vagina through the cervix; the womb.

vagina: The canal in the female extending from the uterus to the vulva; the birth canal.

vasoconstriction: The narrowing of the diameter of a blood vessel.

vein: Any blood vessel that carries blood from the tissues to the heart.

venom: A poison, usually derived from reptiles or insects.

venous blood: Unoxygenated blood, containing hemoglobin in the carboxyhemoglobin state.

ventilation: Breathing; supplying of fresh air to the lungs.

ventricular fibrillation: A rapid, tremulous, and ineffectual contraction of the cardia myofibrils, producing no cardiac output; cardiac arrest.

vertebrae: The 33 bones of the spinal column.

vertigo: Dizziness; a hallucination of movement; a sensation that the external world is spinning; it may be right or left, upward or downward.

vital signs: The indication of life through values that reflect mental status, blood pressure, pulse rate, and respiration rate.

vitreous fluid: A jellylike, transparent substance filling the inside of the eyeball.

voice box: The larynx.

vomiting: The forceful, active expulsion of stomach contents through the mouth, as opposed to regurgitation, which is passive.

vomitus: The matter ejected from the stomach by vomiting.

wheal: A swelling on the skin, produced by a sting, an injection, external force, or internal reaction.

wheeze: A high-pitched, whistling sound characterizing an obstruction or spasm of the lower airways.

windchill factor: The relationship of wind velocity and temperature in determining the effect of cold on a living organism.

windpipe: The trachea.

womb: The uterus.

wrist: The joint or the region of the joint between the forearm and the hand.

xiphoid process: The sword-shaped cartilaginous process at the lowest portion of the sternum that ossifies in the aged and has no ribs attached to it.

Index

Additional Photo and Illustration Credits

Part 1
Opener © Andrew Sacks, Tony Stone

Chapter 1
Opener Steve Ferry, P & F Communications

Chapter 2
Opener Steve Ferry, P & F Communications

Part II
Opener © Grant Pix, Stock Boston

Chapter 3
Opener Steve Ferry, P & F Communications; ppgs 36-46: **Figures 3.1-3.11** Vincent Perez

Chapter 4
Opener Steve Ferry, P & F Communications

Part III
Opener Steve Ferry, P & F Communications

Chapter 5
Opener © Bruce Ayres, Tony Stone

Chapter 6
Opener Steve Ferry, P & F Communications

Chapter 7
Opener Steve Ferry, P & F Communications

Chapter 8
Opener Steve Ferry, P & F Communications

Chapter 9
Opener Steve Ferry, P & F Communications

Chapter 10
Opener Steve Ferry, P & F Communications

Chapter 11
Opener Steve Ferry, P & F Communications

Chapter 12
Opener Steve Ferry, P & F Communications

Chapter 13
Opener © Bob Daemmrich, Stock Boston

Chapter 14
Opener Steve Ferry, P & F Communications

Chapter 15
Opener © Wedgworth. All rights reserved.

Chapter 16
Opener Steve Ferry, P & F Communications

Chapter 17
Opener Steve Ferry, P & F Communications; **p. 321 Figures 17.10** © Janet Haas, 1993, **17.11** © Kim Taylor, 1989, **17.12** © Ron Sanford, 1994, **17.13** © Ron Sanford, 1981; p. 340, **Figures 17.31** © Eric Popp, 1994, **17.32** © Charles Seaborn, Tony Stone, **17.33** © Doug Perrine, Innerspace Visions; **p. 342, Figure 17.34** © Kevin McDonnell, 1995; **p. 342, Figure 17.35** © M. Mesgleski, 1989

Chapter 18
Opener © Hulton Deutsch, 1994

Chapter 19
Opener Steve Ferry, P & F Communications

Chapter 20
Opener Steve Ferry, P & F Communications

Chapter 21
Opener Steve Ferry, P & F Communications

Chapter 22
Opener Steve Ferry, P & F Communications
p. 416, Figure 22.7 © Ray Nelson, 1994

Chapter 23
Opener Steve Ferry, P & F Communications

Quick Emergency Index